AF364251

Pathophysiology for Pharmacy

A Concise Review

Pathophysiology for Pharmacy

A Concise Review

Sujesh M

M.Pharm, Pharmacology

Dept. of Pharmaceutical Sciences

Centre for Professional and Advanced Studies

Kottayam, Kerala.

and

Prof. Jyoti Harindran

M.Pharm, M.S (U.K.) PhD PGDBM

Principal and Prof. in charge of Research

Dept. of Pharmaceutical Sciences

Centre for Professional and Advanced Studies

Kottayam, Kerala.

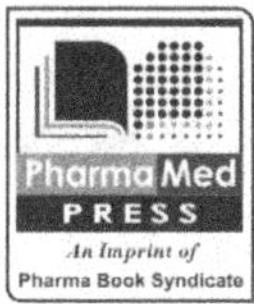

PharmaMed Press

An imprint of Pharma Book Syndicate

A unit of BSP Books Pvt. Ltd.

4-4-309/316, Giriraj Lane,

Sultan Bazar, Hyderabad - 500 095.

Pathophysiology for Pharmacy – A Concise Review
by *Sujesh M and Jyoti Harindran*

Published by

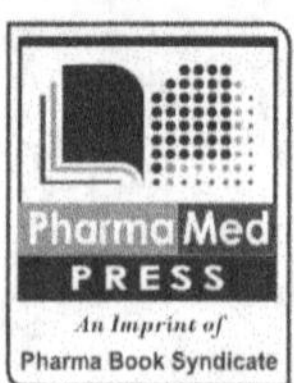

PharmaMed Press

An imprint of Pharma Book Syndicate

A unit of BSP Books Pvt. Ltd.
4-4-309/316, Giriraj Lane, Sultan Bazar, Hyderabad - 500 095.
Phone: 040-23445688, 23445600; Fax: 91+40-23445611
E-mail: info@pharmamedpress.com
www.pharmamedpress.com/pharmamedpress.net

ISBN: 978-93-87593-27-5 (Hardback)

PREFACE

The aim of the authors had been to remove any type of complexity so that there is an easy learning. Students when exposed to classes in tight schedule do understand the matter, but many times the problems come when they have to answer the examination questions. Sometimes it happens that we know all the points but do not know what to write, when to write and how to write. This book will serve as an excellent substitute to class notes and specifically pin points what all can be written in the best way so as to fit as an answer to a question. The book is designed to impart a thorough knowledge of the relevant aspects of pathology of various conditions with reference to its pharmacological applications, and understanding of basic Pathophysiological mechanisms. Hence it will not only help to study the syllabus of pathology, but also to get baseline knowledge of its application in other subject of pharmacy.

Upon going through the book thoroughly the student shall be able to –

A. Describe the etiology and pathogenesis of the selected disease states;
B. Name the signs and symptoms of the diseases; and
C. Mention the complications of the diseases.

It has been a credible attempt to condense out the needed and keep away the unwanted. But this does not mean that other textbooks or reference books are unwanted. This book is a last minute supplement which can add on to your class notes in a well prescribed format so as to serve the needs of an exam going pharmacy students. The book is equally useful for B. Pharm students, Pharm D students, Practicing pharmacists, Pharmacy teachers and Working Pharmacists. It is covered with such a depth and is framed under the vastness of Pharm D syllabus. Our courtesy also goes to the immense help we got from the readily available internet services to give a wider choice to collect and select matter including valuable diagrams which have made understanding Pathophysiology better.

Hope that it is well received and will serve the purpose for which it is meant and for whom it is meant.

- Authors

ACKNOWLEDGEMENT

I take this opportunity to express my sincere gratitude to my research guide and co author of this book Prof. Dr. Jyoti Harindran for guiding me and putting all effort to fulfill this project.

I gratefully remember the help and support given by Dr. A. Abdul Vahab, Mr. Jayachandran T. P., my wife K. Shalini, my father Mr. M. T. Balakrishnan Nair and my mother Mrs. M. Sarada. I would also like to thank M/s Pharma Book Syndicate and PharmaMed Press for their committed effort in bringing out this book.

I honestly remember all the teachers who made their contribution in my life.

I surrender this work at the lotus feet of almighty.

- Sujesh M

CONTENTS

1

Introduction

Pathophysiology

The subject pathophysiology is the study of structural and functional changes occurring in the cell, tissue and organ that underline disease. These changes in the system leads to changes in the biochemical estimation values of the functional tests conducted in order to estimate the functioning levels of various organs in the body say for example liver, kidney, blood parameters, stool, sputum etc., to name a few. The Science of pathophysiology there detects an abnormal functioning organ system in the body and also studies the mechanism of disease, how and why structural and functional changes lead to signs and symptoms of disease.

Importance of Pathophysiology in Clinical Practice

It gives strong base for rational clinical care and therapy. Understanding pathophysiology guides the healthcare professional in planning, selection and evaluation of therapy and treatment. Knowledge of human anatomy and physiology, interrelationship among various organ systems of body, is an essential foundation for study of pathophysiology. Changes in the normal biochemical parameters are the first indication of a disease. The body produces its first form of signaling that "Something is wrong in the body system" by showing changes in the biochemical estimation values. These will be highlighted in the coming chapters and will serve as backbone of Pathophysiology.

Close monitoring of these biochemical parameters will help in early detection of diseases or abnormal body functioning i.e. pathological conditions [Pathos-suffering; logos-study of] needing clinical attention. This will help physicians/clinical pharmacists/clinicians to administer early cure or preventive measures to various diseased conditions which can or otherwise induct serious health hazards.

Dictionary of Terminology with Definitions (Glossary)

1. **ABC:** In its original form it stands for *Airway, Breathing,* and *Circulation*

2. **Acini (acinus):** Small sac like dilation, particularly in a gland.

3. **Actinomyces:** A genus of bacteria (family *Actinomycetaceae*).

4. **Actinomycosis:** An infectious disease causes by Actinomyces; marked by swelling and abscesses in the head and neck region and sometimes in the peritoneum, or in the lung due to aspiration.

5. **Allergen:** An antigenic substance capable of producing immediate hypersensitivity (allergy).

6. **Acute:** Of abrupt onset, in reference to a disease. Acute often also denotes an illness that is of short duration, rapidly progressive and in need of urgent care.

7. **Acute myocardial infarction:** A heart attack. The term focuses on the heart muscle, which is called the myocardium. The death (necrosis) of myocardial tissue occurs due to the sudden deprivation of circulating blood.

8. **Adaptation:** The process by which organisms are modified so as to improve their chances of survival in an environment is called adaptation. These changes could be anatomical, physiological, developmental or behavioral.

9. **Addiction:** A persistent, compulsive dependence on a behavior or substance.

10. **Afebrile:** Without fever, having a normal body temperature.

11. **AIDS:** Acquired immuno deficiency syndrome, a syndrome caused by infection with the human immuno deficiency virus (HIV), there is a visible compromise of the body's immune system.

12. **Alcoholism:** It is a primary, chronic disease arising from drinking of alcohol. It has genetic, psychological and environmental factors influencing its development and manifestations that result in problems.

13. **Allergy:** The hypersensitive response of the immune system of an **allergic** individual to a substance when an **allergen** enters the body. It is a result of hypersensitivity caused by exposure to a particular antigen called allergen.

14. **Allogeneic:** Individuals or tissues that are of the same species but antigenically distinct.

15. **Alloimmunity:** Specifically immune to an allogenic antigen.

16. **Ambulant:** Walking about or able to walk about; denoting a patient who is not confined to bed or hospital as a result of disease or surgery.

17. **Ambulatory care:** It is medical care provided on an outpatient basis, including diagnosis, observation, consultation, treatment, intervention, and rehabilitation services. This care can be provided outside of hospitals. (Also called **outpatient care).**

18. **Angiotensin:** It is a decapeptide hormone (a. I) formed from, the plasma glycoprotein angiotensinogen by renin secreted by the juxtaglomerular apparatus. It is in turn hydrolyzed by a peptidase in the lungs to form an octapeptide (a. II) which is a powerful vasopressor and stimulator of aldosterone secretion by the adrenal cortex. This is in turn hydrolysed to

form a heptapeptide (a. III) which has less vasopressor activity but more adrenal cortex stimulating activity.

19. **Anemia** refers to a decreased number of circulating red blood cells and is the most common blood disorder.

20. **Angina pectoris** is the sensation of chest pain, pressure, or squeezing, often due to not enough blood flow to the heart muscle as a result of obstruction or spasm of the coronary arteries.

21. **Anorexia:** A serious psychological disorder precipitated as lack or loss of appetite; it is characterized by markedly reduced appetite or total aversion to food.

22. **Anoxia:** The absence, or near absence, of oxygen. It leads to a condition in which there is an abnormally low amount of oxygen in the body tissues.

23. **Anti-anxiety:** Tending to prevent or relieve anxiety.

24. **Antibiotic:** A substance derived from a mould or bacterium, or produced synthetically, that destroys (bactericidal) or inhibits the growth (bacteriostatic) of other microorganisms.

25. **Antibody:** Specialized cells of the immune system which can recognize organisms that invade the body (such as bacteria, viruses, and fungi). They set off a chain of events designed to kill the invaders.

26. **Antidepressant:** Anything used to prevent or treat depression or symptoms of mood disorders.

27. **Antipsychotics:** A class of medicine used to treat psychosis and other mental/emotional conditions. They are used to manage psychosis (including delusions, hallucinations, paranoia or disordered thought), principally in schizophrenia and bipolar disorders.

28. **Anxiety:** Is a collective term for several disorders that cause nervousness, fear, apprehension, and worrying. These disorders affect how we feel and behave.

29. **Appendicitis** is inflammation of the appendix (which is the worm-shaped pouch attached to the cecum) at the beginning of the large intestine. Symptoms commonly include right lower abdominal pain, nausea, vomiting, and decreased appetite.

30. **Arachidonic acid:** A poly unsaturated 20 carbon essential fatty acid occurring in animal fats and formed by biosynthesis from linoleic acid; it is a precursor of leukotrienes, prostaglandins, and thromboxane.

31. **Arrest:** Indicates a sudden stop in effective manner, due to failure of a normal function.

32. **Arthritis:** Inflammation of one or more of your joints. The main symptoms are joint pain and stiffness.

33. **Ataxia:** Lack of muscle coordination which may affect speech, eye movements, ability to swallow, walking, picking up objects, and other voluntary movements.

34. **Aura:** Related to the ear or to the sense of hearing.

35. **Autoimmunity:** A condition characterised by a specific humoral or cell mediated immune response against the constituents of the body's own tissues (auto antigens); it may result in hypersensitivity reaction or if severe, in autoimmune disease.

36. **Autologous:** Related to self; belonging to the same organism.

37. **Autolysis:** Spontaneous disintegration of cells or tissues by autologous enzymes, as occurs after death and in some pathologic conditions.

38. **Azotemia:** (uremia) An excess of nitrogenous compounds (blood urea nitrogen, creatinine) in blood.

39. **Azure:** One of three metachromatic basic dyes (A, B and C).

40. **Azuresin:** A complex combination of azure dye and carbacrylic cationic exchange resin used as adiagnostic aid in detection of gastric secretion.

41. **Azurophil:** A tissue constituent staining with azure or a similar metachromatic thiazine.

42. **Bacteria:** Pathogenic microorganisms that proliferate, resulting in tissue injury that can progress to disease **bacterial infection**.

43. **Bradykinin:** A non apeptide kinin formed from HMW kininogen by the action of kallikrein; it is a very powerful vasodilator and increases capillary permeability; in addition, it constricts smooth muscle and stimulates pain receptors.

44. **Baseline blood test:** Any test that measures current or pre-treatment parameters (e.g., chemistries, cell counts, enzyme levels, etc.), against which responses to therapy are evaluated.

45. **BCG:** An effective immunization against tuberculosis. **BCG** stands for **Bacille Calmette Guerin**. It consists of a weakened (attenuated) version of *Mycobacterium bovis* which is closely related to *Mycobacterium tuberculosis*, responsible to cause tuberculosis.

46. **Bereavement:** A deprivation causing grief and desolation, especially the death or loss of a loved one.

47. **Bronchitis:** An inflammation of the air passages between the nose and the lungs, including trachea and air tubes of the lung that bring air in from the trachea (bronchi).

48. **Burden of disease:** Is a comprehensive regional and global assessment of mortality and disability from diseases and injuries.

49. **Cardiomyopathy:** A general diagnostic term designating primary non inflammatory disease of the heart. More restrictively, only those disorders in which the myocardium alone is involved, and in which the cause is unknown and not part of a disease affecting other organs.

50. **Care:** (primary, secondary, tertiary) **Primary care** is the day-to-day healthcare given by a health care provider. **Secondary care**: Medical care that is provided by a specialist or facility upon referral by a primary care physician **Tertiary care** is specialized consultative health **care**, usually for inpatients and on referral from a primary or secondary health professional.

51. **Chaemotaxis/Chemotaxis:** Movement of a cell or organism in response to differences in concentration of a dissolved substance, either in the direction of increasing concentration (positive) or in the direction of decreasing concentration (negative).

52. **Cholecystitis:** Inflammation of gall bladder

53. **Collagenase:** An enzyme that catalyses the hydrolysis of peptide bonds in triple helical regions of collagen.

54. **Creatinine:** An anhydride of creatine, the end product of phosphocreatine metabolism; measurements of its rate of urinary excretion are used as diagnostic indicators of kidney function and muscle mass.

55. **Cytokine:** A generic term for non-antibody proteins released by one cell population on contact with specific antigen, which act as intercellular mediators, as in the generation of an immune response.

56. **Chronic care** management encompasses the oversight and education activities conducted by healthcare professionals to help patients with chronic diseases and health conditions such as diabetes, high blood pressure, lupus, multiple sclerosis and sleep apnea.

57. **Cirrhosis** is disease in which healthy liver tissue is replaced with scar tissue, eventually preventing the liver from functioning properly. The scar tissue blocks the flow of blood through the liver and slows the processing of nutrients, hormones, drugs, and naturally produced toxins.

58. **Clinical care:** Classification (CCC) System is a standardized, coded nursing terminology. It is a nursing care component which is defined as a cluster of elements that represents a unique pattern of clinical care nursing practice. The CCC provides a unique framework and coding structure for documenting

59. **Clinical pathways**: One of the main tools used to manage the quality in healthcare concerning the standardization of care processes. Clinical pathways promote organized and efficient patient care based on evidence based practice.

60. **Clinical practice guidelines** are statements that include recommendations intended to optimize patient care that are informed by a systematic review of evidence and an assessment of the benefits and harms of alternative care options.

61. **Clinical significance:** A change in a patient's/subject's clinical status that is regarded as important, whether or not it is due to an intervention in the context of a clinical trial.

62. **Clinical trials** are trials conducted to evaluate the effectiveness and safety of medications or medical devices by monitoring their effects on large groups of people.

63. **Cognitive tests** are assessments of the cognitive capabilities of humans and other animals. The tests administered to humans include various forms of IQ tests.

64. **Coma:** A **coma** is a state of prolonged unconsciousness that can be caused by a variety of problems - traumatic head injury, stroke, brain tumor, drug or alcohol intoxication, or even an underlying illness, such as diabetes or an infection. It is a state of deep sleep, it is a state of extreme unresponsiveness, in which an individual exhibits no voluntary movement or behavior.

65. **Concurrent review:** Review of the medical necessity of hospital or other health facility admissions, upon or within a short time following an admission, and periodic review. Reviewers monitor appropriateness of the care, the setting, and the progress of discharge plans.

66. **Concussion** is a clinical syndrome characterized by immediate and transient alteration in brain function, including alteration of mental status and level of consciousness, resulting from mechanical force or trauma. This traumatic injury to soft tissue, usually the brain, as a result of a violent blow, shaking, or spinning.

67. **Contraindication:** It is a specific situation in which a drug, procedure, or surgery should not be used because it may be harmful to the person. A condition which makes a particular treatment or procedure potentially inadvisable.

68. **Conventional medicine:** A system in which **medical** doctors and other **healthcare** professionals (such as nurses, pharmacists, and therapists) treat symptoms and diseases.

69. **Cost of illness:** The personal cost of acute or chronic disease. The cost to the patient may be an economic, social, or psychological cost or personal loss to self, family, or immediate community. Core direct costs are those connected with the use of medical care in the prevention, diagnosis, and treatment of disease Cost of illness (COI), known as burden of disease (BOD).

70. **CPR:** Cardiopulmonary resuscitation (CPR) is a procedure to support and maintain breathing and circulation for a person who has stopped breathing (respiratory arrest) and/or whose heart has stopped (cardiac arrest).

71. **CVD:** Any disease of the heart or blood vessels, including atherosclerosis, cardiomyopathy, coronary artery disease, peripheral vascular disease. Cardiovascular diseases also include arteriosclerosis, coronary artery disease, heart valve disease, arrhythmia, heart failure, hypertension, orthostatic hypotension, shock, endocarditis, diseases of the aorta and its branches, disorders of the peripheral vascular system, and congenital heart disease.

72. **Critical pathways:** They describe pivotal steps in the clinical processes of care which include combining information about process and outcomes to improve medical care.

73. **Devascularisation:** Interruption of circulation of blood to a part due to obstruction of vessels supplying it.

74. **Delirium:** is a syndrome, or group of symptoms, caused by a disturbance in the normal functioning of the brain. Delirium is often marked by hallucinations, delusions, and a dream-like state. A sudden state of severe confusion and rapid changes in brain function

75. **Delusion:** A delusion is an unshakable belief in something untrue. These irrational beliefs defy normal reasoning, and remain firm even when overwhelming proof is presented to dispute them.

76. **Dementia** is a general term for a decline in mental ability severe enough to interfere with daily life. Memory loss is an example. Alzheimer's is the most common type of dementia.

77. **Dependency** is a psychologic craving for, habituation to, or addiction to a chemical substance; or drug dependence.

78. **Depersonalization:** Loss of the sense of personal identity; especially: a psychopathological syndrome characterized by loss of identity and feelings of unreality or strangeness about one's own behavior. Also called self-alienation.

79. **Depression:** It is a mood disorder that causes a persistent feeling of sadness and loss of interest. It affects how you feel, think and behave and can lead to a variety of emotional and physical problems.

80. **Dermatitis:** Inflammation of the skin, either due to an inherent skin defect, direct contact with an irritating substance, or to an allergic reaction. Symptoms include redness, itching, and in some cases blistering.

81. **Detoxification:** To remove a toxic substance or the effects of such a substance. It is the physiological or medicinal removal of toxins.

82. **Diabetes** is a chronic disease associated with abnormally high levels of the sugar glucose in the blood.

83. **Diagnosis:** The process of determining, through examination and analysis, the nature of illness. It is therefore a process of identifying a disease by signs and symptoms.

84. **Diapedesis:** The outward passage of cellular elements of the blood through intact vessel walls.

85. **Direct patient care:** Care of a patient provided personally by a staff member. Direct patient care may involve any aspects of the health care of a patient, including treatments, counseling, self-care, patient education, and administration of medication.

86. **Disability:** It is the inability of an individual to engage in any substantial gainful activity by reason of any medically determinable physical or mental impairment which can be expected to last for a continuous period of not less than 12 months. It may reduce the individual's quality of life and cause clear disadvantages to the individual.

87. **Disability Adjusted Life Years (DALY)** is a measure of overall disease burden, expressed as the number of years lost due to ill-health, disability or early death.

88. **Disability adjusted life expectancy** is the number of years lost due to ill-health disability or early death and a subsequent gain in the number of years due to adjustments made during DALY.

89. **Disease:** A condition of abnormal vital function involving any structure, part, or system of an organism. It is a specific illness or disorder characterized by a recognizable set of signs and symptoms.

90. **Disease control:** Measures taken to reduce the spread of a disease.

91. **Disease management:** It is defined as a system of coordinated healthcare interventions and communications for populations with conditions in which patient self-care efforts are significant.

92. **Disease prevention:** Medical practices that are designed to avert and avoid disease.

93. **Disorder:** A physical or mental condition that is not normal or healthy. A lack of order or regular arrangement; confusion. It hence is a condition characterized by lack of normal functioning of physical or mental processes: (kidney disorders; a psychiatric disorder).

94. **Disorientation:** A usually transient state of confusion especially as to time, place, or identity often as a result of disease or drugs.

95. **Dissemination:** Widely dispersed in a tissue, organ, or the entire body

96. **Drug utilization** Review an authorized, structured, ongoing program that collects, analyzes, and interprets drug use patterns to improve the quality of pharmacotherapy and patient outcomes.

97. **Drug withdrawal:** Abrupt discontinuation of a drug leading to withdrawal symptoms like abnormal physical or psychological features that follow the abrupt discontinuation of a drug. Example, common opiates withdrawal symptoms include sweating, goose bumps, vomiting, anxiety, insomnia, and muscle pain.

98. **Dyspnea:** Breathlessness or shortness of breath; laboured or difficult breathing.

99. **Elastase:** An endopeptidase catalysing the cleavage of specific peptide bonds in protein.

100. **Endocarditis:** Exudative and proliferative inflammatory alterations in the endocardium, usually characterised by the presence vegetations on the surface of endocardium or in the endocardium itself, and most commonly involving a heart valve, but also affecting the inner lining of the cardiac chambers or the endocardium elsewhere.

101. **Endocardium:** The endothelial lining membrane of the cavities of the heart and the connective tissue bedon which it lies.

102. **Eosinophil:** A granular leukocyte having a nucleus with two lobes connected by a thread of chromatin, and cytoplasm containing coarse, round granules of uniform size.

103. **ECG:** Electro Cardio Gram (ECG) A record of the electrical activity of the heart showing certain waves called P, Q, R, S, and T waves. The Q, R, S, T waves are associated with contraction of the ventricles, the lower two chambers of the heart.

104. **ECT:** Electroconvulsive therapy (ECT) is a medical treatment for severe mental illness in which a small, carefully controlled amount of electricity is introduced into the brain. This electrical stimulation, used in conjunction with anesthesia and muscle relaxant medications, produces a mild generalized seizure or convulsion.

105. **Efficacy** is a social cognitive theory, a person's belief in their ability to execute the behaviours necessary to achieve desired outcomes. In contrast to self-confidence, self-efficacy refers to beliefs about specific behaviours in specific situations.

106. **Emphysema:** A pathological condition of the lungs marked by an abnormal increase in the size of the air spaces, resulting in labored breathing and an increased susceptibility to infection. It can be caused by irreversible expansion of the alveoli or by the destruction of alveolar walls.

107. **End of life care:** Refers to health care, not only of patients in the final hours or days of their lives, but more broadly care of all those with a terminal illness or terminal disease condition that has become advanced, progressive and incurable.

108. **End point:** A point marking the completion of a process or stage of a process: eg: a point in a titration. In a clinical research trial, a clinical endpoint generally refers to occurrence of a disease, symptom, sign or laboratory abnormality that constitutes one of the target outcomes of the trial, but may also refer to any such disease or sign that strongly motivates the withdrawal of that individual or entity.

109. **Epilepsy:** A pattern of repeated seizures is referred to as epilepsy. A seizure is defined as an abnormal, disorderly discharging of the brain's nerve cells, resulting in a temporary disturbance of motor, sensory, or mental function.

110. **Epistaxis:** It is medical term for nose bleed. The nose is very rich in blood vessels (vascular) and is situated in a vulnerable position on the face. As a result, any trauma to the face can cause bleeding, which may be profuse.

111. **Ethics** is a system of moral principles that apply values and judgments to the practice of medicine.

112. **Euthanasia:** The act or practice of causing or permitting the death of hopelessly sick or injured individuals (including persons or domestic animals) in a relatively painless way for reasons of mercy. This term is also called mercy killing.

113. **Evidence based care:** It is the integration of putting into use the clinical expertise, patient values and the best research evidence for the decision making process of patient care. Clinical expertise refers to the clinician's cumulated experience, education and clinical skills.

114. **Evidence based decision-making:** It is an approach to medical practice intended to optimize decision-making by emphasizing the use of evidence from well-designed and well -conducted research. It promotes the use of formal, explicit methods to analyze evidence and makes it available to decision makers.

115. **Expectation of life:** It is an epidemiological expression of the probability of dying between one age and the next. It is calculated based on the human cohort life table which describes the actual mortality experience of a group of animals which were all born at the same time.

116. **Febrile** means "related to fever." It can be used in a medical sense when someone is sick and running a temperature.

117. **Fever:** Although a fever technically is any body temperature above the normal of 98.6 °F (37 °C), in practice a person is considered to have a significant fever when the temperature is above 100.4 °F (38°C).

118. **Facultative** Not obligatory; pertaining to the ability to adjust to particular circumstances or to assume a particular role.

119. **Fibrinopeptide:** Either of two peptides (A and B) split off from fibrinogen during coagulation by the action of thrombin.

120. **Fibronectin:** An adhesive glycoprotein; one form circulates in plasma and acts as an opsonin another is a cell surface protein that mediates cellular adhesive interactions.

121. **Fistula:** A fistula is an abnormal anastomosis or an abnormal connection between two hollow epithelialized surfaces such as blood vessels, intestines, or other hollow organs.

122. **Fits:** Also known as seizures. A person having a seizure may experience convulsions and/or lose consciousness. It is caused by disturbances in the electrical activity of the brain, which can be due to conditions such as epilepsy.

123. **Fracture:** A break in bone or cartilage due to accident or due to acquired disease of bone.

124. **Gall bladder:** A pear-shaped organ that stores bile salts until they are needed to help digest fatty foods.

125. **Gall stones:** It is a solid crystal deposit that forms in the gallbladder. Gallstones can migrate to other parts of the digestive tract and cause severe pain with life-threatening complications.

126. **Gastritis:** It describes a group of conditions with inflammation of the lining of the stomach. [Inflammation of the colon and rectum], and may progress to ulcerations, rectal strictures, rectovaginal fistulas, and genital elephantiasis.

127. **Gastroenteritis:** Inflammation of the stomach and the intestines caused mainly by infections (viruses, bacteria, and parasites), food poisoning, and stress.

128. **Glomerulo nephritis:** Nephritis with inflammation of the capillary loops in the renal glomeruli.

129. **Hematemesis:** Is vomiting of blood. The source of this blood is generally from the upper gastrointestinal tract, typically above the suspensory muscle of duodenum.

130. **Haematuria:** It is the medical term for the presence of red blood cells in the urine which can come from the kidney (where urine is made) or anywhere in the urinary tract.

131. **Haemoglobin:** Is the oxygen-carrying pigment. It is a predominant protein in the red blood cells.

132. **Haemoptysis:** Spitting up blood or blood-tinged sputum from the respiratory tract because of breaking of tiny blood vessels that line the lung airways.

133. **Haemorrhage:** Escape of blood from a ruptured vessel either external or internal.

134. **Hallucination:** It is a perception of something as a visual image or a sound with no external cause usually arising from a disorder of the nervous system or in response to drugs.

135. **Harm:** Anything that impairs or adversely affects the safety of patients in clinical care, drug therapy, research investigations or public health is termed as harm. Harms include adverse drug reactions, side effects of treatments, and other undesirable consequences of health care products and services.

136. **Hazard:** Is a condition or phenomenon that increases the probability of a loss. A hazard increases the chances of a loss that does not necessarily result from illness or injury.

137. **Haematoma:** Extravasation of blood into the tissues with resultant swelling is known as haematoma.

138. **Healing:** A process of cure or restoration of integrity of injured tissue.

139. **Healing by first intention** that in which union or restoration of continuity occurs directly without intervention of granulations.

140. **Healing by second intention:** Union by closure of wound with granulations.

141. **Hyperaemia:** Engorgement; an excess of blood in a part.

142. **Hypercalcemia:** An excess of calcium in blood.

143. **Hypersensitivity:** A state of altered reactivity in which the body reacts with an exaggerated immune response to what is perceived as a foreign substance.

144. **Health care:** The prevention, treatment, and management of illness and the preservation of mental and physical well-being through the services offered by the medical and allied health professions is called Health Care.

145. **Health expectancy** is the number of years a person could expect to live in good health.

146. **Health Related Quality of Life: (HRQoL)** is an assessment of how the individual's well-being may be affected over time by a disease, disability, or disorder.

147. **Heart attack:** The loss of blood supply caused by complete blockage of a coronary artery, supplying blood to the heart muscle because of which the heart is starved of oxygen and heart cells die. The medical term for this is myocardial infarction.

148. **Heart disease:** Any disorder that affects the heart. Heart disease is synonymous with cardiac disease but not with cardiovascular disease which is any disease of the heart or blood vessels.

149. **Heart failure:** Is is a condition in which the heart has lost the ability to pump enough blood to the body's tissues thereby being unable to maintain adequate circulation of blood in the tissues of the body because of which the tissues do not receive enough oxygen and nutrients to function properly.

150. **Hematoma:** A localized swelling filled with blood caused by a break in the wall of a blood vessel. The blood is usually clotted or partially clotted, and it exists within an organ or in a soft tissue space, such as muscle.

151. **Hepatitis:** It refers to an inflammatory condition of the liver. It is commonly caused by a viral infection, but there are other possible causes of hepatitis. These include autoimmune hepatitis and hepatitis that occurs as a secondary result of medications, drugs, toxins, and alcohol.

152. **Hernia:** It is a protrusion of an organ or part through connective tissue or through a wall of the cavity in which it is normally enclosed.

153. **HIV:** Human Immunodeficiency Virus (HIV) is the cause of AIDS (Acquired immunodeficiency syndrome) which is a chronic, potentially life-threatening condition caused by damaging the immune system.

154. **Homeostasis:** The processes through which such bodily equilibrium is maintained is referred to as homeostasis. It is the state of equilibrium or balance between opposing pressures in the body with respect to various functions and to the chemical compositions of the fluids and tissues.

155. **Hospice care:** The word "hospice" comes from the Latin "hospitium" meaning guest house. Hospice care is hence a care designed to give supportive care to people in the final phase of a terminal illness and focus on comfort and quality of life, rather than cure. Volunteer care is part of hospice philosophy.

156. **Hyperglycaemia:** An abnormally high concentration of glucose in the circulating blood, seen especially in patients with diabetes mellitus.

157. **Hypertension:** High blood pressure, defined as a repeatedly elevated blood pressure exceeding 140 over 90 mmHg i.e. a systolic pressure above 140 or a diastolic pressure above 90 mmHg.

158. **Hyperventilation:** Excessive ventilation; specifically: excessive rate and depth of respiration leading to abnormal loss of carbon dioxide from the blood—called also over ventilation.

159. **Hypoglycaemia:** The condition with low blood sugar. Hypoglycemia occurs when blood sugar or blood glucose concentrations fall below a level necessary to properly support the body's need for energy and stability throughout its cells.

160. **Hypotension:** It is characterized by diminished blood pressure i.e. Abnormally low blood pressure.

161. **Hypothermia** a potentially fatal condition, occurs when body temperature falls below 95°F (35°C).

162. **Illness:** Is an abnormal condition of a part, organ, or system of an organism resulting from various causes, such as infection, inflammation, environmental factors, or genetic defects etc. It is characterized by an identifiable group of signs, symptoms, or both.

163. **Ileitis:** Inflammation of the ileum, regional ileitis: Crohn's disease affecting the ileum.

164. **Immunoglobulin:** A protein of animal origin with known antibody activity synthesised by lymphocytesand plasma cells and found in serum and in other body fluids and tissues; abbreviated 'Ig'. There are five distinct classes based on structural and antigenic properties: Ig-A, Ig-D, Ig-E, Ig-G, and Ig-M.

165. **Important growth factors:** Epithelial growth factor (EGF), FGF -Fibroblast growth factor (FGF), Platelet derived growth factor (PDGF), Colony stimulating factor (CSF), Transforming growth factor-β (TGF- β), Interleukin (IL), Basic fibroblast growth factor (6 FBG).

166. **Ischaemia:** Deficiency of blood in a part due to functional constriction or actual obstruction of blood vessel.

167. **Impact:** The forcible striking of one body against another or to press two bodies, parts, or fragments closely together.

168. **Impairment:** Is any loss or abnormality of psychological, physiologic, or anatomic structure or function. A physical or mental defect at the level of a body system or organ.

169. **Incontinence:** Unable to restrain natural discharges or evacuations of urine or feces.

170. **Independence:** Is a process or activity that can be implemented without the assistance of another. It is freestanding and capable of functioning in an autonomous fashion.

171. **Indication:** A symptom or particular circumstance that indicates the advisability or necessity of a specific medical treatment or procedure a condition which makes a particular treatment or procedure advisable.

172. **Infection:** The invasion and multiplication of microorganisms such as bacteria, viruses, and parasites that are not normally present within the body.

173. **Inflammation:** It is a local response to cellular injury that is marked by capillary dilatation, leukocytic infiltration, redness, heat, pain, swelling, and often loss of function and that serves as a mechanism initiating the elimination of noxious agents and of damaged tissue.

174. **Insomnia**: Is the inability to obtain an adequate amount or quality of sleep. The difficulty can be in falling asleep, remaining asleep, or both.

175. **Insulin:** A natural hormone produced by the pancreas that controls the level of the sugar or glucose in the blood.

176. **Integrated care:** Collaborative care is a related healthcare philosophy and movement that has many names, models, and definitions that often includes the provision of mental-health, behavioral-health and substance-use services in primary care.

177. **Intensive care:** The specialized care of patients whose conditions are life-threatening and who require comprehensive care and constant monitoring, usually in intensive care units.

178. **Intravenous:** Into a vein. Intravenous (IV) medications are a solutions administered directly into the venous circulation via a syringe or intravenous catheter.

179. **Ischemia:** Deficient supply of blood to body parts like the heart or brain that is due to obstruction of the inflow of arterial blood because of the narrowing of arteries by spasm or disease.

180. **Jaundice:** Yellow staining of the skin and sclerae (the whites of the eyes) by abnormally high blood levels of the bile pigment bilirubin.

181. **Jacksonian epilepsy:** Epilepsy marked by focal motor seizure with unilateral clonic movements that start in one muscle group and spread systematically to adjacent groups, reflecting the march epileptic activity through the motor cortex.

182. **Kinin:** Any of group of vasoactive straight chain polypeptides formed by kallikrein-catalysed cleavage of kininogen; causing vasodilation and also altering vascular permeability.

183. **Leukotriene:** Any of a group of biologically active compounds derived from arachidonic acid thatfunctions as regulators of allergic and inflammatory reactions. They are identified by the letters A, B, C, D, and E, with subscript numerals indicating the number of double bonds in each molecule.

184. **Lipo-oxygenase:** An enzyme that catalyses the oxidation of polyunsaturated fatty acids to form a peroxide of the acid.

185. **Lumen:** The cavity or channel within a tube or tubular organ.

186. **Lymphogranuloma venereum: (Hodgkin's disease):** A venereal infection due to strains of *Chlamydiatrachomatis*, marked by a primary transient ulcerative lesion of the genitals, followed by acute lymphadenopathy. In men, primary infection on the penis usually leads to inguinal lymphadenitis; in women, primary infection often labia, vagina, or cervix often leads to haemorrhagic proctocolitis.

187. **Lymphokine:** A general term for soluble protein mediators postulated to be released by sensitized lymphocytes on contact with antigen, and believed to play a role in macrophage activation, lymphocyte transformation, and cell mediated immunity.

188. **Margination:** Accumulation and adhesion of leukocytes to the endothelial cells of blood vessel walls at the site of injury in the early stages of inflammation.

189. **Monocytes:** A mono nuclear, phagocytic leukocyte, 13μ to $25\,\mu$ in diameter, with an ovoid or kidney shaped nucleus, and azurophilic cytoplasmic

granules. Formed in the bone marrow from promonocytes. Monocytes are transported to tissues, such as the lung and liver, where they develop into macrophages.

190. **Monokine:** A general term for soluble mediators of immune responses that are not antibodies or complement components and that are produced by mononuclear phagocytes (monocytes or macrophages).

191. **Mucoid:** Resembling mucus.

192. **Mucopurulent:** Containing both mucus and pus.

193. **Multiple myeloma:** A tumor composed of cells of the type normally found in the bone marrow. A disseminated type of plasma cell dyscrasia characterised by multiple bone marrow tumor foci and secretion of an M component, manifested by skeletal destruction, pathologic fractures, bone pain. The presence of anomalous circulating immunoglobulins. Bence Jones proteinuria and anemia.

194. **Myofibroblast:** An atypical fibroblast combing the ultra-structural features of a fibroblast and a smooth muscle cell.

195. **Managed care:** Any system that manages health care delivery to control costs. By typically relying on a primary care physician.

196. **Mania:** Excitement of psychotic proportions manifested by mental and physical hyperactivity, disorganization of behavior, and elevation of mood.

197. **Manipulation:** It is an act, process, or an instance of manipulating / adjustment of faulty structural relationships by manual means as in the reduction of fractures or dislocations.

198. **Montoux test:** An intradermal test for hypersensitivity to tuberculin that indicates past or present infection with tubercle bacilli. A small quantity of a sterile liquid derived from a culture of tubercle bacilli (tuberculin) is injected into the skin and the local reaction noted.

199. **Medical error** is a preventable adverse effect of care, whether or not it is evident or harmful to the patient. This might include an inaccurate or incomplete diagnosis or treatment of a disease, injury, syndrome, behavior, infection, or other ailment.

200. **Meningitis:** It is an inflammation of the meninges. Meninges is the collective name for the three membranes (called the dura mater, the arachnoid mater, and the pia mater) that envelope the brain and spinal cord.

201. **Mental health:** refers to a wide range of mental health conditions/disorders that affect the mood, thinking and behavior. It is a state of psychological well-being with an appropriate balance of love, work.

202. **Migraine:** A throbbing headache that usually affects only one side of the head. Nausea, vomiting, increased sensitivity to light, and other symptoms often accompany migraine.

203. **Morbidity:** Is a term used to describe a focus on death. It is a diseased condition or state.

204. **Multiple risk/causation** Fundamentally, the issue of *causation* in clinical negligence cases, *Multiple*(cumulative) causes sometimes *several* symptoms always appear to explain *multiple* epidemiological associations or *risk* factors.

205. **Neovascularisation:** New blood vessel formation in abnormal tissue or in abnormal positions.

206. **Neutrophil:** a granular leukocyte having a nucleus with three to five lobes connected by threads of chromatin and cytoplasm containing very fine granules. Any cell, structure, or histological element readily stainable with neutral dyes.

207. **Nausea:** Is the sensation of being about to vomit. Vomiting, or emesis, is the expelling of undigested food through the mouth.

208. **Nebulization:** A method of administering a drug by spraying it into the respiratory passages of the patient. The medication may be given with or without oxygen to help carry it into the lungs.

209. **Neuritis:** Neuritis and neuralgia attack the peripheral nerves, the nerves that link the brain and spinal cord with the muscles, skin, organs, and all other parts of the body. It causes inflammation of a nerve; but also denote certain non-inflammatory lesions of the peripheral nervous system.

210. **Nutrition:** Is the process of taking in food and using it for growth, metabolism and repair.

211. **Oedema/edema:** An abnormal accumulation of fluid in intercellular spaces of the body.

212. **Oliguric/oliguria:** Diminished urine production and excretion in relation to fluid intake.

213. **Opsonisation:** The rendering of bacteria and other cells subject to phagocytosis.

214. **Perineum:** The region and associated structures occupying the pelvic outlet and beneath the pelvic diaphragm.

215. **Phagosome:** A membrane bound vesicle in a phagocyte containing the phagocytised material.

216. **Plasma cell dyscrasia:** A diverse group of neoplastic diseases involving proliferation of a single clone of cells producing a serum M component (a monoclonal immunoglobulin or immunoglobulin fragment) and usually having a plasma cell morphology; it includes multiple myeloma and heavy chain diseases.

217. **Polymorphonuclear:** Having a nucleus so deeply lobed or so divided as to appear to be multiple.

218. **Prostaglandin:** Any of a group of naturally occurring, chemically related fatty acids that stimulate contractility of the uterine and other smooth muscle and have the ability to lower blood pressure, regulate acid secretion of the stomach, regulate body temperature and platelet aggregation, and control inflammation and vascular permeability; they also affect the action of certain hormones. Nine primary types are labelled A through I, the degree of saturation of the side chain of each being designated by subscripts 1, 2, and 3. The types of prostaglandins are abbreviated PGE_2, $PGF_{2\alpha}$, and so on.

219. **Pyelonephritis:** Inflammation of the kidney and its pelvis due to bacterial infection.

220. **Pyogenesis:** Suppuration, the formation of pus.

221. **Occupational health services:** The Basic Occupational Health Services are an application of the primary health care principles in the sector of occupational health. These services include a statutory preventive occupational health care services, namely occupational health physician, occupational health nurse, an occupational physiotherapist and psychologist services, as well as the general level medical treatment, including laboratory and X-ray examinations.

222. **Occupational therapy:** It is the therapy based on engagement in meaningful activities of daily life as self-care skills, education, work, or social interaction especially to enable or encourage participation of the clients in such activities despite impairments or limitations in their physical or mental functioning.

223. **Oedema:** It is a buildup of fluid in the body which causes swelling in the affected tissue. The swelling can occur in one particular part of the body or may be general depending on the cause.

224. **Oesophagus:** Is the tube that connects the pharynx (throat) with the stomach. Oesophagus lies between the trachea (windpipe) and the spine. It passes down the neck, pierces the diaphragm just to the left of the midline, and joins the cardiac (upper) end of the stomach. It is also known as the gullet or swallowing tube.

225. **Orientation:** Is awareness of one's environment, with reference to place, time, and people. It is the act or process of orienting or of being oriented, the state of being oriented.

226. **Outcome:** A result, new condition or event occurring in individual study subjects which is used to assess efficacy.

227. **Overdose:** Is the accidental or intentional use of a drug or medicine in an amount that is higher than is normally used.

228. **Palliative care:** Is medical and related care provided to a patient with a serious, life-threatening, or terminal illness to manage symptoms, relieving

pain and discomfort, improve quality of life, and meet the emotional, social, and spiritual needs of the patient.

229. **Palpitations:** A sensation in which a person is aware of an irregular, hard or rapid, fluttering or pounding heart. Heart palpitations can be triggered by stress, exercise, medication or, a medical condition.

230. **Pancreatitis:** It is an inflammation of the pancreas, an organ that is important in digestion.

231. **Paralysis** is defined as complete loss of voluntary movements i.e. motor functions/ strength of an affected limb or muscle group. Paralysis that affects only one muscle or limb is partial paralysis, also known as palsy; paralysis of all muscles is total paralysis.

232. **Paranoia:** It is an unfounded or exaggerated distrust for others, sometimes reaching delusional proportions. Paranoid individuals constantly suspect the motives of those around them, and believe that certain individuals, or people in general, are dangerous for them.

233. **Pediculosis:** Infestation with lice. *Pediculosis corporis* is infestation of the skin of the body with lice. *Pediculosis palpebrarum* is infestation of the eyelids and eyelashes with lice. *Pediculosis pubis* is infestation of the pubic hair region with lice.

234. **Peptic ulcer:** Ulcer in the wall of the stomach or duodenum resulting from the digestive action of the gastric juice on the mucous membrane when the latter is rendered susceptible to its action or from infection with the bacterium Helicobacter pylori or the chronic use of NSAIDs.

235. **Personality disorder:** A personality disorder is a type of mental disorder in which you have a rigid and unhealthy pattern of thinking, functioning and behaving. A person with a personality disorder has trouble perceiving and relating to situations and people.

236. **Phlebitis:** It is a condition in which a vein becomes inflamed. The inflammation may cause pain and swelling. When the inflammation is caused by a blood clot or thrombus, it is called **thrombophlebitis.**

237. **Phobia:** Is an extreme separation anxiety disorder of children, usually in the elementary grades, characterized by a persistent irrational fear.

238. **Pneumonia:** Inflammation of one or both lungs. Pneumonia is frequently due to infection. The infection may be bacterial, viral, fungal, or parasitic. Symptoms may include fever, chills, cough with sputum production, chest pain, and shortness of breath.

239. **Pneumothorax:** Results from a wound in the chest wall which acts as a valve that permits air to enter the pleural cavity but prevents its escape. Air enters the pleural cavity and is trapped there during expiration so the air pressure within the thorax mounts higher than atmospheric pressure,

compresses the lung and may displace the mediastinum and its structures, including the lung, toward the opposite side.

240. **Prognosis** is often used as a general term for predicting the unfolding of events: The forecast of the probable outcome or course of a disease and improving the chances of patient recovery.

241. **Psychosis** Means a loss of contact with reality; it is a symptom of mental illness. Generally, there are two types of psychiatric disorder that produce psychotic symptoms: schizophrenia and mood disorders like bipolar disorder.

242. **Psychiatry:** It is a branch of medicine that deals with the science and practice of treating mental, emotional, or behavioral disorders especially as originating in endogenous causes or resulting from faulty interpersonal relationships.

243. **Psychosomatic:** A descriptive term for the relationship between the mind and body. Psychosomatic disorders are thought to be caused by emotional or psychological factors.

244. **Psychotherapy:** It is a general term for the treatment of mental (i.e., emotional, behavioral, personality and psychiatric) disorders through verbal and nonverbal communication with the patient.

245. **Public health:** It is the art and science dealing with the protection and improvement of community health by organized community effort. It also includes preventive medicine, sanitary and social science. It also assures that all population have access to appropriate cost-effective care, health promotion and disease prevention services.

246. **Pulmonary embolism:** It is an obstruction of a blood vessel in the lungs, usually due to a blood clot, which blocks a coronary artery.

247. **Pulse:** The rhythmic dilation of an artery that results from beating of the heart. Pulse is often measured by feeling the arteries of the wrist or neck.

248. **Quality of life:** Subjective well-being is the central component in the evaluation of Quality of Life. It is therefore the patient's ability to enjoy normal life activities. It is an overall assessment of a person's well-being, which may include physical, emotional, and social dimensions, as well as stress level, sexual function, and self-perceived health status.

249. **Rapport:** A conscious feeling of harmonious accord, trust, empathy, and mutual responsiveness between two or more people including physician and patient that fosters the therapeutic process.

250. **Rehabilitation:** They are set of treatments designed to facilitate the process of recovery from injury, illness or disease to as normal a condition as possible.

251. **Resuscitation:** A procedure designed to restore normal breathing that includes the clearance of air passages to the lungs, the mouth-to-mouth

method of artificial respiration, and cardiac massage by the exertion of pressure on the chest. It is abbreviated as CPR. (Cardiopulmonary resuscitation).

252. **Scabies:** It is an itchy skin condition caused by a tiny burrowing mite called *Sarcoptes scabiei*. The presence of the mite leads to intense itching in the area of its burrows. The urge to scratch may be especially strong at night.

253. **Schizophrenia:** It is a psychotic disorder marked by severely impaired thinking, emotions, and behaviors. Schizophrenic patients are typically unable to filter sensory stimuli and may have enhanced perceptions of sounds, colors, and other features of their environment.

254. **Schistosomiasis:** The blood flukes, a genus of parasitic trematodes. Species that cause schistosomiasis in humans include- S. haematobium and S. intercalatum in Africa, S. japonicum in East Asia and nearby islands, and S. mansoni in Africa, South America, and the West Indies. The invertebrate hosts are snails. Infection follows penetrating the skin of those coming in contact with infected waters.

255. **Serotonin:** A hormone and neurotransmitter, 5-hydroxytryptamine (5-HT), found in many tissues, including blood platelets, intestinal mucosa, the pineal body, and the central nervous system; it has many physiologic properties including inhibition of gastric secretion, stimulation of smooth muscle, and production of vasoconstriction.

256. **Suppurative:** Agent that cause pyogenesis [formation of pus].

257. **Sepsis:** The presence of bacteria (bacteremia), other infectious organisms, or toxins created by infectious organisms in the bloodstream with spread throughout the body. Sepsis may be associated with clinical symptoms of systemic illness, such as fever, chills, malaise, low blood pressure, and mental-status changes.

258. **Shock:** Is a critical condition that is brought on by a sudden drop in blood flow through the body. The circulatory system fails to maintain adequate blood flow, sharply curtailing the delivery of oxygen and nutrients to vital organs.

259. **Sinus:** Is a channel permitting the passage of blood or lymph fluid that is not a blood or lymphatic vessel.

260. **Spleen:** Is largest lymphatic organ in the body that is located in the upper-left part of the abdomen, not far from the stomach, that produces lymphocytes, which are important elements in the immune system.

261. **Sputum:** Mucous material from the lungs that is produced and brought up by coughing.

262. **Sternum:** It is a plate of bone forming the middle of the anterior wall of the thorax and articulating with the clavicles and the cartilages of the first seven

ribs. It consists of three parts, the manubrium, the body, and the xiphoid process.

263. **Steroid:** One of a large group of chemical substances classified by a specific carbon structure. Steroids include drugs used to relieve swelling and inflammation, such as prednisone and cortisone; vitamin D; and some sex hormones, such as testosterone and estradiol.

264. **Stomach ulcer:** An ulcer in the wall of the stomach or duodenum resulting from the digestive action of the gastric juice on the mucous membrane when the latter is rendered susceptible to its action (*as from infection with the bacterium Helicobacter pylori* or the chronic use of NSAIDs).

265. **Syndrome:** A syndrome is a set of medical signs and symptoms that are correlated with each other. It basically means "running together".

266. **Terminal care:** Care designed to give supportive care to people in the final phase of a terminal illness and focus on comfort and quality of life, rather than cure. Palliative care is a multidisciplinary approach to specialized medical care for people with life-limiting illnesses. It focuses on providing people with relief from the symptoms, pain, physical stress, and mental stress of the terminal diagnosis.

267. **Terminal illness:** Terminal illness is a disease that cannot be cured or adequately treated and that is reasonably expected to result in the death of the patient within a short period of time.

268. **Tetanus:** Is an acute infectious disease characterized by tonic spasm of voluntary muscles and especially of the muscles of the jaw and caused by an exotoxin produced by a bacterium of the genus Clostridium.

269. **Thiamine:** Thiamine (vitamin B1) acts as a coenzyme in the metabolism of the body. Its deficiency causes beriberi, a syndrome characterized by inflammation of multiple nerves (polyneuritis), heart disease (cardiopathy), and edema (swelling).

270. **Tolerance:** Is the capacity of the body to endure or become less responsive to a substance (as a drug) or a physiological environment especially by repeated use / exposure.

271. **Transference:** In psychiatry, the unconscious tendency of a patient to assign to others, the environment feelings and attitudes associated with significant persons in one's life.

272. **Tuberculosis:** A specific disease caused by infection with *Mycobacterium tuberculosis*, the most common site of the disease being the lungs although it can affect any organ of the body.

273. **Tuberculous:** Pertaining to or affected with tuberculosis.

274. **Traditional medicine:** Any system of healthcare that has ancient cultural bonds, trained healer it include Ayurvedic medicine, ethno medicine and traditional Chinese medicine.

275. **Transitional care:** Transitional care refers to the coordination and continuity of health care during a movement from one healthcare setting to either another or to home, called care transition, between health care practitioners.

276. **Ulcer:** A lesion of the skin or a mucous membrane like the lining of the stomach or duodenum that is accompanied by formation of pus and necrosis of surrounding tissue, usually resulting from inflammation or ischemia.

277. **Urgency:** It is the quality or state requiring immediate action or attention.

278. **Urological manifestations:** Clinical disturbances of the urinary system.

279. **Vacuole:** Any membrane bound space or cavity within a cell.

280. **Vasodilation:** Increase in caliber of blood vessels.

281. **Viral infection:** Infection caused by the presence of a virus in the body.

282. **Vital signs:** Signs of life; specifically: the pulse rate, respiratory rate, body temperature, and often blood pressure of a person.

283. **Wheeze:** A wheeze is a continuous, coarse, whistling sound produced in the respiratory airways during breathing.

284. **Withdrawal:** Act of removal or retreat. It is highlighted as psychological and/or physical syndrome caused by abrupt cessation of use of a drug in a habituated person.

2

Cellular Injury and Adaptation

Syllabus: Cause, Pathogenesis, Morphology of cell injury and cell death-Reversible and irreversible cell injury-Apoptosis- adaptations-Modification of cell growth to various stimuli (dysplasia, hyperplasia etc.). Abnormalities in lipoproteinaemia, Glycogen infiltration and Glycogen storage diseases.

Cell injury can occur because of an adverse stimulus which disrupts the normal homeostasis of affected cells. Among other causes, this can be due to physical, chemical, infectious, biological, nutritional or immunological factors. Physical agents such as heat or radiation damage a cell by coagulating their contents. Impaired nutrient supply, lack of oxygen or glucose, impaired ATP production may deprive the cell of essential materials needed to survive thereby leading to cell death.

Any type of cell injury changes the fluid volume **total body water (TBW).** Extracellular fluid (**ECF**) or extracellular fluid volume (ECFV) usually denotes all body fluid outside the cells. The remainder is called intracellular fluid (**ICF**). The **ECF and ICF** are the two major fluid compartments, which together account for **total body water (TBW).**

Extracellular fluid (**ECF**) is found in blood plasma, lymph, body cavities lined with serous (moisture-exuding) membranes, the cavities and channels of the brain and spinal cord, and as interstitial fluid between the cells of all the other organs of the body.

Cell injury and Adaptation

Cell: A cell is the smallest living unit in human body. In multicellular living organism, cells are in close contact with other cells and are surrounded by body fluids and extra cellular matrix- which provide internal environment.

Cell injury: May be defined as variety of stress a cell encounter because of change in internal/external environment.

Cellular adaptation: Cellular adaptation is a reversible adjustment to environmental condition. That includes change in cell function, morphology or both. When stimulus is reversed cell revert to their normal state. When limit of adaptive response to stimulus are exceeded, adaption is not possible and lead to cell injury.

Reversible cell injury: when the stress is mild to moderate injured cell may recover.

Irreversible cell injury: If stimulus persists or severe, cell reaches the point of no return and cell death occurs.

Cell death: It is the ultimate result of cell injury. There are two morphological patterns of cell death-necrosis and apoptosis.

Necrosis: Pathological cell death is called necrosis. It is the common type of cell death after exogenous stimuli. It occurs after stress like ischemia, chemical injury etc. It is characterized by severe cell swelling, cell rupture, denaturation and coagulation of cytoplasmic proteins, breakdown of cell organelles etc.

Apoptosis: More regulated form of cell death. It is designed for normal elimination of unwanted cells, during embryogenesis and in various physiologic processes. Chief morphological features are chromatin condensation and fragmentation. It may also occur in pathological conditions.

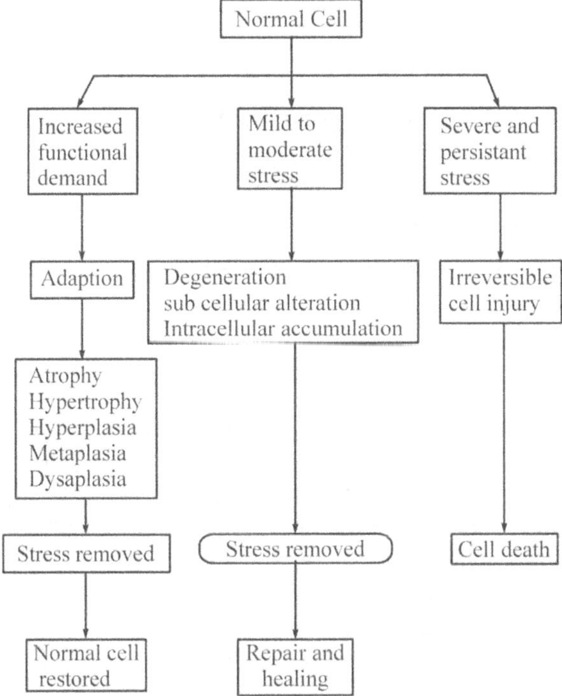

Fig. 2.1 Cellular response to injury.

Etiology (causes) of Cell Injury

(a) **Hypoxia:** It is an extremely important and common cause for cell injury and cell death. Loss of blood supply (ischemia) is the common cause of hypoxia. Hypoxia also occurs from cardio respiratory failure, loss of oxygen carrying capacity of blood (anemia, C, O poisoning etc.). Hypoxia impairs the acrobic oxidative respiration.

(b) Physical agents: These include mechanical trauma, extreme temperature (burns, deep cold) sudden change in atmospheric pressure, radiation, electric shock etc.

(c) Chemical agents: Ever increasing list of chemical agents and drugs cause cell injury. Important examples are chemical poisons-cyanide, arsenic, mercury, strong acids, alkalis etc.

(d) Infectious agents: Injuries caused by microbes include infection caused by bacteria, rickettsiae, virus, fungi, protozoa, parasites etc.

(e) Immunologic reactions: Immunity is a double-edged sword, it protects the host against various injurious agents, but it may also turn lethal and cause cell injury. e.g.: hypersensitivity reaction, anaphylactic reaction, autoimmune disease etc.

(f) Genetic derangement: Many inborn errors in metabolism may be due to enzyme abnormalities. e.g.: Sickle cell anemia, congenital malformation in Down's syndrome etc.

(g) Nutritional imbalance: Deficiency or excess of nutrition may cause nutritional imbalance. Nutritional deficiency diseases may be due to overall deficiency of nutrients like- proteins (marasmus, kwashiorkor), minerals (anemia) or trace elements. Nutritional excess results in obesity, atherosclerosis, heart disease, hypertension etc.

(h) Psychological factors: Drug addiction, alcoholism, smoking result in various organic disease like liver damage, chronic bronchitis, lung cancer, peptic ulcer, hypertension, ischemic heart disease etc.

Pathogenesis (Mechanism) of Cell Injury

Pathology is the study of suffering. Pathologist uses a variety of molecular, microbiologic, immunologic techniques to understand the biochemical, structural, and functional changes that occur in cells, tissues, and organs. To render (perform/judge) diagnoses and guide therapy, pathologists identify changes in the gross or microscopic appearance (morphology) of cells and tissues, and biochemical alterations in body fluids.

Cell Response to Stress and Noxious Stimuli

Cell constantly adjust their structure and functions to accommodate changing demands and extracellular stress. Cells maintain normal homeostasis (steady state).As cells encounter physiologic stresses/ pathologic stimuli, they can undergo adaptation, achieving a new steady state and preserving viability and function.

The principal adaptive responses –hypertrophy, hyperplasia, atrophy and metaplasia. If the adaptive capability is exceeded or if the external stress is inherently (fundamentally) harmful cell injury develops. Within certain limit injury is reversible and cells return to stable baseline. Severe or persistent stress results in irreversible injury and death of the affected cells. Whether a specific form of stress induce adaptation, reversible or irreversible injury also depends on nature of the cells, cellular metabolism, blood supply, and nutritional status of the cell.

Cellular Adaptations to Stress

Adaptations are reversible changes in the number, size, phenotype, metabolic activity or function of cells in response to changes in their environment.Physiologic adaptations usually represent responses of cells to normal stimulation by hormones or endogenous chemical mediators. (E.g.: hormone induced enlargement of breast and uterus during pregnancy).Pathologic adaptations are responses to stress that allow cells to modulate (modify) their structure and functions so as to escape from injury.

Hypertrophy

Hypertrophy is an increase in size of cells resulting in increase in the size of the organ. In hypertrophy, there are no new cells, but just bigger cells, enlarged by an increased amount of structural proteins and organelles. Hypertrophy occurs in cells incapable of replication (post mitotic cells). Hypertrophy and hyperplasia can also occur together. E.g.: pregnancy, increased workload on skeletal muscle, in weightlifters causes hypertrophy of skeletal muscles.

Cardiac muscle enlargement due to hypertension or aortic valve disease is an example for pathologic hypertrophy. In cardiac hypertrophy, two type of signals such as; mechanical triggers (stretch) and trophic triggers (activation of α – adrenergic receptors) turn on signal transduction pathway, that lead to induction of several genes, which in turn stimulate synthesis of numerous cellular proteins, including growth factors and structural proteins. This cause synthesis of more proteins and myofilaments in the cell, which improve performance and help the heart to balance the demand and cell's functional capacity.

There is a limit; beyond which enlargement of muscle mass cannot compensate increased functional demand. At this stage, several degenerative changes occur in myocardial fibres like fragmentation and loss of myofibrillar contractile elements. The variables that limit continued hypertrophy and cause the regressive changes are incompletely understood. There may be finite limits of the vasculature to adequately supply the enlarged fibres of the mitochondria to supply adenosine triphosphate (ATP) or of the biosynthetic machinery to provide the contractile proteins or other cytoskeletal elements. The net result of these changes is ventricular dilation and ultimately cardiac failure.

Hyperplasia

As discussed above, hyperplasia takes place if the cell population is capable of replication; it may occur with hypertrophy and often in response to the same stimuli. The two types of physiologic hyperplasia are –

1. Hormonal hyperplasia, exemplified by the proliferation of the glandular epithelium of the female breast at puberty and during pregnancy; and

2. Compensatory hyperplasia, that is, hyperplasia that occurs when a portion of the tissue is removed or diseased. For example, when a liver is partially resected, mitotic activity in the remaining cells begins as early as 12 hours later, eventually restoring the liver to its normal weight.

The stimuli for hyperplasia in this setting are polypeptide growth factors produced by remnant hepatocytes as well as non-parenchymal cells in the liver. After restoration of the liver mass, cell proliferation is "turned off" by various growth inhibitors.

Most forms of pathologic hyperplasia are caused by excessive hormonal or growth factor stimulation. For example, normal menstrual period is tightly regulated by stimulation through pituitary hormones and ovarian oestrogen and progesterone. If the balance between oestrogen and progesterone is disturbed, endometrial hyperplasia causes abnormal menstrual bleeding.

Hyperplasia is also an important response of connective tissue cells in wound healing. In this process, growth factors are produced by white blood cells (leukocytes) responding to the injury and by cells in the extracellular matrix.

Papillomaviruses cause skin warts and mucosal lesions composed of masses of hyperplastic epithelium. Here the growth factors may be produced by the virus or by infected cells.

It is important to note that in all these situations, the hyperplastic process remains controlled; if hormonal or growth factor stimulation abates (subsides/ decreases), the hyperplasia disappears. It is this sensitivity to normal regulatory control mechanisms that distinguishes benign pathologic hyperplasias from cancer, in which the growth control mechanisms become dysregulated or ineffective.

Nevertheless, pathologic hyperplasia constitutes a fertile soil in which cancerous proliferation may eventually arise. Thus, patients with hyperplasia of the endometrium are at increased risk of developing endometrial cancer, and certain papillomavirus infections predispose to cervical cancers.

Atrophy

Shrinkage in the size of the cell by the loss of cell substance is known as atrophy. When a sufficient number of cells is involved, the entire tissue or organ diminishes in size, becoming atrophic. It should be emphasized that although atrophic cells may have diminished function, they are not dead. Causes of atrophy include,

- decreased workload (e.g., immobilization of a limb to permit healing of a fracture),
- loss of innervation,
- diminished blood supply,
- inadequate nutrition,
- loss of endocrine stimulation,
- and aging (senile atrophy).

Although some of these stimuli are physiologic (e.g., the loss of hormone stimulation in menopause) and others pathologic (e.g., denervation), the fundamental cellular changes are identical. They represent-

- A retreat (recoil/withdrawal) by the cell to a smaller size at which survival is still possible;

- A new equilibrium is achieved between cell size and diminished blood supply, nutrition, or trophic stimulation.

Atrophy results from decreased protein synthesis and increased protein degradation in cells. Protein synthesis decreases because of reduced metabolic activity. The degradation of cellular proteins occurs mainly by the ubiquitin-proteasome pathway. Nutrient deficiency and disuse may activate ubiquitin ligases, which attach multiple copies of the small peptide ubiquitin to cellular proteins and target these proteins for degradation in proteasomes. In many situations, atrophy is also accompanied by increased autophagy, with resulting increases in the number of autophagic vacuoles. Autophagy ("self-eating") is the process in which the starved cell eats its own components in an attempt to find nutrients and survive.

Metaplasia

Metaplasia is a change in phenotype of differentiated cells, often a response to chronic irritation that makes cells better able to withstand the stress; may result in reduced functions or increased propensity for malignant transformation. Metaplasia is a reversible change in which one adult cell type (epithelial or mesenchymal) is replaced by another adult cell type. In this type of cellular adaptation, cells sensitive to a particular stress are replaced by other cell types better able to withstand the adverse environment. Metaplasia is thought to arise by genetic "reprogramming" of stem cells rather than trans-differentiation of already differentiated cells.

E.g.: In habitual cigarette smokers in respiratory epithelium the normal ciliated columnar epithelial cells of the trachea and bronchi are focally or widely replaced by stratified squamous epithelial cells.

The "rugged (rough)" stratified squamous epithelium may be able to survive circumstances that the more fragile specialized epithelium (like ciliated columnar epithelium) would not tolerate. But important protective mechanisms, such as mucus secretion and ciliary clearance of particulate matter are lost.

Epithelial metaplasia is therefore a double-edged sword; moreover, the influences (stimulus) that induce metaplastic transformation, persistent, may predispose to malignant transformation of the epithelium.

It is thought that cigarette smoking initially causes squamous metaplasia, and cancers arise later in some of these altered foci.

In chronic gastric reflux, the normal stratified squamous epithelium of the lower oesophagus may undergo metaplastic transformation to gastric or intestinal-type columnar epithelium.

Metaplasia may also occur in mesenchymal cells. For example, bone is occasionally formed in soft tissues, particularly in foci of injury.

The Morphology of Cell and Tissue Injury

All stresses and noxious influences exert their effects first at the molecular or biochemical level. Cellular function may be lost long before cell death occurs. For example, myocardial cells become non-contractile after 1 to 2 minutes of ischemia, although they do not die until 20 to 30 minutes of ischemia have elapsed. Morphologic changes of lag far behind cell injury (or death).The cellular derangements of reversible injury can be repaired and, if the injurious stimulus abates (decreases), the cell will return to normalcy.

Persistent or excessive injury, however, causes cells to pass the nebulous (vague/not clear) "point of no return" into irreversible injury and cell death. The events that determine when reversible injury becomes irreversible and progresses to cell death remain poorly understood. The clinical relevance of this question is obvious; if we can answer it we may be able to devise strategies for preventing cell injury from having permanent deleterious consequences.

Two phenomena consistently characterize irreversibility:

- The inability to reverse mitochondrial dysfunction (lack of oxidative phosphorylation and ATP generation) even after resolution of the original injury, and

- Profound disturbances in membrane function. As mentioned earlier, injury to lysosomal membranes results in the enzymatic dissolution of the injured cell that is characteristic of necrosis.

Reversible Injury

The two main morphologic correlates of reversible cell injury are cellular swelling and fatty change. Cellular swelling is the result of failure of energy-dependent ion pumps in the plasma membrane, leading to an inability to maintain ionic and fluid homeostasis.

Fatty change occurs in hypoxic injury and various forms of toxic or metabolic injury, and is manifested by the appearance of small or large lipid vacuoles in the cytoplasm. It occurs mainly in cells involved in and dependent on fat metabolism, such as hepatocytes and myocardial cells. Fatty change is also reversible.

Morphology

Cellular swelling, the first manifestation of almost all forms of injury to cells, when it affects many cells in an organ it causes some pallor, increased turgor, and increase in weight of the organ. Microscopic examination may reveal small, clear vacuoles within the cytoplasm; these are distended and pinched off segments of the ER. This pattern of nonlethal (reversible) injury is called vacuolar degeneration.

The ultrastructural changes of reversible cell injury are:

- Plasma membrane alterations such as blebbing, blunting or distortion of microvilli, and loosening of intercellular attachments;
- Mitochondrial changes such as swelling and the appearance of phospholipid-rich amorphous densities;
- Dilation of the ER with detachment of ribosomes and dissociation of polysomes;
- Nuclear alterations, with clumping of chromatin.

Necrosis

Necrosis involve cell death caused by degrading action of enzymes on lethally injured cells. Necrotic cells are unable to maintain membrane integrity, and their contents often leak out. The enzymes responsible for digestion of the cell are derived either from the lysosomes of the dying cells themselves or from the lysosomes of leukocytes that are recruited as part of the inflammatory reaction to the dead cells.

Morphology

In cell death caused by hypoxia, the necrotic cells show increased eosinophilia (i.e., pink staining from the eosin dye, the "E" in "H&E"). This is attributable in part to increased binding of eosin to denatured cytoplasmic proteins and in part to loss of the basophilia that is normally imparted by (given by) the ribonucleic acid (RNA) in the cytoplasm (basophilia is the blue staining from the hematoxylin dye, the "H" in "H&E").

When enzymes have digested the cytoplasmic organelles, the cytoplasm becomes vacuolated. Dead cells may be replaced by large, whorled phospholipid masses, called myelin figures that are derived from damaged cellular membranes.

By electron microscopy, necrotic cells are characterized by:
- Discontinuities in plasma and organelle membranes,
- Marked dilation of mitochondria with the appearance of large amorphous densities,
- Disruption of lysosomes,
- Intra-cytoplasmic myelin figures,
- And profound nuclear changes culminating in nuclear dissolution.

Nuclear changes assume one of three patterns, all due to breakdown of DNA and chromatin.
- The basophilia of the chromatin may fade (karyolysis), presumably secondary to deoxyribonuclease (DNase) activity,
- A second pattern is, characterized by nuclear shrinkage and increased basophilia (pyknosis); the DNA condenses into a solid shrunken mass,

- In the third pattern, karyorrhexis, the pyknotic nucleus undergoes fragmentation. In 1 to 2 days, the nucleus in a dead cell completely disappears.

Patterns of Tissue Necrosis

Necrosis of a collection of cells in a tissue or an organ has morphologically distinct patterns, which may provide clues about the underlying cause.

Morphology

- **Coagulative necrosis** is a form of tissue necrosis in which the component cells are dead but the basic tissue architecture is preserved for at least several days. Presumably the injury denatures structural proteins and enzymes and so blocks (stops) the proteolysis of the dead cells; as a result, eosinophilic, anucleated cell may persist for days or weeks. Ultimately, the necrotic cells are removed by phagocytosis of the cellular debris by infiltrating leukocytes and by digestion of the dead cells by the action of lysosomal enzymes of the leukocytes. Coagulative necrosis is characteristic of ischemic necrosis (infarcts) in all solid organs except the brain.

- **Liquefactive necrosis** is seen in focal bacterial or, occasionally, fungal infections, because microbes stimulate the accumulation of inflammatory cells and the enzymes of leukocytes digest ("liquefy") the tissue. For obscure reasons, hypoxic death of cells within the central nervous system often evokes liquefactive necrosis. Whatever the pathogenesis, liquefaction completely digests the dead cells, resulting in transformation of the tissue into a liquid viscous mass. If the process was initiated by acute inflammation, the material is frequently creamy yellow and is called pus.

- **Gangrenous necrosis** is not a distinctive pattern of cell death the term is still commonly used in clinical practice. It is usually applied to a limb, generally the lower leg that has lost its blood supply and has undergone coagulative necrosis involving multiple tissue layers. When bacterial infection is superimposed, coagulative necrosis is modified by the liquefactive action of the bacteria and the attracted leukocytes (so called wet gangrene).

- **Caseous necrosis** is encountered most often in foci of tuberculous infection. The term "caseous" (cheese like) is derived from the friable yellow-white appearance of the area of necrosis. On microscopic examination, the necrotic focus appears as a collection of fragmented or lysed cells with an amorphous granular appearance. Unlike coagulative necrosis, the tissue architecture is completely obliterated (destroyed) and cellular outlines cannot be discerned (distinguished/ detected). Caseous necrosis is often enclosed within a distinctive inflammatory border; this appearance is known as a granuloma.

- **Fat necrosis,** refers to focal areas of fat destruction, typically resulting from release of activated pancreatic lipases into the substance of the pancreas and the peritoneal cavity. This occurs in the acute pancreatitis. In this disorder, pancreatic enzymes that have leaked out of acinar cells and ducts liquefy the membranes of fat cells in the peritoneum, and lipases split the triglyceride esters contained within fat cells. The released fatty acids combine with calcium to produce grossly visible chalky white areas (fat saponification), which enable the surgeon and the pathologist to identify the lesions. On histologic examination, the foci of necrosis contain shadowy outlines of necrotic fat cells with basophilic calcium deposits, surrounded by an inflammatory reaction.

- **Fibrinoid necrosis** is a special form of necrosis usually seen in immune reactions involving blood vessels. This pattern of necrosis is prominent (obvious) when complexes of antigens and antibodies are deposited in the walls of arteries. Deposits of these "immune complexes," together with fibrin that has leaked out of vessels, result in a bright pink and amorphous appearance in H&E stains, called "fibrinoid" (fibrin-like) by pathologists. The immunologically mediated diseases (e.g., polyarteritis nodosa) shows this type of necrosis.

Leakage of intracellular proteins through the damaged cell membrane and ultimately into the circulation provides a means of detecting tissue-specific necrosis using blood or serum samples. Cardiac muscle, for example, contains a unique isoform of the enzyme creatine kinase and of the contractile protein troponin, whereas hepatocytes contain transaminases. Irreversible injury and cell death in these tissues are reflected in increased serum levels of such proteins, and measurement of serum levels is used clinically to assess damage to these tissues.

Subcellular Responses to Injury

Certain agents and stresses induce distinctive alterations involving only subcellular organelles.

Autophagy

Autophagy refers to lysosomal digestion of the cell's own components and is contrasted with heterophagy, in which a cell (usually a macrophage) ingests substances from the outside for intracellular destruction. Autophagy is thought to be a survival mechanism in times of nutrient deprivation, such that the starved cell lives by eating its own contents.

In this process, intracellular organelles and portions of cytosol are first sequestered from the cytoplasm in an autophagic vacuole formed from ribosome-free regions of the rough ER (RER). The vacuole fuses with lysosomes to form an autophagolysosome, and the cellular components are digested by lysosomal enzymes. Autophagy is initiated by several proteins that sense nutrient deprivation. If it is not corrected, autophagy may also signal cell death by apoptosis.

Certain indigestible pigments, such as Lipofuscin, carbon particles inhaled from the atmosphere or inoculated pigment in tattoos, can persist in phagolysosomes of macrophages for decades. Lysosomes are also repositories (store houses) wherein cells sequester materials that cannot be completely degraded.

Hereditary lysosomal storage disorders, caused by deficiencies of enzymes that degrade various macromolecules, result in abnormal collections of intermediate metabolites in the lysosomes of cells all over the body; neurons are particularly susceptible to lethal injury from such accumulations.

Induction (Hypertrophy) of Smooth ER

The smooth ER (SER) is involved in the metabolism of various chemicals, and cells exposed to these chemicals show hypertrophy of the ER as an adaptive response that may have important functional consequences.

For instance, barbiturates are metabolized in the liver by the cytochrome P-450 mixed-function oxidase system found in the SER. Protracted (prolonged) use of barbiturates leads to a state of tolerance, with a decrease in the effects of the drug and the need to use increasing doses. This adaptation is due to increased volume (hypertrophy) of the SER of hepatocytes and increased P-450 enzymatic activity. Although P -450–mediated modification produces "detoxification," many compounds are rendered (made) more injurious by this process. Cells adapted to one drug have increased capacity to metabolize other compounds handled by the same system.

Mitochondrial Alterations

Mitochondrial dysfunction plays an important role in acute cell injury and death. In some nonlethal pathologic conditions, however, there may be alterations in the number, size, shape, and presumably function of mitochondria. For example, in cellular hypertrophy there is an increase in the number of mitochondria in cells; conversely, mitochondria decrease in number during cellular atrophy (probably via autophagy).

Mitochondria may assume extremely large and abnormal shapes (megamito-chondria), as seen in hepatocytes in various nutritional deficiencies and alcoholic liver disease. In certain inherited metabolic diseases of skeletal muscle, (e.g.: mitochondrial myopathies), defects in mitochondrial metabolism are associated with increased numbers of unusually large mitochondria containing abnormal cristae.

Cytoskeletal Abnormalities

The cytoskeleton consists of actin and myosin filaments, microtubules, and various classes of intermediate filaments; several other non-polymerized and non-filamentous forms of contractile proteins also contribute to the cellular scaffold (framework / skeleton).

The cytoskeleton is important for many cellular functions, including:

- Intracellular transport of organelles and molecules
- Maintenance of basic cell architecture (e.g., cell polarity, distinguishing up and down)

- Transmission of cell-cell and cell–extracellular matrix signals to the nucleus
- Maintenance of mechanical strength for tissue integrity
- Cell mobility
- Phagocytosis

Cells and tissues respond to environmental stresses (e.g., shear stress in blood vessels or increased pressures in the heart) by constantly remodelling their intracellular scaffolding (frame work).Abnormalities of the cytoskeleton occur in a variety of pathologic states. These abnormalities may be manifested as-

- an abnormal appearance and function of cells (hypertrophic cardio-myopathy),
- aberrant (atypical /abnormal) movements of intracellular organelles,
- defective cell locomotion, or
- intracellular accumulations of fibrillar material as in alcoholic liver disease.

Perturbations in the organization of microtubules can cause sterility by inhibiting sperm motility, defective mobility of cilia in the respiratory epithelium, resulting in chronic infections due to impaired clearance of inhaled bacteria (Kartagener, or the immotile cilia, syndrome).Microtubules are also essential for leukocyte migration and phagocytosis.

Drugs that prevent microtubule polymerization (e.g., colchicine) are useful in treating gout, in which symptoms are due to movement of macrophages toward urate crystals with subsequent frustrated (unsatisfied /unsuccessful) attempts at phagocytosis and inflammation. Since microtubules form the mitotic spindle, drugs that bind to microtubules (e.g., vinca alkaloids) are also anti-proliferative and may therefore be useful as antitumor agents.

Mechanisms of Cell Injury

The cellular response to injurious stimuli depends on the type of injury, its duration, and its severity. Thus, low doses of toxins or a brief duration of ischemia may lead to reversible cell injury, whereas larger toxin doses or longer ischemic intervals may result in irreversible injury and cell death.

The consequences of an injurious stimulus depend on the type, status, adaptability, and genetic makeup of the injured cell. The same injury has vastly different outcomes depending on the cell type; thus, striated skeletal muscle in the leg accommodates complete ischemia for 2 to 3 hours without irreversible injury, whereas cardiac muscle dies after only 20 to 30 minutes.

The nutritional (or hormonal) status can also be important; clearly, a glycogen-replete (full) hepatocyte will tolerate ischemia much better than one that has just burned its last glucose molecule.

Genetically determined diversity in metabolic pathways can also be important. For instance, when exposed to the same dose of a toxin, individuals who inherit variants in genes encoding cytochrome P-450 may catabolize the toxin at different rates, leading to different outcomes.

Much effort is now directed toward understanding the role of genetic polymorphisms in responses to drugs and toxins and in disease susceptibility. The study of such interactions is called pharmacogenomics.

Cell injury results from functional and biochemical abnormalities in one or more of several essential cellular components. The most important targets of injurious stimuli are:

1. mitochondria, the sites of ATP generation;

2. cell membranes, on which the ionic and osmotic homeostasis of the cell and its organelles depends;

3. protein synthesis;

4. the cytoskeleton; and

5. the genetic apparatus of the cell.

Depletion of ATP

ATP, the energy store of cells, is produced mainly by oxidative phosphorylation of adenosine diphosphate (ADP) during reduction of oxygen in the electron transport system of mitochondria. In addition, the glycolytic pathway can generate ATP in the absence of oxygen using glucose derived either from the circulation or from the hydrolysis of intracellular glycogen. The major causes of ATP depletion are –

- reduced supply of oxygen and nutrients,

- mitochondrial damage,

- actions of some toxins (e.g., cyanide).

Tissues with a greater glycolytic capacity (e.g., the liver) can survive loss of oxygen and decreased oxidative phosphorylation better than are tissues with limited capacity for glycolysis (e.g., the brain). High-energy phosphate in the form of ATP is required for virtually all synthetic and degradative processes within the cell, including membrane transport, protein synthesis, lipogenesis, and the deacylation /reacylation reactions necessary for phospholipid turnover. Depletion of ATP to less than 5% to 10% of normal levels has widespread effects on many criticalcellular systems.

- The activity of the plasma membrane energy dependent sodium pump is reduced, resulting in intracellular accumulation of sodium and efflux of potassium. The net gain of solute is accompanied by iso-osmotic gain of water, causing cell swelling and dilation of the ER.

- There is a compensatory increase in anaerobic glycolysis in an attempt to maintain the cell's energy sources. As a consequence, intracellular glycogen stores are rapidly depleted, and lactic acid accumulates, leading to decreased intracellular pH and decreased activity of many cellular enzymes.

- Failure of the Ca^{2+} pump leads to influx of Ca^{2+}, with damaging effects on numerous cellular components, described below.

- Prolonged or worsening depletion of ATP causes structural disruption of the protein synthetic apparatus, manifested as detachment of ribosomes from the rough endoplasmic reticulum (RER) and dissociation of polysomes into monosomes, with a consequent reduction in protein synthesis. Ultimately, there is irreversible damage to mitochondrial and lysosomal membranes, and the cell undergoes necrosis.

Damage to Mitochondria

Mitochondria are the cell's suppliers of life-sustaining energy in the form of ATP, but they are also critical players in cell injury and death. Mitochondria can be damaged by:

- Increases of cytosolic Ca^{2+},
- Reactive oxygen species (free radicles)
- Oxygen deprivation.

They are sensitive to virtually all types of injurious stimuli, including hypoxia and toxins. There are two major consequences of mitochondrial damage:

- Formation of a high-conductance channel in the mitochondrial membrane, called the mitochondrial permeability transition pore. The opening of this channel leads to the loss of mitochondrial membrane potential and pH changes, resulting in failure of oxidative phosphorylation and progressive depletion of ATP, culminating in necrosis of the cell.

- The mitochondria also contain several proteins that are capable of activating apoptotic pathways, including cytochrome c (the major protein involved in electron transport). Increased permeability of the mitochondrial membrane may result in leakage of these proteins into the cytosol and death by apoptosis.

Thus, cytochrome c plays a key dual role in cell survival and death; in its normal location inside mitochondria, it is essential for energy generation and the life of the cell, but when mitochondria are damaged so severely that cytochrome c leaks out, it signals cells to die.

Influx of Calcium

Cytosolic free calcium is normally maintained by ATP dependent calcium transporters at concentrations that are as much as 10,000 times lower than the concentration of extracellular calcium or calcium sequestered in mitochondria or ER.

Ischemia and certain toxins cause an increase in cytosolic calcium concentration, initially because of release of Ca^{2+} from the intracellular stores, and later resulting from increased influx across the plasma membrane. Increased cytosolic Ca^{2+} activates a number of enzymes, with potentially deleterious cellular effects. These enzymes include:

- Phospholipases (which cause membrane damage),

- Proteases (which break down both membrane and cytoskeletal proteins),

- Endonucleases (which are responsible for DNA and chromatin fragmentation),

- Adenosinetriphosphatases (ATPases; thereby hastening ATP depletion).

Increased intracellular Ca^{2+} levels also result in the induction of apoptosis, by direct activation of caspases and by increasing mitochondrial permeability.

Accumulation of Oxygen-Derived Free Radicals (Oxidative Stress)

Free radicals are chemical species with a single unpaired electron in an outer orbital. Such chemical states are extremely unstable and readily react with inorganic and organic chemicals. When generated in cells they avidly (actively) attack nucleic acids as well as a variety of cellular proteins and lipids.

In addition, free radicals initiate autocatalytic reactions; molecules that react with free radicals are in turn converted into free radicals, thus propagating the chain of damage. Reactive oxygen species (ROS) are a type of oxygen-derived free radical whose role in cell injury is well established. They are produced normally in cells during mitochondrial respiration and energy generation, but they are degraded and removed by cellular defense systems.

When the production of ROS increases or the scavenging systems are ineffective, the result is an excess of these free radicals, leading to a condition called oxidative stress. Cell injury in many circumstances involves damage by free radicals; these situations include ischemia-reperfusion, chemical and radiation injury, toxicity from oxygen and other gases, cellular aging, microbial killing by phagocytic cells, and tissue injury caused by inflammatory cells.

The accumulation of free radicals is determined by their rates of production and removal. Several reactions are responsible for the generation of free radicals –

- The reduction-oxidation (redox) reactions that occur during normal mitochondrial metabolism. During normal respiration, for example, molecular oxygen is sequentially reduced in mitochondria by the addition of four electrons to generate water. In the process, small amounts of toxic intermediate species are generated by partial reduction of oxygen; these include superoxide radicals ($O_2 \bullet-$), hydrogen peroxide (H_2O_2), and OH•.

  Transition metals such as copper and iron also accept or donate free electrons during certain intracellular reactions and thereby catalyse free-radical formation, .as in the- Fenton reaction ($Fe^{2+} + H_2O_2 \rightarrow Fe^{3+} + OH\bullet + OH-$).

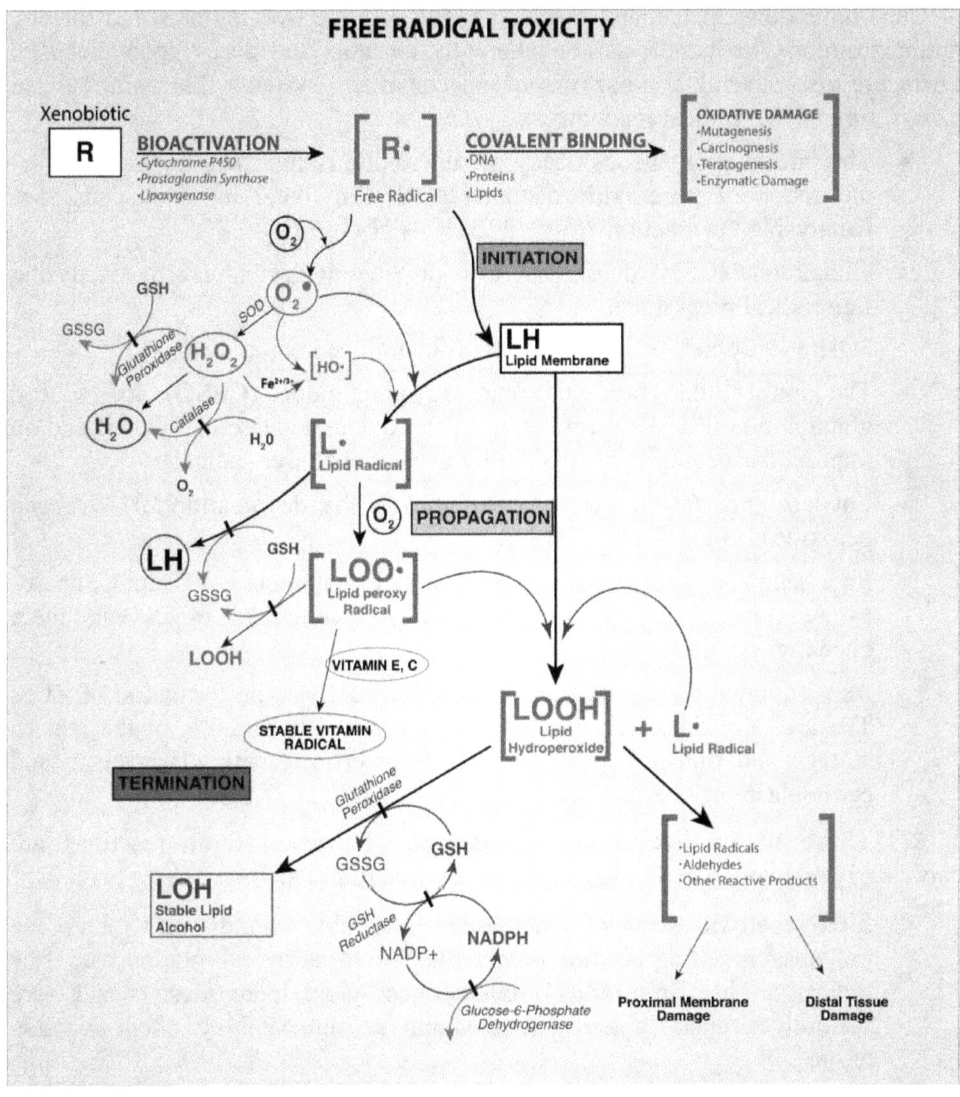

- The absorption of radiant energy (e.g., ultraviolet light, x-rays). Ionizing radiation can hydrolyse water into hydroxyl (OH•) and hydrogen (H•) free radicals.

- The enzymatic metabolism of exogenous chemicals (e.g., carbon tetrachloride).

- Inflammation, since free radicals are produced by leukocytes that enter tissues.

- Nitric oxide (NO), an important chemical mediator normally synthesized by a variety of cell types, can act as a free radical or can be converted into highly reactive nitrite species.

Cells have developed many mechanisms to remove free radicals and thereby minimize injury. Free radicals are inherently unstable and decay spontaneously. There are also several non-enzymatic and enzymatic systems that contribute to inactivation of free-radical reactions:

- The rate of spontaneous decay of superoxide is significantly increased by the action of superoxide dismutases (SODs) found in many cell types (catalysing the reaction $2O_2 \bullet - + 2H + \rightarrow H_2O_2 + O_2$).

- Glutathione (GSH) peroxidase also protects against injury by catalysing free-radical breakdown:

  $2OH \bullet - + 2GSH \rightarrow 2H_2O + GSSG$ (glutathione homodimer).

- The intracellular ratio of oxidized glutathione (GSSG) to reduced glutathione (GSH) is a reflection of the oxidative state of the cell and an important aspect of the cell's ability to catabolize free radicals.

- Catalase, present in peroxisomes, directs the degradation of hydrogen peroxide ($2H_2O_2 \rightarrow O_2 + 2H_2O$).

- Endogenous or exogenous antioxidants (e.g., vitamins E, A, and C, and β-carotene) may either block the formation of free radicals or scavenge them once they have formed.

- As mentioned above, iron and copper can catalyse the formation of ROS. The levels of these reactive metals are reduced by binding of the ions to storage and transport proteins (e.g., transferrin, ferritin, lactoferrin, and ceruloplasmin), thereby decreasing the formation of ROS.

ROS have many diverse effects on cells. However, three reactions are particularly relevant to cell injury mediated by free radicals:

- Lipid peroxidation of membranes: Double bonds in membrane polyunsaturated lipids are vulnerable to attack by oxygen-derived free radicals. The lipid-radical interactions yield peroxides, which are themselves unstable and reactive, and an autocatalytic chain reaction ensues.

- Cross-linking of proteins: Free radicals promote sulfhydryl-mediated protein cross-linking, resulting in enhanced degradation or loss of enzymatic activity. Free-radical reactions may also directly cause polypeptide fragmentation.

- DNA fragmentation. Free-radical reactions with thymine in nuclear and mitochondrial DNA produce single-strand breaks. Such DNA damage has been implicated in cell death, aging, and malignant transformation of cells.

Defects in Membrane Permeability

Early loss of selective membrane permeability leading ultimately to overt membrane damage is a consistent feature of most forms of cell injury (except apoptosis).

The plasma membrane can be damaged by ischemia, various microbial toxins, lytic complement components, and a variety of physical and chemical agents.Several biochemical mechanisms may contribute to membrane damage:

- ***Decreased phospholipid synthesis:*** The production of phospholipids in cells may be reduced whenever there is a fall in ATP levels. The reduced phospholipid synthesis may affect all cellular membranes including the mitochondria themselves, thus exacerbating the loss of ATP.

- ***Increased phospholipid breakdown:*** Severe cell injury is associated with increased degradation of membrane phospholipids, probably due to activation of endogenous phospholipases by increased levels of cytosolic Ca2+.

- ***ROS:*** Oxygen free radicals cause injury to cell membranes by lipid peroxidation.

- ***Cytoskeletal abnormalities:*** Cytoskeletal filaments serve as anchors connecting the plasma membrane to the cell interior. Activation of proteases by increased cytosolic Ca^{2+} may cause damage to elements of the cytoskeleton.

- ***Lipid breakdown products:*** These include un-esterified free fatty acids, acyl carnitine, and lysophospholipids, catabolic products that are known to accumulate in injured cells because of phospholipid degradation. They have detergent effect on membranes. They also either insert into the lipid bilayer of the membrane or exchange with membrane phospholipids, potentially causing changes in permeability and electro-physiologic alterations. The most important sites of membrane damage during cell injury are the mitochondrial membrane, the plasma membrane, and membranes of lysosomes.

- ***Mitochondrial membrane damage:*** damage to mitochondrial membranes results in decreased production of ATP, culminating in necrosis, and release of proteins that trigger apoptotic death.

- ***Plasma membrane damage:*** plasma membrane damage leads to loss of osmotic balance and influx of fluids and ions, as well as loss of cellular contents. The cells may also leak metabolites that are vital for the reconstitution of ATP, thus further depleting energy stores.

- Injury to lysosomal membranes results in leakage of their enzymes into the cytoplasm and activation of the acid hydrolases in the acidic intracellular pH of the injured (e.g., ischemic) cell. Lysosomes contain RNases, DNases, proteases, glucosidases, and other enzymes. Activation of these enzymes leads to enzymatic digestion of cell components, and the cells die by necrosis.

Damage to DNA and Proteins

Cells have mechanisms that repair damage to DNA, but if this damage is too severe to be corrected (e.g., after radiation injury or oxidative stress), the cell initiates its suicide program and dies by apoptosis. A similar reaction is triggered by improperly folded proteins, which may be the result of inherited mutations or external triggers such as free radicals.

Examples of cell injury and necrosis

Ischemic and Hypoxic Injury

Ischemia, or diminished blood flow to a tissue, is the most common cause of cell injury in clinical medicine. Ischemia injures tissues faster than does hypoxia. The fundamental biochemical abnormality in hypoxic cells that leads to cell injury is reduced intracellular generation of ATP, as a consequence of reduced supply of oxygen. Loss of ATP leads to the failure of many energy-dependent cellular systems, including –

1. ion pumps (leading to cell swelling, and influx of Ca^{2+}, with its deleterious consequences);

2. depletion of glycogen stores, with accumulation of lactic acid, thus lowering the intracellular pH;

3. reduction in protein synthesis.

The functional consequences may be severe at this stage. For instance, heart muscle ceases to contract within 60 seconds of coronary occlusion. However, loss of contractility does not mean cell death. If hypoxia continues, worsening ATP depletion causes further deterioration, with loss of microvilli and the formation of "blebs". At this time, the entire cell and its organelles (mitochondria, ER) are markedly swollen, with increased concentrations of water, sodium, and chloride and a decreased concentration of potassium. If oxygen is restored, all of these disturbances are reversible.

If ischemia persists, irreversible injury and necrosis ensue. Irreversible injury is associated with severe swelling of mitochondria, extensive damage to plasma membranes, and swelling of lysosomes. Massive influx of calcium into the cell may occur. Death is mainly by necrosis. But apoptosis also contributes; the apoptotic pathway is activated probably by release of pro-apoptotic molecules from leaky mitochondria. The cell's components are progressively degraded, and there is widespread leakage of cellular enzymes into the extracellular space.

Finally, the dead cells may become replaced by large masses composed of phospholipids in the form of myelin figures. These are then either phagocytosed by leukocytes or degraded further into fatty acids that may become calcified.

Ischemia-Reperfusion Injury

If cells are reversibly injured, the restoration of blood flow can result in cell recovery. However, under certain circumstances, the restoration of blood flow to ischemic but otherwise viable tissues result, paradoxically (ironically/ surprisingly), in exacerbated and accelerated injury. This so-called ischemia-reperfusion injury is a clinically important process that may contribute significantly to tissue damage in myocardial and cerebral infarctions.

Several mechanisms may account for the exacerbation of cell injury resulting from reperfusion into ischemic tissues:

- New damage may be initiated during re-oxygenation by increased generation of ROS from parenchymal and endothelial cells and from infiltrating leukocytes. When the supply of oxygen is increased, there may be a corresponding increase in the production of ROS, especially because mitochondrial damage leads to incomplete reduction of oxygen, and because of the action of oxidases in leukocytes, endothelial cells, or parenchymal cells. Cellular antioxidant defense mechanisms may also be compromised by ischemia, favouring the accumulation of free radicals.

- Ischemic injury is associated with inflammation, which may increase with reperfusion because of increased influx of leukocytes and plasma proteins. The products of activated leukocytes may cause additional tissue injury. Activation of the complement system may also contribute to ischemia-reperfusion injury. Some antibodies have a propensity to deposit in ischemic tissues for unknown reasons, and when blood flow is resumed, complement proteins bind to the deposited antibodies, are activated, and exacerbate the cell injury and inflammation.

Chemical (Toxic) Injury

Chemicals induce cell injury by one of two general mechanisms-

- Some chemicals act directly by combining with a critical molecular component or cellular organelle. For example, in mercuric chloride poisoning, mercury binds to the sulfhydryl groups of various cell membrane proteins, causing inhibition of ATP-dependent transport and increased membrane permeability. Many antineoplastic chemotherapeutic agents also induce cell damage by direct cytotoxic effects. In such instances, the greatest damage is sustained by the cells that use, absorb, excrete, or concentrate the compounds.

- Many other chemicals are not intrinsically biologically active but must be first converted to reactive toxic metabolites, which then act on target cells. This modification is usually accomplished by the P-450 mixed function oxidases in the smooth endoplasmic reticulum of the liver and other organs.

Although the metabolites might cause membrane damage and cell injury by direct covalent binding to protein and lipids, the most important mechanism of cell injury involves the formation of free radicals. Carbon tetrachloride (CCl_4) and the analgesic acetaminophen belong in this category. CCl_4, for example, is converted to the toxic free radical $CCl_3\bullet$, principally in the liver. The free radicals cause autocatalytic membrane phospholipid peroxidation, with rapid breakdown of the ER.

In less than 30 minutes after exposure to CCl_4, there is a decline in hepatic protein synthesis of enzymes and plasma proteins; within 2 hours, swelling of the smooth endoplasmic reticulum and dissociation of ribosomes from the smooth endoplasmic reticulum have occurred. There is reduced lipid export from the hepatocytes, as a result of their inability to synthesize apoprotein to form complexes with triglycerides and thereby facilitate lipoprotein secretion; the result is the "fatty liver" of CCl_4 poisoning.

Mitochondrial injury follows, and subsequently diminished ATP stores result in defective ion transport and progressive cell swelling; the plasma membranes are further damaged by fatty aldehydes produced by lipid peroxidation in the ER. The result can be calcium influx and eventually cell death.

APOPTOSIS , ("falling off")

Apoptosis is a pathway of cell death that is induced by a tightly regulated suicide program. Cells activate enzymes capable of degrading the cells' own nuclear DNA and nuclear and cytoplasmic proteins. The fragments of apoptotic cells then break off. The plasma membrane of the apoptotic cell remains intact, but the membrane is altered in such a way that the cell and its fragments become avid power full) targets for phagocytes.

The dead cell is rapidly cleared before its contents have leaked out, and therefore cell death by this pathway does not elicit an inflammatory reaction in the host. Thus, apoptosis differs from necrosis, which is characterized by loss of membrane integrity, enzymatic digestion of cells, leakage of cellular contents, and frequently a host reaction.

Causes of Apoptosis

Apoptosis occurs normally in many situations, and serves to eliminate potentially harmful cells and cells that have outlived their usefulness. It is also a pathologic event when cells are damaged beyond repair, especially when the damage affects the cell's DNA or proteins; in these situations, the irreparably damaged cell is eliminated.

Apoptosis in Physiologic Situations

Death by apoptosis is a normal phenomenon that serves to eliminate cells that are no longer needed and to maintain a steady number of various cell populations in tissues. It is important in the following physiologic situations:

- The programmed destruction of cells during embryogenesis, including implantation, organogenesis, developmental involution, and metamorphosis.

- Involution of hormone-dependent tissues upon hormone deprivation, such as endometrial cell breakdown during the menstrual cycle, and regression of the lactating breast after weaning (stopping).

- Cell loss in proliferating cell populations, such as intestinal crypt epithelia, so as to maintain a constant number.

- Death of cells that have served their useful purpose, such as neutrophils in an acute inflammatory response, and lymphocytes at the end of an immune response. In these situations, cells undergo apoptosis because they are deprived of necessary survival signals, such as growth factors.

- Elimination of potentially harmful self-reactive lymphocytes, either before or after they have completed their maturation, in order to prevent reactions against one's own tissues.

- Cell death induced by cytotoxic T lymphocytes, a defence mechanism against viruses and tumors that serves to kill and eliminate virus-infected and neoplastic cells.

Apoptosis in Pathologic Conditions

Apoptosis eliminates cells that are genetically altered or injured beyond repair without eliciting a severe host reaction, thus keeping the damage as contained (controlled /restricted) as possible.

Death by apoptosis is responsible for loss of cells in a variety of pathologic states:

- ***DNA damage:*** Radiation, cytotoxic anticancer drugs, extremes of temperature, and even hypoxia can damage DNA, either directly or via production of free radicals. If repair mechanisms cannot cope with the injury, the cell triggers intrinsic mechanisms that induce apoptosis. In these situations, elimination of the cell may be a better alternative than risking mutations in the damaged DNA, which may progress to malignant transformation. These injurious stimuli cause apoptosis if the insult is mild, but larger doses of the same stimuli result in necrotic cell death. Inducing apoptosis of cancer cells is a desired effect of chemotherapeutic agents, many of which work by damaging DNA.

- ***Accumulation of misfolded proteins:*** Improperly folded proteins may arise because of mutations in the genes encoding these proteins or because of extrinsic factors, such as damage caused by free radicals. Excessive accumulation of these proteins in the ER leads to a condition called ER stress, which culminates in apoptotic death of cells.

- Cell injury in certain infections, particularly viral infections, in which loss of infected cells is largely due to apoptotic death that may be induced by the virus (as in adenovirus and human immunodeficiency virus infections) or by the host immune response (as in viral hepatitis).

- Pathologic atrophy in parenchymal organs after duct obstruction, such as occurs in the pancreas, parotid gland, and kidney.

Mechanisms of Apoptosis

Apoptosis is an active enzymatic process in which nucleoproteins are broken down and then the cell is fragmented. Before discussing the molecular mechanisms, it is useful to review the morphology of this pathway of cell death.

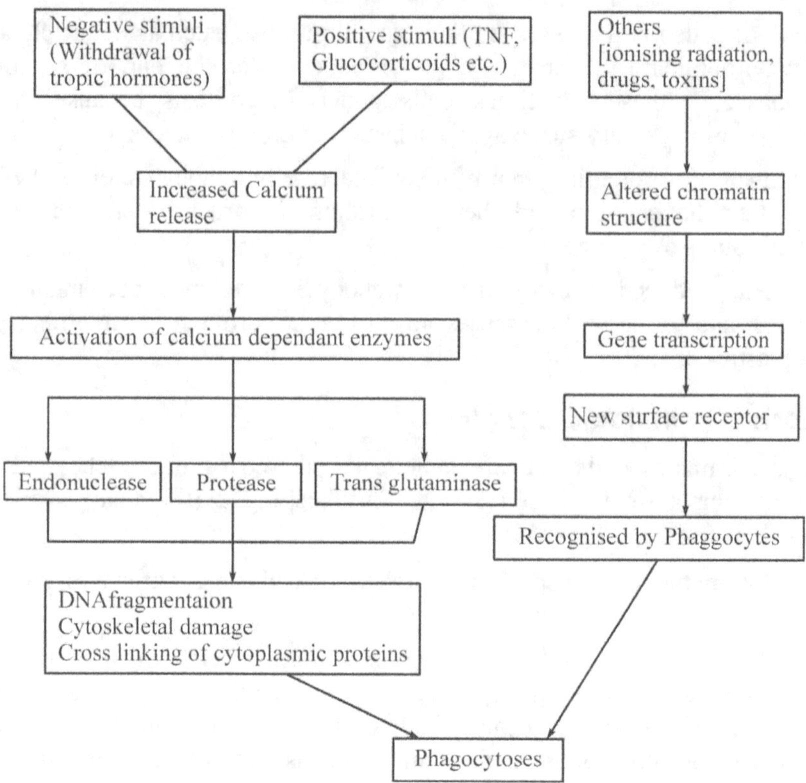

Fig. 2.2 Mechanism of apoptosis.

Morphology

In H&E-stained tissue sections, apoptotic cells may appear as round or oval masses with intensely eosinophilic cytoplasm. Nuclei show various stages of chromatin condensation and aggregation and, ultimately, karyorrhexis; at the molecular level, this is reflected in fragmentation of DNA into nucleosome sized pieces.

The cells rapidly shrink, form cytoplasmic buds, and fragment into apoptotic bodies composed of membrane-bound vesicles of cytosol and organelles. Because these fragments are quickly extruded and phagocytosed without eliciting an inflammatory response, even substantial apoptosis may be histologically undetectable.

The fundamental event in apoptosis is the activation of enzymes called caspases (so named because they are cysteine proteases that cleave proteins after aspartic residues). Activated caspases cleave numerous targets, culminating in activation of nucleases that degrade DNA and other enzymes that presumably destroy nucleoproteins and cytoskeletal proteins.

The activation of caspases depends on a finely tuned balance between pro- and antiapoptotic molecular pathways. Two distinct pathways converge on caspase activation, called the mitochondrial pathway and the death receptor pathway.

Although these pathways can interact, they are generally induced under different conditions, involve different molecules, and serve distinct roles in physiology and disease.

The Mitochondrial (Intrinsic) Pathway of Apoptosis

Mitochondria contain several proteins that are capable of inducing apoptosis; these proteins include cytochrome c and antagonists of endogenous cytosolic inhibitors of apoptosis. The choice between cell survival and death is determined by the permeability of mitochondria, which is controlled by a family of more than 20 proteins, the prototype of which is Bcl-2. When cells are deprived of growth factors and trophic hormones, or are exposed to agents that damage DNA, or accumulate unacceptable amounts of misfolded proteins, a group of sensors is activated.

Some of these sensors, which are members of the Bcl-2 family, in turn activate two pro-apoptotic members of the family called Bax and Bak, which dimerise, insert into the mitochondrial membrane, and form channels through which cytochrome c and other mitochondrial proteins escape into the cytosol.

Other related sensors inhibit the anti-apoptotic molecules Bcl-2 and Bcl-xL (see below), with the same result—the leakage of mitochondrial proteins. Cytochrome c, together with some cofactors, activates caspase-9, while other proteins block the activities of caspase antagonists that function as physiologic inhibitors of apoptosis.

The net result is the activation of the caspase cascade, ultimately leading to nuclear fragmentation. If cells are exposed to growth factors and other survival signals, they synthesize antiapoptotic members of the Bcl-2 family, the two main ones of which are Bcl-2 itself and Bcl-xL. These proteins antagonize Bax and Bak, and thus limit the escape of mitochondrial pro-apoptotic proteins.

Cells deprived of growth factors not only activate the pro-apoptotic proteins but also show reduced levels of Bcl-2 and Bcl-xL, thus further tilting the balance toward death. The mitochondrial pathway seems to be the pathway that is responsible for most situations of apoptosis, as we shall discuss below.

The Death Receptor (Extrinsic) Pathway of Apoptosis

Many cells express surface molecules, called death receptors, that trigger apoptosis. Most of these are members of the tumor necrosis factor (TNF) receptor family that contain in their cytoplasmic regions a conserved "death domain," so named because it mediates interaction with other proteins.

The prototypic death receptors are the type I TNF receptor and Fas (CD95). Fas-ligand (FasL) is a membrane protein expressed mainly on activated T lymphocytes. When these T cells recognize Fas-expressing targets, Fas molecules are cross-linked by the FasL and they bind adapter proteins, which in turn bind caspase-8.

Clustering of many caspase molecules leads to their activation, thus initiating the caspase cascade. In many cell types caspase-8 may cleave and activate a pro-apoptotic member of the Bcl-2 family called Bid, thus feeding into the mitochondrial pathway. The combined activation of both pathways delivers a lethal blow to the cell.

Cellular proteins, notably a caspase antagonist called FLIP, block activation of caspases downstream of death receptors. Interestingly, some viruses produce homologues of FLIP, and it is suggested that this is a mechanism that viruses use to keep infected cells alive. The death receptor pathway is involved in elimination of self-reactive lymphocytes and in killing of target cells by some cytotoxic T lymphocytes.

Clearance of Apoptotic Cells

Apoptotic cells undergo several changes in their membranes that promote their phagocytosis. In normal cells phosphatidylserine is present on the inner leaflet of the plasma membrane, but in apoptotic cells this phospholipid "flips" out and is expressed on the outer layer of the membrane, where it is recognized by macrophages.

Cells that are dying by apoptosis also secrete soluble factors that recruit phagocytes. This facilitates prompt clearance of the dead cells before they undergo secondary membrane damage and release their cellular contents (which can result in inflammation).Some apoptotic bodies express adhesive glycoproteins that are recognized by phagocytes, and macrophages themselves may produce proteins that bind to apoptotic cells (but not to live cells) and target the dead cells for engulfment.

Numerous macrophage receptors have been shown to be involved in the binding and engulfment of apoptotic cells. This process of phagocytosis of apoptotic cells is so efficient that dead cells disappear without leaving a trace, and inflammation is virtually absent. Although we have emphasized the distinctions between necrosis and apoptosis, these two forms of cell death may coexist and be related mechanistically.

For instance, DNA damage (seen in apoptosis) activates an enzyme called poly-ADP(ribose) polymerase, which depletes cellular supplies of nicotinamide adenine dinucleotide, leading to a fall in ATP levels and ultimately necrosis.

In fact, even in common situations such as ischemia, it has been suggested that early cell death can be partly attributed to apoptosis, and necrosis is the dominant type of cell death late, with worsening ischemia.

Examples of Apoptosis

Cell death in many situations is known to be caused by apoptosis, and the selected examples listed below illustrate the role of this death pathway in normal physiology and in disease.

Growth factor deprivation: Hormone-sensitive cells deprived of the relevant hormone, lymphocytes that are not stimulated by antigens and cytokines, and neurons deprived of nerve growth factor, die by apoptosis.

In all these situations, apoptosis is triggered by the mitochondrial pathway and is attributable to activation of proapoptotic members of the Bcl-2 family and decreased synthesis of Bcl-2 and Bcl-xL.

DNA damage: Exposure of cells to radiation or chemotherapeutic agents induces DNA damage, and if this is too severe to be repaired it triggers apoptotic death. When DNA is damaged, the p53 protein accumulates in cells. It first arrests the cell cycle (at the G1 phase) to allow time for repair. However, if the damage is too great to be repaired successfully, p53 triggers apoptosis, mainly by activating sensors that ultimately activate Bax and Bak, and by stimulating synthesis of proapoptotic members of the Bcl-2 family. When p53 is mutated or absent (as it is in certain cancers), it is incapable of inducing apoptosis, so that cells with damaged DNA are allowed to survive. In such cells, the DNA damage may result in mutations or translocations that lead to neoplastic transformation.

Accumulation of misfolded proteins: During normal protein synthesis, chaperones in the ER control the proper folding of newly synthesized proteins, and misfolded polypeptides are targeted for proteolysis. If, however, unfolded or misfolded proteins accumulate in the ER because of inherited mutations or stresses, they induce "ER stress" that triggers a number of cellular responses, collectively called the unfolded protein response. This response activates signaling pathways that increase the production of chaperones and retard protein translation, thus reducing the levels of misfolded proteins in the cell.

However, if this response is unable to cope with the accumulation of misfolded proteins, the result is the activation of caspases that lead to apoptosis. Intracellular accumulation of abnormally folded proteins, caused by mutations, aging, or unknown environmental factors, is now recognized as a feature of several neurodegenerative diseases, including Alzheimer, Huntington, and Parkinson diseases, and possibly type II diabetes. Deprivation of glucose and oxygen, and stress such as heat, also result in protein misfolding, culminating in cell injury and death.

Apoptosis of self-reactive lymphocytes: Lymphocytes capable of recognizing self-antigens are normally produced in all individuals. If these lymphocytes encounter self-antigens, the cells die by apoptosis. Both the mitochondrial pathway and the Fas death receptor pathway have been implicated in this process. Failure of apoptosis of self-reactive lymphocytes is one of the causes of autoimmune diseases.

Cytotoxic T lymphocyte–mediated apoptosis: Cytotoxic T lymphocytes (CTLs) recognize foreign antigens presented on the surface of infected host cells and tumor cells. Upon activation, CTL granule proteases called granzymes enter the target cells. Granzymes cleave proteins at aspartate residues and are able to activate cellular caspases.

In this way, the CTL kills target cells by directly inducing the effector phase of apoptosis, without engaging mitochondria or death receptors. CTLs also express FasL on their surface and may kill target cells by ligation of Fas receptors.

Intracellular Accumulations

Under some circumstances cells may accumulate abnormal amounts of various substances, which may be harmless or associated with varying degrees of injury. The substance may be located in the cytoplasm, within organelles (typically lysosomes), or in the nucleus, and it may be synthesized by the affected cells or may be produced elsewhere.

There are three main pathways of abnormal intracellular accumulations:

- A normal substance is produced at a normal or an increased rate, but the metabolic rate is inadequate to remove it. An example of this type of process is fatty change in the liver.

- A normal or an abnormal endogenous substance accumulates because of genetic or acquired defects in its folding, packaging, transport, or secretion. Mutations that cause defective folding and transport may lead to accumulation of proteins (e.g., α1-antitrypsin deficiency).

- An inherited defect in an enzyme may result in failure to degrade a metabolite. The resulting disorders are called storage diseases.

- An abnormal exogenous substance is deposited and accumulates because the cell has neither the enzymatic machinery to degrade the substance nor the ability to transport it to other sites. Accumulations of carbon or silica particles are examples of this type of alteration.

Fatty Change (Steatosis)

Fatty change refers to any abnormal accumulation of triglycerides within parenchymal cells. It is most often seen in the liver, since this is the major organ involved in fat metabolism, but it may also occur in heart, skeletal muscle, kidney, and other organs. Steatosis may be caused by toxins, protein malnutrition, diabetes mellitus, obesity, and anoxia. Alcohol abuse and diabetes associated with obesity are the most common causes of fatty change in the liver (fatty liver) in industrialized nations.

Free fatty acids from adipose tissue or ingested food are normally transported into hepatocytes, where they are esterified to triglycerides, converted into cholesterol or phospholipids, or oxidized to ketone bodies. Some fatty acids are synthesized from acetate within the hepatocytes as well.

Egress (outlet) of the triglycerides from the hepatocytes requires the formation of complexes with apoproteins to form lipoproteins, which are able to enter the circulation. Excess accumulation of triglycerides may result from defects at any step from fatty acid entry to lipoprotein exit, thus accounting for the occurrence of fatty liver after diverse hepatic insults.

Hepatotoxins (e.g., alcohol) alter mitochondrial and SER function and thus inhibit fatty acid oxidation; CCl_4 and protein malnutrition decrease the synthesis of apoproteins; anoxia inhibits fatty acid oxidation; and starvation increases fatty acid mobilization from peripheral stores. The significance of fatty change depends on the cause and severity of the accumulation. When mild it may have no effect on cellular function. More severe fatty change may transiently impair cellular function, but unless some vital intracellular process is irreversibly impaired (e.g., in CCl_4 poisoning), fatty change is reversible. In the severe form, fatty change may precede cell death, and may be an early lesion in a serious liver disease called non-alcoholic steatohepatitis.

Morphology

In any site, fatty accumulation appears as clear vacuoles within parenchymal cells. Special staining techniques are required to distinguish fat from intracellular water or glycogen, which can also produce clear vacuoles but have a different significance. To identify fat microscopically, tissues must be processed for sectioning without the organic solvents typically used in sample preparation.

Usually, portions of tissue are therefore frozen to enable the cutting of thin sections for histologic examination; the fat is then identified by staining with Sudan IV or oil red O (these stain fat orange-red).Glycogen may be identified by staining for polysaccharides using the periodic acid–Schiff stain (which stains glycogen red-violet).If vacuoles do not stain for either fat or glycogen, they are presumed to be composed mostly of water. Fatty change is most commonly seen in the liver and the heart.

Mild fatty change in the liver may not affect the gross appearance. With increasing accumulation, the organ enlarges and becomes progressively yellow until, in extreme cases, it may weigh 3 to 6 kg (1.5–3 times the normal weight) and appear bright yellow, soft, and greasy. Early fatty change is seen by light microscopy as small fat vacuoles in the cytoplasm around the nucleus. In later stages, the vacuoles coalesce to create cleared spaces that displace the nucleus to the cell periphery.

Occasionally contiguous cells rupture, and the enclosed fat globules unite to produce so-called fatty cysts. In the heart, lipid is found in the form of small droplets, occurring in one of two patterns-

- Prolonged moderate hypoxia (as in profound anaemia) results in focal intracellular fat deposits, creating grossly apparent bands of yellowed myocardium alternating with bands of darker, red-brown, uninvolved heart ("tigered effect").

- The other pattern of fatty change is produced by more profound hypoxia or by some forms of toxic injury (e.g., diphtheria) and shows more uniformly affected myocytes.

Cholesterol and cholesteryl Eesters: Cellular cholesterol metabolism is tightly regulated to ensure normal cell membrane synthesis without significant intracellular accumulation.

However, phagocytic cells may become overloaded with lipid (triglycerides, cholesterol, and cholesteryl esters) in several different pathologic processes.

Macrophages in contact with the lipid debris of necrotic cells or abnormal (e.g., oxidized) forms of lipoproteins may become stuffed with phagocytosed lipid. These macrophages may be filled with minute, membrane-bound vacuoles of lipid, imparting a foamy appearance to their cytoplasm (foam cells).

In atherosclerosis, smooth muscle cells and macrophages are filled with lipid vacuoles composed of cholesterol and cholesteryl esters; these give atherosclerotic plaques their characteristic yellow colour and contribute to the pathogenesis of the lesion.

In hereditary and acquired hyperlipidemic syndromes, macrophages accumulate intracellular cholesterol; when present in the sub-epithelial connective tissue of skin or in tendons, clusters of these foamy macrophages form masses called xanthomas.

Proteins: Morphologically visible protein accumulations are much less common than lipid accumulations; they may occur because excesses are presented to the cells or because the cells synthesize excessive amounts. In the kidney, for example, trace amounts of albumin filtered through the glomerulus are normally reabsorbed by pinocytosis in the proximal convoluted tubules.

However, in disorders with heavy protein leakage across the glomerular filter (e.g., nephrotiic syndrome), there is a much larger reabsorption of the protein. Pinocytic vesicles containing this protein fuse with lysosomes, resulting in the histologic appearance of pink, hyaline cytoplasmic droplets. The process is reversible; if the proteinuria abates (subsides), the protein droplets are metabolized and disappear.

Another example is the marked accumulation of newly synthesized immunoglobulins that may occur in the RER of some plasma cells, forming rounded, eosinophilic Russell bodies. Accumulations of intracellular proteins are also seen in certain types of cell injury. For example, the Mallory body, or "alcoholic hyalin," is an eosinophilic cytoplasmic inclusion in liver cells that is highly characteristic of alcoholic liver disease.

Such inclusions are composed predominantly of aggregated intermediate filaments that presumably resist degradation. The neurofibrillary tangle found in the brain in Alzheimer disease is an aggregated protein inclusion that contains microtubule-associated proteins and neurofilaments, a reflection of a disrupted neuronal cytoskeleton.

Glycogen: Excessive intracellular deposits of glycogen are associated with abnormalities in the metabolism of either glucose or glycogen. In poorly controlled diabetes mellitus, the prime example of abnormal glucose metabolism, glycogen accumulates in renal tubular epithelium, cardiac myocytes, and β cells of the islets of Langerhans.

Glycogen also accumulates within cells in a group of closely related genetic disorders collectively referred to as glycogen storage diseases, or glycogenoses. In these diseases, enzymatic defects in the synthesis or breakdown of glycogen result in massive stockpiling, with secondary injury and cell death.

Pigments: Pigments are coloured substances that are either exogenous, coming from outside the body, or endogenous, synthesized within the body itself.

- The most common exogenous pigment is carbon (an example is coal dust), a ubiquitous (abundant) air pollutant of urban life. When inhaled, it is phagocytosed by alveolar macrophages and transported through lymphatic channels to the regional tracheobronchial lymph nodes. Aggregates of the pigment blacken the draining lymph nodes and pulmonary parenchyma (anthracosis). Heavy accumulations may induce emphysema or a fibroblastic reaction that can result in a serious lung disease called coal workers' pneumoconiosis.

- Endogenous pigments include lipofuscin, melanin, and certain derivatives of hemoglobin. Lipofuscin, or "wear-and-tear pigment," is an insoluble brownish yellow granular intracellular material that accumulates in a variety of tissues (particularly the heart, liver, and brain) as a function of age or atrophy. Lipofuscin represents complexes of lipid and protein that derive from the free radical–catalysed peroxidation of polyunsaturated lipids of subcellular membranes. It is not injurious to the cell but is important as a marker of past free-radical injury.

The brown pigment, when present in large amounts, imparts an appearance to the tissue that is called brown atrophy. By electron microscopy, the pigment appears as perinuclear electron-dense granules.

- Melanin is an endogenous, brown-black pigment produced in melanocytes following the tyrosinase catalysed oxidation of tyrosine to dihydroxyphenylalanine. It is synthesized exclusively by melanocytes located in the epidermis and acts as a screen against harmful ultraviolet radiation. Although melanocytes are the only source of melanin, adjacent basal keratinocytes in the skin can accumulate the pigment (e.g., in freckles), as can dermal macrophages.

- Hemosiderin is a hemoglobin-derived granular pigment that is golden yellow to brown and accumulates in tissues when there is a local or systemic excess of iron. Iron is normally stored within cells in association with the protein apoferritin, forming ferritin micelles. Hemosiderin pigment represents large aggregates of these ferritin micelles, readily visualized by light and electron microscopy; the iron can be unambiguously (clearly) identified by the Prussian blue histochemical reaction.

Although hemosiderin accumulation is usually pathologic, small amounts of this pigment are normal in the mononuclear phagocytes of the bone marrow, spleen, and liver, where there is extensive red cell breakdown.

- Local excesses of iron, and consequently of hemosiderin, result from haemorrhage. The best example is the common bruise. After lysis of the erythrocytes at the site of haemorrhage, the red cell debris is phagocytosed by macrophages; the haemoglobin content is then catabolized by lysosomes with accumulation of the haeme iron in hemosiderin.

The array of colours through which the bruise passes reflects these transformations. The original red-blue colour of haemoglobin is transformed to varying shades of green-blue by the local formation of biliverdin (green bile) and bilirubin (red bile) from the haeme moiety; the iron ions of haemoglobin accumulate as golden-yellow hemosiderin.

- Whenever there is systemic overload of iron, hemosiderin is deposited in many organs and tissues, a condition called haemosiderosis. It is found at first in the mononuclear phagocytes of the liver, bone marrow, spleen, and lymph nodes and in scattered macrophages throughout other organs. With progressive accumulation, parenchymal cells throughout the body (but principally the liver, pancreas, heart, and endocrine organs) become "bronzed" with accumulating pigment.

Hemosiderosis occurs in the setting of-

1. increased absorption of dietary iron,
2. impaired utilization of iron,
3. haemolytic anaemias, and
4. transfusions (the transfused red cells constitute an exogenous load of iron).

In most instances of systemic hemosiderosis, the iron pigment does not damage the parenchymal cells or impair organ function despite an impressive accumulation. However, more extensive accumulations of iron are seen in hereditary hemochromatosis, with tissue injury including liver fibrosis, heart failure, and diabetes mellitus.

Pathologic Calcification

Pathologic calcification is a common process in a wide variety of disease states; it implies the abnormal deposition of calcium salts, together with smaller amounts of iron, magnesium, and other minerals. When the deposition occurs in dead or dying tissues, it is called dystrophic calcification; it occurs in the absence of calcium metabolic derangements (i.e., with normal serum levels of calcium).

In contrast, the deposition of calcium salts in normal tissues is known as metastatic calcification and almost always reflects some derangement in calcium metabolism (hypercalcaemia).It should be noted that while hypercalcaemia is not a prerequisite for dystrophic calcification, it can exacerbate it.

Dystrophic calcification: Dystrophic calcification is encountered in areas of necrosis of any type. It is virtually inevitable in the atheromas of advanced atherosclerosis, associated with intimal injury in the aorta and large arteries and characterized by accumulation of lipids.

Although dystrophic calcification may be an incidental finding indicating insignificant past cell injury, it may also be a cause of organ dysfunction. For example, calcification can develop in aging or damaged heart valves, resulting in severely compromised valve motion. Dystrophic calcification of the aortic valves is an important cause of aortic stenosis in the elderly.

Morphology

Regardless of the site, calcium salts are grossly seen as fine white granules or clumps, often felt as gritty deposits. Sometimes a tuberculous lymph node is essentially converted to radio-opaque stone. Histologically, calcification appears as intracellular and/or extracellular basophilic deposits. In time, heterotopic bone may be formed in the focus of calcification.

The pathogenesis of dystrophic calcification involves initiation (or nucleation) and propagation, both of which may be either intracellular or extracellular; the ultimate end product is the formation of crystalline calcium phosphate. Initiation in extracellular sites occurs in membrane bound vesicles about 200nm in diameter; in normal cartilage and bone they are known as matrix vesicles, and in pathologic calcification they derive from degenerating cells.

It is thought that calcium is initially concentrated in these vesicles by its affinity for membrane phospholipids, while phosphates accumulate as a result of the action of membrane-bound phosphatases. Initiation of intracellular calcification occurs in the mitochondria of dead or dying cells that have lost their ability to regulate intracellular calcium.

After initiation in either location, propagation of crystal formation occurs. This is dependent on the concentration of Ca^{2+} and PO_4^- in the extracellular spaces, the presence of mineral inhibitors, and the degree of collagenisation, which enhances the rate of crystal growth.

Metastatic calcification: Metastatic calcification can occur in normal tissues whenever there is hypercalcaemia.

The four major causes of hypercalcemia are:

1. Increased secretion of parathyroid hormone, due to either primary parathyroid tumours or production of parathyroid hormone-related protein by other malignant tumours;

2. Destruction of bone due to the effects of accelerated turnover (e.g., Paget disease), immobilization, or tumours (increased bone catabolism associated with multiple myeloma, leukemia, or diffuse skeletal metastases);

3. Vitamin D–related disorders including vitamin D intoxication and sarcoidosis (in which macrophages activate a vitamin D precursor); and

4. Renal failure, in which phosphate retention leads to secondary hyperparathyroidism.

Morphology

Metastatic calcification can occur widely throughout the body but principally affects the interstitial tissues of the vasculature, kidneys, lungs, and gastric mucosa. The calcium deposits morphologically resemble those described in dystrophic calcification.

Although they do not generally cause clinical dysfunction, extensive calcifications in the lungs may produce remarkable radiographs and respiratory deficits, and massive deposits in the kidney (nephrocalcinosis) can cause renal damage.

Cellular Aging

Cellular aging is the result of a progressive decline in the proliferative capacity and life span of cells and the effects of continuous exposure to exogenous factors that cause accumulation of cellular and molecular damage.

Several mechanisms are known or suspected to be responsible for cellular aging:

- *DNA damage:* Cellular aging is associated with increasing DNA damage, which may happen during normal DNA replication and can be enhanced by free radicals. Although most DNA damage is repaired by DNA repair enzymes, some persists and accumulates as cells age.

  In fact, the intervention that has most consistently prolonged life span in most species is calorie restriction. Recently, it has been proposed that calorie restriction imposes a level of stress that activates proteins of the Sirtuin family, such as Sir2, that function as histone deacetylases. These proteins may deacetylate and thereby activate DNA repair enzymes, thus stabilizing the DNA; in the absence of these proteins, DNA is prone to damage.

- **Decreased cellular replication:** All normal cells have a limited capacity for replication, and after a fixed number of divisions cells become arrested in a terminally non-dividing state, known as replicative senescence (showing the effect of being old).Aging is associated with progressive replicative senescence of cells.

  Cells from children have the capacity to undergo more rounds of replication than do cells from older people. In contrast, cells from patients with Werner syndrome, a rare disease characterized by premature aging, have a markedly reduced in vitro life span. In human cells, the mechanism of replicative senescence involves incomplete replication and progressive shortening of telomeres, which ultimately results in cell cycle arrest.

Telomeres are short repeated sequences of DNA present at the linear ends of chromosomes that are important for ensuring the complete replication of chromosome ends and for protecting the ends from fusion and degradation. When somatic cells replicate, a small section of the telomere is not duplicated, and telomeres become progressively shortened.

As the telomeres become shorter, the ends of chromosomes cannot be protected and are seen as broken DNA, which signals cell cycle arrest. The lengths of the telomeres are normally maintained by nucleotide addition mediated by an enzyme called telomerase. Telomerase is a specialized RNA-protein complex that uses its own RNA as a template for adding nucleotides to the ends of chromosomes.

Telomerase activity is expressed in germ cells and is present at low levels in stem cells, but it is usually absent in most somatic tissues. Therefore, as cells age their telomeres become shorter and they exit the cell cycle, resulting in an inability to generate new cells to replace damaged ones. Conversely (on other hand/in opposition), in immortal cancer cells, telomerase is reactivated and telomeres are not shortened, suggesting that telomere elongation might be an important—possibly essential—step in tumour formation.

Despite such alluring (attractive/ fascinating) observations, however, the relationship of telomerase activity and telomere length to aging and cancer has yet to be fully established.

- Reduced regenerative capacity of tissue stem cells: Recent studies suggest that with age, the p16(CDKN2A) protein accumulates in stem cells, and they progressively lose their capacity to self-renew.p16 is a physiological inhibitor of cell cycle progression; deletion or loss-of-function mutations of p16 are associated with cancer development.

- Accumulation of metabolic damage: Cellular life span is also determined by a balance between damage resulting from metabolic events occurring within the cell and counteracting molecular responses that can repair the damage.

One group of potentially toxic products of normal metabolism is reactive oxygen species. These by-products of oxidative phosphorylation cause covalent modifications of proteins, lipids, and nucleic acids.

Increased oxidative damage could result from repeated environmental exposure to such influences as ionizing radiation along with progressive reduction of antioxidant defense mechanisms. Damaged cellular organelles accumulate as cells age. This may also be the result of declining function of the proteasome, the proteolytic machine that serves to eliminate abnormal and unwanted intracellular proteins.

- Studies in model organisms, like the worm *Caenorhabditiselegans*, have shown that growth factors, such as insulin-like growth factor, and intracellular signaling pathways triggered by these hormones, tend to reduce life span. The underlying mechanisms are not fully understood, but these growth factors may attenuate Sir2 responses to cellular stress and thus reduce the stability of the DNA.

Summary

Morphologic Alterations in Injured Cells

- Reversible cell injury: cell swelling, fatty change, plasma membrane blebbing and loss of microvilli, mitochondrial swelling, dilation of the ER, eosinophilia (due to decreased cytoplasmic RNA)

- Necrosis: increased eosinophilia; nuclear shrinkage, fragmentation, and dissolution; breakdown of plasma membrane and organellar membranes; myelin figures; leakage and enzymatic digestion of cellular contents

- Apoptosis: nuclear chromatin condensation; formation of apoptotic bodies (fragments of nuclei and cytoplasm).

Subcellular Alterations in Cell Injury:

Effects of Injurious Agents on Organelles and Cellular Components:

- Autophagy: In nutrient-deprived cells, organelles are enclosed in vacuoles that fuse with lysosomes. The organelles are digested but in some cases indigestible pigment (e.g. lipofuscin) remains.

- Hypertrophy of SER: Cells exposed to toxins that are metabolized in the SER show hypertrophy of the ER, a compensatory mechanism to maximize removal of the toxins.

- Mitochondrial alterations: Changes in the number, size, and shape of mitochondria are seen in diverse adaptations and responses to chronic injury.

- Cytoskeletal alterations: Some drugs and toxins interfere with the assembly and functions of cytoskeletal filaments or result in abnormal accumulations of filaments.

Mechanisms of Cell Injury:

- ATP depletion: failure of energy-dependent functions → reversible injury → necrosis

- Mitochondrial damage: ATP depletion → failure of energy-dependent cellular functions → ultimately, necrosis; under some conditions, leakage of proteins that cause apoptosis.

- Influx of calcium: activation of enzymes that damage cellular components and may also trigger apoptosis.

- Accumulation of reactive oxygen species: covalent modification of cellular proteins, lipids, nucleic acids.

- Increased permeability of cellular membranes: may affect plasma membrane, lysosomal membranes, mitochondrial membranes; typically culminates in necrosis.
- Accumulation of damaged DNA and misfolded proteins: triggers apoptosis

Apoptosis

- Regulated mechanism of cell death that serves to eliminate unwanted and irreparably damaged cells, with the least possible host reaction.
- Characterized by: enzymatic degradation of proteins and DNA, initiated by caspases; and recognition and removal of dead cells by phagocytes.
- Initiated by two major pathways:
- Mitochondrial (intrinsic) pathway is triggered by loss of survival signals, DNA damage and accumulation of misfolded proteins (ER stress); associated with leakage of pro-apoptotic proteins from mitochondrial membrane into the cytoplasm, where they trigger caspase activation; inhibited by anti-apoptotic members of the Bcl family, which are induced by survival signals including growth factors.
- Death receptor (extrinsic) pathway is responsible for elimination of self-reactive lymphocytes and damage by cytotoxic T lymphocytes; is initiated by engagement of death receptors (members of the TNF receptor family) by ligands on adjacent cells.

Abnormal Intracellular Depositions and Calcifications

Abnormal deposits of materials in cells and tissues are the result of excessive intake or defective transport or catabolism.

- **Depositions of lipids**

  Fatty change: accumulation of free triglycerides in cells, resulting from excessive intake or defective transport (often because of defects in synthesis of transport proteins); manifestation of reversible cell injury.

  Cholesterol deposition: result of defective catabolism and excessive intake; in macrophages and smooth muscle cells of vessel walls in atherosclerosis.

- ***Deposition of proteins:*** reabsorbed proteins in kidney tubules; immunoglobulins in plasma cells.

- ***Deposition of glycogen:*** in macrophages of patients with defects in lysosomal enzymes that break down glycogen (glycogen storage diseases).

- ***Deposition of pigments:*** typically, indigestible pigments, such as carbon, lipofuscin (breakdown product of lipid peroxidation), iron (usually due to overload, as in haemosiderosis).

- **Pathologic calcifications:**

  Dystrophic calcification: deposition of calcium at sites of cell injury and necrosis.

Metastatic calcification: deposition of calcium in normal tissues, caused by hypercalcaemia (usually a consequence of parathyroid hormone excess).

Cellular Aging

- Results from combination of accumulating cellular damage (e.g., by free radicals), reduced capacity to divide (replicative senescence), and reduced ability to repair damaged DNA.

- *Accumulation of DNA damage:* defective DNA repair mechanisms; DNA repair may be activated by calorie restriction (known to prolong aging in model organisms).

- *Replicative senescence:* reduced capacity of cells to divide because of decreasing amounts of telomerase and progressive shortening of chromosomal ends (telomeres).

- *Other factors:* progressive accumulation of metabolic damage; possible roles of growth factors that promote aging in simple model organisms.

3

Inflammation

Syllabus: Pathogenesis and clinical significance of acute inflammation, chronic inflammation, Chemical mediators in inflammation, Wound healing, Repairs of wounds in the skin, factors influencing healing of wounds.

Definition: Self-defense is a property of living organism. Inflammation is a direct tissue response to noxious or injurious external/internal stimuli. Inflammation can occur in response to any thing that damages the tissue, e.g.:

- Toxic chemicals: acid, alkali etc.

- Physical factors: heat, cold, electricity, radiation, trauma – microorganism and their metabolic by-product

- Immune response: hypersensitivity, immune complex, auto immune reactions

Every organ/tissue type is susceptible to inflammation.

Degree and nature of the inflammatory response depends on person's state of health, nutrition, immunity, nature and severity of noxious stimuli.

Some of the Cardinal signs of inflammation:

- Ruber   :   Redness
- Tumour   :   Swelling
- Calor   :   Heat
- Dolor   :   Pain, Loss of function

Classification

(a) *Latent Inflammation:* When trauma or injury is extremely mild, the response may be immediate and brief. Inflammation subsides before it is noticeable.

(b) *Acute Inflammation:* To certain type of trauma (injury) tissue react sharply by undergoing severe changes, such response is acute inflammation. Tissue changes occurring in acute inflammation may subside partly, completely after overcoming the trauma.

(c) *Chronic Inflammation:* Inflammation of prolonged duration. Trauma continues to elicit response in subsidised form. The resultant inflammation is called chronic inflammation. Chronic inflammation may be the result of acute inflammation or have separate entity.

Advantages and Disadvantages of Inflammation

Advantages

- Inflammation serves to localise and isolate infected tissue/injured tissue area and protect the surrounding healthy tissue.
- It neutralises and inactivates toxic substance
- Destroy or limit the growth of infecting microorganism
- Prepare the area for wound healing and repair by removing devitalised tissue and cell debris
- Normalisation of injured tissue.

Disadvantages

- Pain and swelling associated with inflammation lead to varying degree of disability
- Inflammation may lead to rapture of viscera, e.g. perforation of appendix in appendicitis
- Severe haemorrhage, e.g. from pulmonary tuberculous granuloma
- It can lead to formation of scar tissue; e.g. Scar tissue may hamper vital organs
- It may result in fistula formation, e.g. abdominal perineal fistula (abnormal passage), joint stiffness (pain and swelling)
- Development of crippling diseases [rheumatoid arthritis, glomerulo nephritis, allergic reaction etc.,] − it may propagate further by destructing healthy surrounding tissue

Acute Inflammation

Salient features of acute inflammation:

- It is the immediate and early response to injurious agent
- Acute inflammation is a stereotypical (same type), response to all forms of injury irrespective of the type of causative agent
- Acute inflammation involves changes that occur within minutes and last for several hours or days it may resolve spontaneously or with treatment

Acute inflammation has three major components:

(a) Alteration in vascular calibre (vasodilation) that leads to increased blood flow

(b) Structural changes in the microvasculature that permits plasma proteins and leukocytes to leave the circulation

(c) Emigration of leukocytes from microvasculature and their accumulation in the focus of injury Inflammatory response involves vascular and cellular events that are mediated by various chemical agents.

A. Vascular Phase of Acute Inflammatory Reaction (Vascular Phenomenon)

- *Vasodilation:* Transient vasoconstriction followed by vasodilation in capillaries and arterioles in injured area. It allows increased blood flow to the site (hyperaemia), which is reflected clinically by heat and erythema (flare phenomenon).Vasodilation induced by action of several mediators mainly nitric oxide (NO), histamine on vascular smooth muscle.

- *Increased vascular permeability:* Vasodilation is followed by increased vascular permeability. Increased vascular permeability leads to escape of protein rich fluid into interstitium (exudation), which is hall mark of acute inflammation. Outflow of fluid and its accumulation in interstitial tissue cause oedema (wheel).Endothelial leakage is caused by endothelial cell contraction, which forms wide intercellular junction, direct endothelial injury, leucocyte mediated injury during transcytosis (movement of leukocytes).

- *Exudation:* Escape of fluid (plasma), blood cells and proteins into interstitial tissue space or body cavities. Exudation of fluid helps to dilute toxic/irritant substance, act as bacteriostatic, bactericidal, involve in opsonisation, oedema etc.

- *Stasis:* Loss of fluid result in increased viscosity of blood which lowers blood flow.

B. Cellular Phase of Acute Inflammatory Response

Critical function of inflammation is to deliver leukocytes to site of injury and to activate leukocytes to perform their normal function in hostdefense. Leukocytes ingest offending agent, kill bacteria and other microorganism, and remove necrotic tissue and foreign substances.

Extravasation: Sequence of events in the journey of leukocytes from blood vessel lumen to interstitial tissue is called extravasation. It is divided into following steps:

(a) *Margination:* Leukocytes (mainly neutrophils and monocytes) assume peripheral position along the endothelial surface

(b) *Rolling and adhesion:* Individual and rows of leukocytes tumble slowly along endothelium, finally come to rest at some point, where they adhere firmly

(c) *Pavementing:* Endothelium becomes virtually lined by leukocytes

(d) *Diapedesis (emigration):* Transmigration across endothelium. After firm adhesion leukocytes insert pseudopods into junction between endothelial cells and squeeze through inter endothelial junction. They traverse the basement membrane and escape into extra vascular space. All leukocytes (neutrophils, monocytes, eosinophils, basophils) use the same pathway to migrate from blood to tissue.

Chemotaxis: Process by which leukocytes directed to site of injury. [Locomotion oriented along chemical gradient].

(a) All granulocytes, monocytes, and to lesser extend lymphocytes respond to chemotactic stimuli

(b) Both exogenous and endogenous agent can act as chemoattractants

(c) Most common exogenous agents are bacterial products

(d) Endogenous agents include, complement components (C5a), product of lipoxygenase pathway (leukotrienes), cytokines, histamine etc.

Leukocyte activation: Microbes, product of necrotic cell, antigen-antibody complex, cytokines, chemotactic factors, induce several responses in leukocytes, referred as leukocyte activation [activation of neutrophils, monocytes, macrophages]. It causes:

(a) Production of arachidonic acid metabolites [leukotrienes] –

degranulation and secretion of lysosomal enzymes

(b) Secretion of cytokines

(c) Modulation of leukocyte adhesion molecule [increased expression of adhesion molecule on endothelium]

Phagocytosis: Process by which phagocytic cells (neutrophils, monocytes/macrophages) recognise, engulf and dispose of foreign particles. Phagocytosis involves three distinct but interrelated steps:

(a) *Recognition and attachment:* Recognition and attachment of particle to be ingested by the leukocytes. Phagocytosis of microbes and dead cells is initiated by recognition of particle by receptor expressed on the surface of leukocyte. Mannose receptors and scavenger receptors are two important receptors that function to bind and ingest microbes. Efficiency of phagocytosis greatly enhanced by opsonisation, (microbes/particle coated with specific proteins like Ig-G antibodies, C3b component of complement etc.).

(b) *Engulfment:* Engulfment with phagocytes and subsequent formation of phagocytic vacuoles. During engulfment, extension of cytoplasm (pseudopods) flow around the particle to be engulfed, eventually complete enclosure of particle within phagosome. Phagocytic vacuoles (Phagosomes) fuse with lysosomal granules resulting in discharge of granular content into phagolysosome. During this process neutrophils and monocytes become progressively degranulated.

(c) *Killing or degradation of ingested material:* It is the ultimate step in elimination of infectious agent and necrotic cell is their killing and degradation within neutrophils and macrophages.

Microbial killing is accomplished by oxygen dependent mechanism. Phagocytes stimulate production of reactive oxygen intermediates (ROI). e.g.: superoxide anion ($O_2.$), Hydrogen peroxide (H_2O_2), Hydroxyl radicle (OH^-), Hypochlorite ($HOCl^-$). Membrane oxidase [NADPH oxidase] reduces oxygen to superoxide anion, superoxide then converted to hydrogen peroxide, hydrogen peroxide further reduced to reactive hydroxyl radical(OH^-).

Myeloperoxidase [MPO] in presence of halide convert H_2O_2 to hypochlorite [HOCl], which is a potent antimicrobial agent that destroys microbes by halogenation. Bacterial killing can also occur by oxygen independent mechanism:

- bacterial permeability increasing proteins.
- enzymes like lysozymes, lactoferrin, iron binding protein etc., After killing acid hydrolases degrade microbes within phagolysosomes.

During phagocytosis leukocytes release microbial and other product not only within phagolysosomes but also to the extra cellular space. e.g.: lysosomal enzymes, reactive oxygen intermediates [ROI], prostaglandins, leukotrienes etc. These products can cause tissue damage, thus amplifying the effect of initial injurious agent.

Outcome of Acute Inflammation

- Complete restoration.
- Neutralisation of injurious stimulus and restoration of site of acute inflammation to normal by regeneration.
- Healing by connective tissue replacement (fibrosis) -it occurs after substantial tissue destruction or in tissue that do not regenerate. A mass of connective tissue develops in the area.
- Abscess formation -occurs in infection with pyogenic bacteria.
- Progression to chronic inflammation -when acute inflammation cannot be cured/resoled due to persistence of injurious agent or interference in process of healing.

Chemical mediators of inflammation: A variety of chemical substances are synthesised and released during inflammatory process. These substances are responsible for controlling the inflammatory response:

Vasoactive Amines: Histamine and Serotonin

- *Histamine:* It is present in mast cells, basophils, platelets etc. It is released by cell degranulation caused by physical injury, immune reaction, C3a, C5a (fragments of complement) etc. Histamine release proteins form leukocytes. Dilate arteries and venules. Chemotactic for eosinophils.
- *Serotonin [5-Hydorxy tryptamine]*: Its action similar to histamine. Stored in platelets, enterochromaffin cells. Platelet aggregation stimulate release of 5-HT.

Plasma derived mediators (Plasma proteases):
Kinin system, complement system, clotting system.

- *Kinin System:* It is triggered by Hageman factor (factor XII). When activated lead to formation of bradykinin (nanopeptide) which is a potent vasodilator. It increases vascular permeability, smooth muscle contraction, pain etc. It is inactivated by kininase.

- *Complement system:* It consists of 20 complement components present in plasma. It is a defense against microbial agents. It increases vascular permeability, chemotaxis and opsonisation. Complement fragments C3a, C5a are most important mediators of inflammation. C3a and C5a -cause release of histamine and increase vascular permeability. C5a -powerful chemotactic agent for neutrophils, monocytes, eosinophils and basophils. Phagocytosis happens when fixed to bacterial cell wall (opsonisation), C3b and C5a favour phagocytosis by neutrophils and macrophages

- *Clotting system:* It is a series of plasma proteins activated by Hageman factor (XII). The final step is conversion of fibrinogen to fibrin. Fibrinopeptides induce increased vascular permeability and chemotactic activity. Thrombin causes leukocyte adhesion, fibroblast proliferation.

Arachidonic Acid Metabolites: Prostaglandins and Leukotrienes (Eicosanoids)

They are autocoids [local or short-range hormones]. Arachidonic acid [20 carbon polyunsaturated fatty acid], formed from linoleic acid (essential fatty acid) and are released from phospholipids by phospholipase.

- *Cyclooxygenase pathway:* Gives prostaglandins [PGE2, PGD2, PGF2α, PGI2 (Prostacyclin] and Thromboxane A2 [Tx A2]. Tx A2 (Thromboxane A2) is a potent platelet aggregating agent and vasoconstrictor. PGI2 (Prostacyclin) is a potent vasodilator and inhibit platelet aggregation. PGD2, PGE2 and PGF2 -cause vasodilation, potentiate oedema formation. Prostaglandins are involved in pain and fever (PGE2)

- *Lipoxygenase pathway:* (predominant in neutrophils) gives 5-HETE which is chemotactic for neutrophils.5- HETE converted to leukotrienes [LTB4, LTC4, LTD4 and LTE4]. LTB4 is a potent chemotactic for neutrophils. LTC4, LTD4 and LTE4 -cause vasodilation, bronchospasm and increase vascular permeability. Aspirin and indomethacin suppress cyclooxygenase. Glucocorticoids release proteins which inhibit phospholipase A2.

Platelet Activating Factor (PAF): Derived from Phospholipids

It causes platelet aggregation, vasoconstriction, bronchoconstriction, increase leukocyte adhesion to endothelium. So PAF elicit most cardinal features of inflammation.

- *Cytokines:* Polypeptides produced by lymphocytes and macrophages. Main cytokines are Interleukin 1 (IL-1), Interleukin-8 (IL-8), Tumour necrosis factor (TNF α and β), and Interleukin-2 (IL-2). Interleukin 1 and TNF α - produced by macrophages, stimulate T-cells. Interleukin 2 (IL-2) produced by activated T-cells, cause amplification of T-cell production. IL-8 is a powerful chemotactic and activator of platelets. Secretion stimulated by endotoxins, immune complex, toxins, physical injury, inflammatory reaction.

- *Nitric oxide [NO]:* This is anendothelium derived relaxing factor [EDRF]. It reduces platelet aggregation, adhesion and cause vasodilation.

Lysosomal Constituents of Leukocytes: include Hydrolytic Enzymes and Proteases

Lysosomal granules contain lactoferrin, lysozyme, alkaline phosphatase, NADPH oxidase, integrins and collagenase

- *Oxygen derived free radicles:* H_2O_2, OH^-etc., are released from leukocytes. It causes endothelial cell damage.Harmful oxygen derived radicles are inactivated by ceruloplasmin, transferrin, superoxide dismutase, catalase (for H_2O_2), glutathione peroxidase etc.
- *Neuropeptides:* Cause vasodilation and increase vascular permeability by stimulating histamine, eicosanoid release (arachidonic acid derivatives). Enhance neutrophil adhesion and chemotaxis.
- *Platelet derived growth factor (PDGF):* It is chemotactic to leukocytes.

Table 3.1 Summary of inflammatory processes

Vasodilation	Prostaglandins, nitric oxide
Vascular permeability	Vasoactive amines (Histamine, Serotonin), C_{3a}, C_{5a}, Bradykinin
Chemotaxis/Leukocyte activation	C_{5a}, Leukotriene B_4, bacterial products, cytokines (IL-8)
Fever	IL-1, IL-6, TNF, Prostaglandin [PGE$_2$]
Pain	Prostaglandins, bradykinin
Tissue damage	Neutrophils, macrophages, lysosomal enzymes, oxygen metabolites, nitric oxide

Cellular Elements of Inflammatory Exudate [Cells involved in inflammation]

- Neutrophils
- Eosinophils
- Basophils and mast cells
- Monocytes and macrophages
- Lymphocytes and plasma cells
- Giant cells

Neutrophils [Polymorphonuclear neutrophils]

Morphology: They are granular with multi lobbed nucleus, stained by neutral dyes. They are the predominant cells in acute inflammation as well as in abscess.

Neutrophils forms first line defense of body against pyogenic bacteria. Neutrophils digest them by enzymes. Neutrophils are the chief constituent of pus.

Functions: Neutrophils are the first cells to arrive the injured area. They enter the tissue space by diapedesis and they are attracted to injured site by chemotaxis. Their main function is phagocytosis of the invading bacterial cell and destruction of the cell by release of lysosomal enzymes.

Eosinophils [Eosinophilic granulocytes]

Morphology: They have Bi lobed nucleus and granules stain red orange with eosin. Granules contain hydrolytic enzymes. Eosinophils on breaking down release histamine which increases capillary permeability.

Function: Important function of eosinophils is Phagocytosis. Eosinophilia may be a reaction to foreign proteins. In bronchial asthma, bronchial mucosa often crowded with eosinophils. Marked eosinophilia is characteristic of many parasitic infestations.

Basophils and Mast cells [Basophilic granulocytes]

Morphology: They have granules which stain blue with wright's stain. The granules contain heparin, histamine, slow reacting substance of Anaphylaxis [SRS-A], 5-HT etc. Basophils in tissue are called mast cells.

Function: Both cells (Basophils and Mast cells) are involved in hypersensitivity reaction mediated by Ig-E immunoglobulin. Surface of these cells have Ig-E antibody. Interaction of specific antigen with Ig-E antibody causes degranulation of mast cells and basophils which release histamine and other mediators. Basophils also play role in type IV hypersensitivity (Delayed Hypersensitivity) reaction, e.g. contact dermatitis.

Monocytes and Macrophages

Monocytes and macrophages belong to mono nuclear phagocyte system (MPS), also called reticuloendothelial system. Macrophages involved in inflammation are derived from monocytes. Different types of macrophages: Pulmonary, alveolar macrophages, peritoneal macrophages, Kupffercells, Mesangial cells of kidney, Fixed and mobile macrophages of lymph node, monocytes in bone marrow.

Functions:

- *Phagocyte function:* Macrophages dispose of noxious matter within tissue (microbes, necrotic tissue, debris etc.).Macrophages contain many digestive enzymes in lysosomes like proteases, hydroxylases etc. Opsonised microorganism (coated with Ig-M or complement C3b) is phagocytised by macrophages.

- *T-cell activation:* Macrophages process antigenic component of foreign matter, present processedantigen and MHC [Major Histocompatibility Complex] to T-cells which is required for activation of T-cells.

- *Macrophage activation:* T-cells once activated cause mobilisation and metabolic activation of macrophages by releasing various lymphokines.

- *B-cell activation:* B-cell activation requires IL-1, which is secreted by macrophages.
- *Secretory function:* Macrophages release interleukin I, colony stimulating factor (CSF), tumournecrosis factor (TNF), which are involved in inflammation and alpha interferon (interferon-α) which block viral infection, precursor prostaglandins etc. Cytokines from macrophages activate lymphocytes.
- *Healing and repair:* Cellular debris is removed by phagocytosis, and release fibroblast proliferating factor.
- Phagocytosis and digestion of invading microorganism/foreign particle – Release of potent enzymes which degrade connective tissue.
- Release of chemotactic and permeability factor which prolong inflammation.
- Release of substance causing leukocytosis and fever (like prostaglandins, endogenous pyrogens).
- Release of substance which aid healing.
- Secretion of antibacterial, antiviral proteins etc.

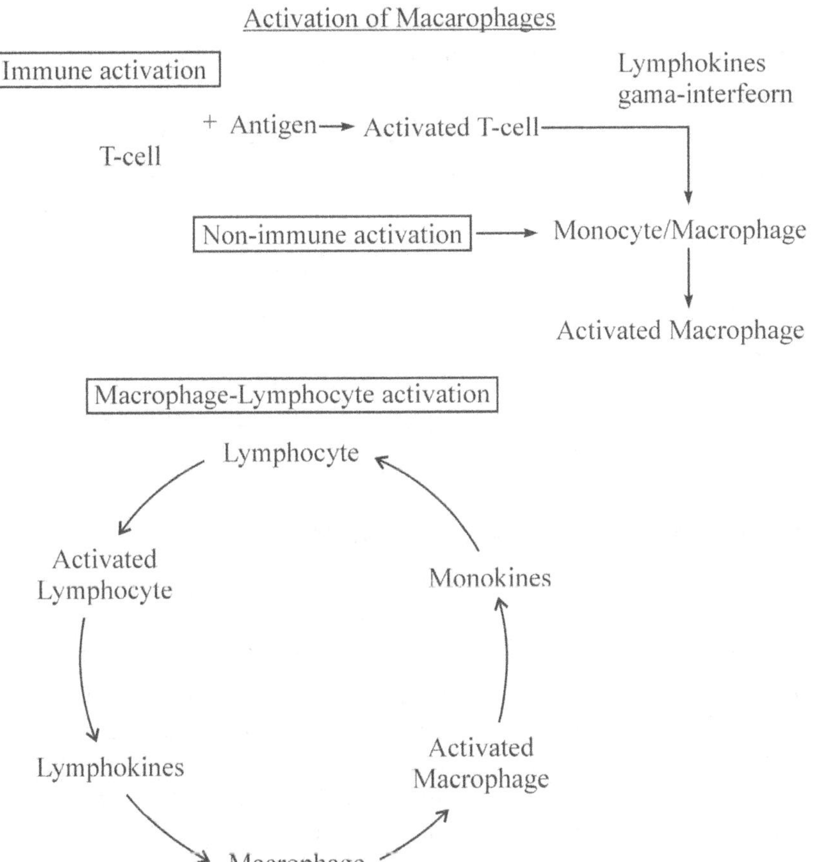

Fig. 3.1. Activation of macrophages.

Lymphocytes and Plasma Cells

T-cells derived from thymus. B-cells named after bursa of fabricious (in chicken). Null Cells Lymphocytes but no character of T-cells / B-cells. T-cells release lymphokines which activate monocytes and macrophages. Cytotoxic T-cells (lyse) kill target cell. B-cells differentiate into immunoglobulin producing plasma cells. Immunoglobulins (anti bodies) neutralise toxins. Ig-G helps in opsonisation. Null cells are lymphocytes, but lack surface antigen that identify T-cells and B-cells, e.g. Killer cells (K-cells), Natural killer cells (NK-cells) Lymphocyte activated Killer cells.

Lymphocytes appear late during chronic phase of inflammation. They are particularly prominent in tuberculosis, syphilis, other granulomus diseases, viral, rickettsial infections.

Giant Cells

When individual macrophages are unable to deal with particle to be removed they fuse together and form multinucleated giant cells. Giant cells are three types:

- *Tumour giant cells*: They are large cells and have one or several nuclei (not numerous). Tumour cells are formed by division of nucleus while cytoplasm fails to divide. Tumour giant cells are found in neoplasm only and are absent in inflammation.

- *Foreign body giant cells*: Cells may be of enormous size. It contains numerous nuclei as many as 50-100. Nuclei are regular in size scattered throughout cytoplasm. In certain conditions like tuberculosis, nuclei may be arranged around periphery [Langerhans giant cells]. Foreign body giant cells are seen in Tuberculosis, Syphilis, Leprosy, Actinomycosis etc.

- *Miscellaneous*: Giant cells of mesodermal origin: e.g.: Ascoff cells of Rheumatic nodule, Reed Stenberg cells of Hodgkin's disease.

  Role of exudate: Dilute irritants, lower the concentration of toxins, bacteriostatic, bactericidal effect, makes bacteria susceptible or phagocytosis by leukocytes.

Morphological Pattern of Acute Inflammation

Pattern of acute and chronic inflammation depends on, severity of reaction, tissue and site involved in reaction and causative agent. Serous inflammation -marked by outpouring of thin fluid, e.g. skin blisters from burn/viral infections.

- *Croupus or fibrinous inflammation:* Occurs with more severe injuries, usually seen in inflammation of body cavities, e.g. pericardium, pleura etc. Also, may occur in epithelia surface e.g. alimentary canal, urinary tract, gall bladder, lungs etc. Exudate more concentrated with excess plasma protein mainly fibrinogen. e.g.: dysentery, lobar pneumonia.

- *Suppurative/purulent inflammation:* It is characterised by production of large amount of pus. Pus consists of neutrophils, necrotised cells etc. It is caused by deep seeding of pyogenic bacteria, e.g. Streptococci. It may form an abscess [localised collection of purulent inflammatory tissue].

- *Ulcers:* Local excavation of surface of an organ or tissue produced by shedding of inflammatory necrotic tissue. Ulcer occurs when inflammatory necrotic area is near the surface, e.g. peptic ulcer, ulcer of mouth.

- *Pseudomembranous inflammation*: Formation of false membrane composed of necrosed epithelium and fibrin, e.g. diphtheria, Dysentery.

- *Catarrhal inflammation:* This affects mucous membrane, acini, duct glands, upper respiratory tract. Mucous secretion is abundant, desquamation surface epithelium, discharge initially mucoid later mucopurulent, e.g. bronchitis, gastritis, colitis etc.

- *Haemorrhagic inflammation:* This is caused by increased fragility of blood vessels and capillaries as in leukaemia, anaemia, various form of purpuras.

- Inflammation with extravasation of red blood cells e.g.: Black small pox, measles, diphtheria, etc.

- *Necrotic inflammation:* Inflammation accompanied by necrosis. e.g.: oriental sore.

Chronic Inflammation

Chronic inflammation is the response of body tissue to persistent traumatic stimuli. Chronic inflammation is the inflammation of prolonged duration (weeks/months), in which active inflammation, tissue destruction and attempts of healing proceed simultaneously. It occurs following acute inflammation or has separate entity.It causes rheumatoid arthritis, atherosclerosis, tuberculosis, chronic lung disease etc.

Etiology

Chronic inflammation arises under following setting:

- Persistent infection by certain microorganism, e.g. Treponema pallidum (Syphilis) – prolonged exposure to certain chemicals, e.g. silica dust, lime salt.

- Autoimmune reaction is an immune reaction against individuals own tissue that result in chronic inflammatory disease, e.g. Rheumatoid arthritis, Systemic lupus erythematosus (SLE).

Pathogenesis

Chronic inflammation of various organs occurs in three ways:

- It may follow an episode of acute inflammation where the inciting stimulus persists in the body

- There may be repeated attack of acute inflammation. e.g.: Cholecystitis, Pyelonephritis

- Chronic inflammation may develop as primary entity without preceding attack of acute inflammation. e.g.: Tuberculosis, Chronic bronchitis, Rheumatoid arthritis.

Chronic inflammation is characterised by:

- Infiltration with mono nuclear cells (Macrophages, Lymphocytes, Plasma cells)
- Tissue destruction (induced by inflammatory cells)
- Attempt to repair (by connective tissue replacement)
- Angiogenesis (development of new blood vessels)
- Fibrosis happens, where replacement of parenchyma by fibrous tissue

Mononuclear infiltration: Macrophage is the prima dona cells (main cells) of chronic inflammation. Macrophages are one component of mononuclear phagocyte system (MPS). They are named as monocytes (blood), macrophage (tissue), kupffer cells (liver), sinus histiocytes (spleen and lymph node), alveolar macrophage (lung) etc.

Monocytes on extravasation transform to phagocytic macrophages. Extravasation of monocytes is governed by same factors involved in neutrophil emigration. Activation signal for macrophage include cytokines (secreted by activated T-cells), bacterial endotoxins, fibronectin etc. After activation macrophages secrete biologically active products which mediate tissue destruction, vascular proliferation and fibrosis.

Chemotactic stimuli [C5a, Cytokines, IL-8] recruit more monocytes from circulation. Cytokines, oxidised lipids immobilise macrophages. Macrophages are central figure of chronic inflammation. Products that are released by macrophages are:

1. Enzymes- neutral proteases, elastase, collagenase, plasminogen activator, acid hydrolase, phosphatase, lipase
2. Plasma proteins [c1 to c5], coagulation factors (V, VIII, tissue factors)
3. Reactive metabolites of oxygen
4. Eicosanoids-cytokines (IL-1, TNF, IL-8), growth factors (PGDFM, EGF, FGF, TGF-β)
5. Nitric oxide

Other types of cells in chronic inflammation are lymphocytes, plasma cells, eosinophils, mast cells. Activated lymphocytes produce lymphokines, which activate monocytes and macrophages.

Monokine [cytokines] - from activated macrophages, stimulate lymphocytes. Plasma cells produce antibody against persistent antigen or altered tissue components.

Fibrosis: [repair by connective tissue]: persistent tissue destruction with damage to both parenchymal cells and stromal frame work are hall mark of chronic inflammation. Process of repair has four stages:

1. Formation of new blood vessel (angiogenesis)
2. Maturation and proliferation of fibroblast
3. Deposition of extracellular matrix
4. Maturation and organisation of fibrous tissue

Factors inducing angiogenesis: Fibroblast growth factor (FGF), vascular endothelial growth factor (VEGF) induce angiogenesis.

Effect of Chronic Inflammation

Contraction of newly formed tissue leads to narrowing of orifices and tubes. e.g.: stenosis of mitral valve, in chronic endocarditis, stenosis of small intestine in regional ileitis. Loss parenchymal cells of organ takes place. Replacement of specialised cells by more resistant connective tissue happens in conditions like liver cirrhosis.

Systemic effect of inflammation: Fever, slow wave sleep, decreased appetite, increased degradation of proteins, hypotension known as acute phase reaction. Leucocytosis is observed with increase in cells, 15,000 to 20,000 cells/cmm., approximately.

Granulomatous inflammation: It is a distinct pattern of chronic inflammation. In Granuloma, focal area of granulomatous inflammation takes place. It consists of macrophages transformed into epithelium like cells (epitheloid cells) surrounded by lymphocytes and plasma cells. Granulomatous inflammation is mainly seen in chronic immune and infectious diseases, e.g. Tuberculosis, leprosy, syphilis, silicosis.

Granulomatous inflammation develops on response to persistent antigen, e.g. Infectious granuloma - formed in response to Mycobacterial infection, Lymphogranuloma venereum, parasitic infestation (e. g. Schistosomiasis), fungal infection (Cryptococcus), Treponema pallidum (syphilis) etc., Foreign body granuloma -formed in presence of particulate matter (glass, soil, metal etc.), surgicalsuture, cellulose etc.

Wound Healing

Healing is a body response to injury. It is an attempt to restore normal structure and function. Healing involves two processes:

1. **Regeneration:** healing by regeneration of parenchymal cells that result in complete restoration of original tissue.
2. **Repair:** healing by proliferation of connective tissue, this result in fibrosis and scarring. Repair involves two processes:

- ***Granulation tissue formation:*** Name due to slightly granular, pink appearance. Active granulation tissue consists of inflammatory cell infiltrate, newly formed blood vessels and young fibrous tissue in loose matrix.

Wound Healing by first intension (Primary Union): Clean uninfected wound, e.g. surgical incision.

Initial Haemorrhage: The space between the wound is filled with blood clot. Acute inflammatory response occurs within 24 hours, with large number of neutrophils. By 3rd day neutrophils are replaced by macrophages.

Epithelial change: Basal cells from epidermis proliferate and migrate towards incision space. Migrated epidermal cells, separate viable dermis form overlying necrotic material and clot, forming scab which cast off (scab = dry blood clot).By 5th day new multi-layered epidermis formed at the site of injury.

Organisation: From 3rdday itself, fibroblasts invade the wound area and proliferate. By fifth day new collagen fibres are synthesised and filled the wound area. In four weeks scar tissue develops with no inflammatory cells and vascular changes.

Healing by second intension (Secondary Union): Healing of wound having large tissue loss, which may be due to infection. Basic events in secondary union are similar to primary union. Healing process in secondary union is by granulation tissue formation. Healing begins from base and progress to the surface. When surface is completely covered by epithelium devascularisation begins. Blood vessels gradually disappear and scar which was red become white.

- ***Contraction of wound:*** Wound contraction is an important feature of secondary union. Due to the action of myofibroblast in granulation tissue, wound contract to 1/3rd or 1/4th of original size. The main bulk of secondary union is granulation tissues. Granulation tissue formation begins from base.

Granulation tissue formed by proliferation of fibroblast and blood vessels (neovascularisation). Granulation tissue consists of inflammatory cells, new blood vessels and young fibrous tissue in loose matrix. Newly formed granulation tissue is deep red, granular and very fragile. With time, scar on maturation become pale and white due to increased collagen and decrease in vascularity.

Factors affecting Wound Healing

General Factors

- *Age:* Healing is quick in children; as age advances, process is impaired due to less blood supply
- *Nutrition:* Nutritional state of the patient, particularly protein intake is very important
- *Vitamin C:* Necessary for formation of intercellular substance and maturation of collagen
- *Vitamin K:* Deficiency cause hypoproteinemia, bleeding tendency, which interfere with normal wound healing
- *Vitamins A, D, E and B complex:* Their deficiency lower rate of phagocytosis and bacterial digestion and thus predisposing to local wound infection
- *Fluid and electrolyte balance:* Dehydration delay wound healing; similarly, water and salt overload also decrease the process of wound healing

Role of Growth Factors in Inflammation and Repair

A growth factor is a naturally occurring substance capable of stimulating cellular growth, proliferation, healing, and cellular differentiation. Usually it is a protein or a steroid hormone. Growth factors are important for regulating a variety of cellular processes.

Growth factors typically act as signaling molecules between cells. Growth factors are biologically active polypeptides affecting the proliferation, chemotaxis and differentiation of cells from epithelium, bone and connective tissue. They express their action by binding to specific cell-surface receptors present on various target cells including osteoblasts, cementoblasts and periodontal ligament fibroblasts.

The observation that growth factors participate in all cell functions led to exogenous application during periodontal tissue repair aiming to their use as an alternative therapeutic approach to periodontal therapy. Cell types and cultures conditions, dose, carrier materials, application requirements are of critical importance in the outcome of periodontal repair. The purpose of this article is to review the literature with respect to the biological actions of PDGF, TGF, FGF, IGF and EGF on periodontal cells and tissues, which are involved in periodontal regeneration. Any body repair whether neurons, renal, liver, injuries, cell damages hence require these growth factors.

Examples are cytokines and hormones that bind to specific receptors on the surface of their target cells. They often promote cell differentiation and maturation, which varies between growth factors. For example, bone morphogenetic proteins stimulate bone cell differentiation, while fibroblast growth factors and vascular endothelial growth factors stimulate blood vessel differentiation (angiogenesis).

Mononuclear cells generate a variety of hormone-like proteins termed growth factors that are instrumental in the evolution and resolution of inflammatory reactions. Many of these growth regulatory molecules have multifunctional properties. For example, the mononuclear cell-derived growth factors, platelet-derived growth factor (PDGF), and transforming growth factor beta (TGF-beta), are potent leukocyte chemo attractants. In addition, TGF-beta, a product of platelets, T lymphocytes, and monocytes, appears to induce the transcription of other monocyte-derived growth hormone genes.

In this regard, picomolar concentrations of TGF-beta stimulate peripheral blood monocytes to transcribe the genes for PDGF (c-sis), basic fibroblast growth factor (FGF), interleukin 1 (IL-1), and tumor necrosis factor (TNF). Furthermore, levels of mRNA for TGF-beta, which is constitutively expressed in resting monocytes, are also increased by exogenous TGF-beta. Each of these monocyte products exhibits a plethora of biological activities on other cell types. T lymphocytes, in response to antigen, contribute to this network by secreting growth factors and lymphokines that regulate monocyte growth factor production.

- Bacterial infection interferes with wound healing process
- Haematomas and serum collection
- Ischaemia
- Foreign bodies
- Desiccation (dryness) of the tissue
- Improper examination

Abscess

Abscess is localised collection of pus caused by suppuration [formation of pus] buried in a tissue, organ or cornified space. Abscess are usually produced by deep seeding of pyogenic (pus producing) bacteria into the tissue. Any organism which can persist in the tissue and can produce their effect can produce suppuration (pus formation).

Digestion and liquefaction of tissue is chiefly due to proteolytic enzymes produced by leukocytes.

4

Diseases Related to Immunity

Syllabus: Introduction to T and B cells, MHC proteins or transplantation antigens, Immune Tolerance hypersensitivity (Allergy, Autoimmunity, Alloimmunity).

Hypersensitivity, Hypersensitivity type I, II, III, IV, Biological significance, Allergy due to food, chemicals and drugs

Autoimmunity Criteria for autoimmunity, Classifications of autoimmune diseases in man, mechanism of autoimmunity, Transplantation and immunologic tolerance, allograft rejections, transplantation antigens, mechanism of rejection of allograft.

Definition: Immune system is like a double-edged sword. Immunodeficiency render human easy prey to infections and tumour, while hyper reactive immune system causes fatal disease like anaphylaxis, autoimmunity etc.

Introduction to T- Cells and B Cells

T Cell

A type of white blood cell that is of key importance to the immune system and is at the core of adaptive immunity. The system tailors the body's immune response to specific pathogens. The T cells are like soldiers who search out and destroy the targeted invaders.

Immature T cells (termed T-stem cells) migrate to the thymus gland in the neck, where they mature and differentiate into various types of mature T cells and become active in the immune system in response to a hormone called thymosin and other factors. T-cells that are potentially activated against the body's own tissues are T cells or T lymphocytes are a type of lymphocyte (in turn, a type of white blood cell) that plays a central role in cell-mediated immunity. They can be distinguished from other lymphocytes, such as B cells and natural killer cells (NK cells), by the presence of a T-cell receptor (TCR) on the cell surface. They are called T cells, because they mature in the thymus (although some also mature in the tonsils).

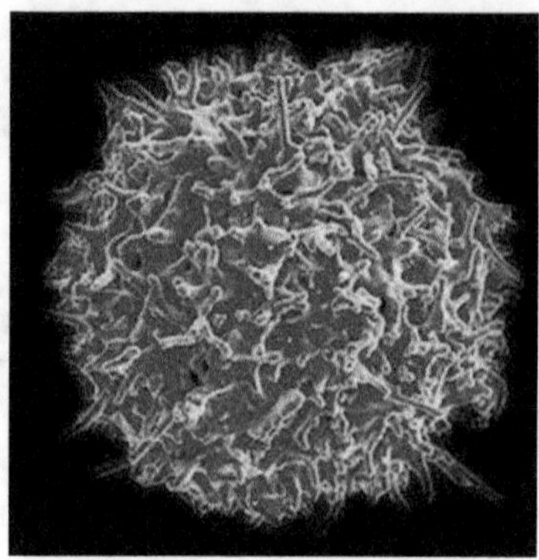

Fig. 4.1 Scanning electron
micrograph of a human T cell.
(Source: https://en.wikipedia.org/wiki/
T cell)

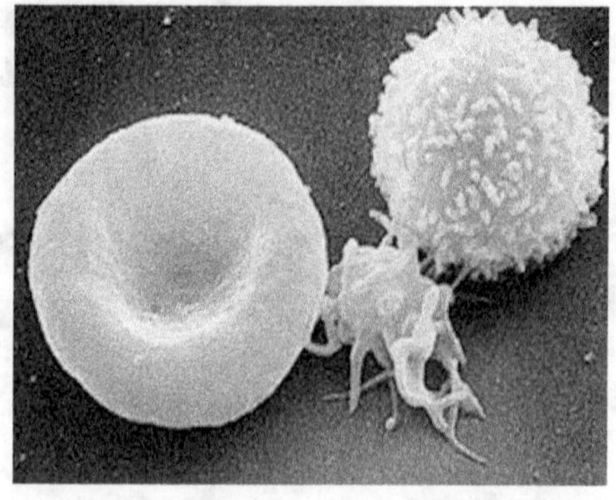

Fig. 4.2 Scanning electron micrograph of
T lymphocyte (right), a platelet (center)
and a red blood cell (left).
(Source: https://en.wikipedia.org/wiki/ T_cell)

B Cells

B cells or B lymphocytes are a type of lymphocyte in the humoral immunity of the adaptive immune system. B cells can be distinguished from other lymphocytes, such as T cells and natural killer cells (NK cells), by the presence of a protein on the B cell's outer surface known as a B cell receptor (BCR).

This specialized receptor protein allows a B cell to bind to a specific antigen. In mammals, immature B cells are formed in the bone marrow. The principal functions of B cells are:

- To make antibodies against antigens,
- To perform the role of antigen-presenting cells (APCs),
- To develop into memory B cells after activation by antigen interaction.
- B cells also release cytokines (proteins), which are used for signaling immune regulatory functions.

Major Histocompatability Complex (MHC) Proteins – Function and Role

They are a set of cell surface molecules encoded by a large gene family which controls a major part of the immune system in all vertebrates. MHC molecules mediate interactions of leukocytes, also called white blood cells (WBCs), which are immune cells, with other leukocytes or with body cells.

The MHC determines compatibility of donors for organ transplant, as well as one's susceptibility to an autoimmune disease via cross reacting immunization. In humans, the MHC is also called the human leukocyte antigen (HLA).

Each MHC molecule on the cell surface displays a molecular fraction of a protein, called epitope. The MHC gene family is divided into three subgroups: class I, class II, and class III. MHC proteins have immunoglobulin-like structure.

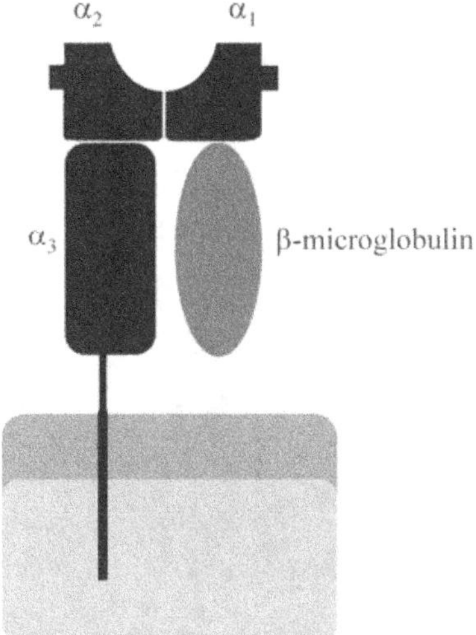

Fig. 4.3 MHC class I protein molecule

(Source: https://en.wikipedia.org/wiki/Major_histocompatibility_complex)

Class I

MHC I occur as α chain composed of three domains—α_1, α_2, and α_3. The α_1 rests upon a unit of the non-MHC molecule β_2 microglobulin (encoded on human chromosome 15). The α_3 subunit is transmembrane, anchoring the MHC class I molecule to the cell membrane. The peptide being presented is held by the floor of the peptide-binding groove, in the central region of the α_1/α_2 hetero dimer (a molecule composed of two nonidentical subunits). The genetically encoded and expressed sequence of amino acids, the sequence of residues, of the peptide-binding groove's floor determines which particular peptide residues it binds.

Function: Sample internal contents of the cell and present endogenously synthesized antigens, e.g. viral. These attract T killer cells (cytotoxic T cells). In MHC class I, any nucleated cell normally presents cytosolic peptides, mostly self-peptides derived from protein turnover and defective ribosomal products. During viral infection, intracellular microorganism infection, or cancerous transformation, such proteins degraded in the proteosome are as well loaded onto MHC class I molecules and displayed on the cell surface.

MHC Class I Pathway: Proteins in the cytosol are degraded by the Proteasomes, liberating peptides internalized by TAP channel in the endoplasmic reticulum, there associating with MHC-I molecules freshly synthesized. MHC-I/peptide complexes enter Golgi apparatus, are glycosylated, enter secretory vesicles, fuse with the cell membrane, and externalize on the cell membrane interacting with T lymphocytes.

Class II

In MHC class II, phagocytes such as macrophages and immature dendritic cells take up entities by phagocytosis into phagosomes—though B cells exhibit the more general endocytosis into endosomes— which fuse with lysosomes whose acidic enzymes cleave the uptaken protein into many different peptides. Via physicochemical dynamics in molecular interaction with the particular MHC class II variants borne by the host, encoded in the host's genome, a particular peptide exhibits immunodominance and loads onto MHC class II molecules. These are trafficked to and externalized on the cell surface.

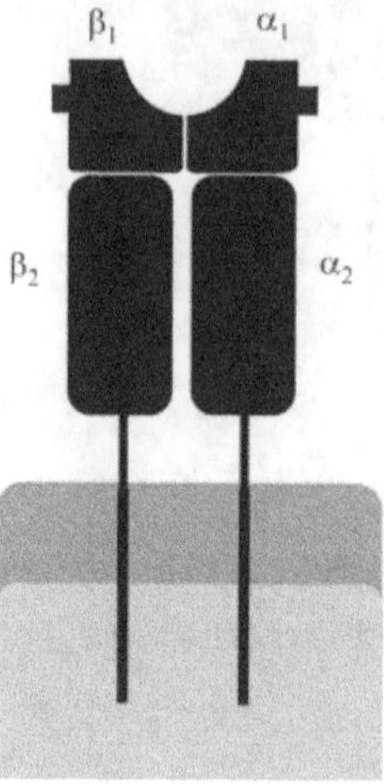

Fig. 4.4 MHC class II protein molecule.
(Source: https://en.wikipedia.org/wiki/Major_histocompatibility_complex)

MHC class II is formed of two chains, α and β, each having two domains—α_1 and α_2 and β_1 and β_2 — each chain having a transmembrane domain, α_2 and β_2, respectively, anchoring the MHC class II molecule to the cell membrane. The peptide-binding groove is formed of the heterodimer of α_1 and β_1. MHC class II molecules in humans have five to six isotypes. Exogenous antigens enter the cell and are presented by MHC II proteins.

Function: When called upon by antigen presenting cells MHC II presents exogenously derived proteins, e.g. bacterial products or viral capsid proteins. These attract T helper cells.

Class III

Class III molecules have physiologic roles unlike classes I and II, but are encoded between them in the short arm of human chromosome 6. Class III molecules include several secreted proteins with immune functions: components of the complement system (such as C2, C4, and B factor), cytokines (such as TNF-α, LTA, and LTB), and heat shock proteins.

MHC proteins play a fundamental role in regulating immune responses. They are a series of genes that code for proteins unique to each individual. MHC proteins and their associated molecules are fundamental in the process of antigen presentation. Class I and II proteins are polymorphic; cell surface proteins which present and help distinguish self and non-self antigens to T cells. By this process they allow the immune system to know if a cell should be killed or repaired.

The evolution of the MHC polymorphism ensures that a population will not succumb to a new pathogen or a mutated one, because at least some individuals will be able to develop an adequate immune response to win over the pathogen. The variations in the MHC molecules (responsible for the polymorphism) are the result of the inheritance of different MHC molecules, and they are not induced by recombination, as it is the case for the antigen receptors.

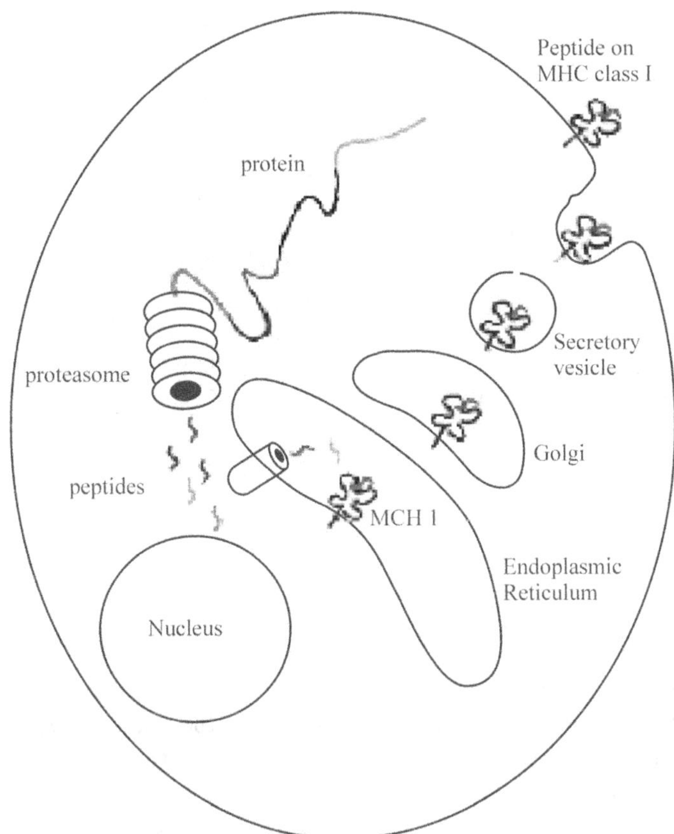

Fig. 4.5 Antigen processing and presentation.
(Source:https://en.wikipedia.org/wiki/Major_histocompatibility_complex)

Antigen Processing and Loading Pathways: Transporter associated with antigen processing (TAP) is a member of the ATP-binding-cassette transporter family. It delivers cytosolic peptides into the endoplasmic reticulum (ER), where they bind to nascent MHC class I molecules.

Proteasomes are processing enzymes capable of generating MHC class I from endogenous antigens by helping cleave antigenic peptides. Resulting peptides are then transported into the ER by a transporter for antigen presentation (TAP) where they become associated with the MHC I in the lumen of the ER. From there they are delivered to the cell surface through the plasma membrane to activate immune system T cells.

Table 4.1 Characteristics of the Antigen Processing Pathways

Characteristic	MHC-I pathway	MHC-II pathway
Composition of the stable peptide-MHC complex	Polymorphic chain α and β2 microglobulin, peptide bound to α chain	Polymorphic chains α and β, peptide binds to both
Types of antigen presenting cells (APC)	All nucleated cells	Dendritic cells, mononuclear phagocytes, B lymphocytes, some endothelial cells, epithelium of thymus
T lymphocytes able to respond	Cytotoxic T lymphocytes (CD8+)	Helper T lymphocytes (CD4+)
Origin of antigenic proteins	cytosolic proteins (mostly synthetized by the cell; may also enter from the extracellular medium via phagosomes	Proteins present in endosomes or lysosomes (mostly internalized from extracellular medium)
Enzymes responsible for peptide generation	Cytosolic proteasome	Proteases from endosomes and lysosomes (for instance, cathepsin)
Location of loading the peptide on the MHC molecule	Endoplasmic reticulum	Specialized vesicular compartment
Molecules implicated in transporting the peptides and loading them on the MHC molecules	TAP (transporter associated with antigen processing)	DM, invariant chain
Source courtesy https://en.wikipedia.org/wiki/Major_histocompatibility_complex		

T lymphocyte recognition restrictions: T lymphocytes are selected to recognize MHC molecules of the host, but not recognize other self-antigens. Following selection, each T lymphocyte shows dual specificity: The TCR recognizes self MHC, but only non-self-antigens.

In sexual mate selection (Genetic matchmaking): MHC molecules enable immune system surveillance of the population of protein molecules in a host cell, and greater MHC diversity permits greater diversity of antigen presentation. There is evidence for non-random mate choice with respect to certain genetic characteristics.

Evolutionary diversity: Most mammals have MHC variants similar to those of humans, who bear great allelic diversity, especially among the nine classical genes—seemingly due largely to gene duplication—though human MHC regions have many pseudo genes.

In cancer: Some HLA- mediated diseases are directly involved in the promotion of cancer. Gluten-sensitive enteropathy is associated with increased prevalence of enteropathy-associated T -cell lymphoma, and DR3-DQ2 homozygotes are within the highest risk group, with close to 80% of gluten-sensitive enteropathy-associated T-cell lymphoma cases. Abnormal cells might be targeted for apoptosis, which is thought to mediate many cancers before diagnosis.

In graft rejection: Any cell displaying some other HLA type is "non-self" and is seen as an invader by the body's immune system, resulting in the rejection of the tissue bearing those cells. This is particularly important in the case of transplanted tissue, because it could lead to transplant rejection.

In transplant rejection: In a transplantation procedure, as of an organ or stem cells, MHC molecules act themselves as antigens and can provoke immune response in the recipient, thus causing transplant rejection. MHC molecules were identified and named after their role in transplant rejection between mice of different strains, though it took over 20 years to clarify MHC's role in presenting peptide antigens to cytotoxic T lymphocytes (CTLs). The T lymphocytes recognition of the foreign MHC as self is allorecognition.

Transplantation antigens (HLA) Human Leukocyte Antigen

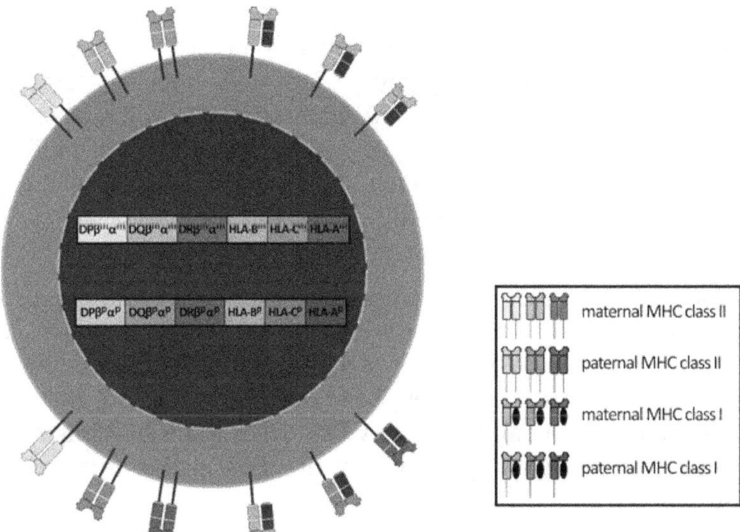

Fig. 4.6 Codominant expression of HLA genes human leukocyte antigen.
(Source https://en.wikipedia.org/wiki/Major_histocompatibility_complex)

Human Leukocyte Antigen: Human MHC class I and II are also called human leukocyte antigen (HLA). The human leukocyte antigen system is the locus of genes that encode for proteins on the surface of cells that are responsible for regulation of the immune system in humans. This group of genes resides on chromosome 6, and encodes cell-surface antigen-presenting proteins and has many other functions. The HLA genes are the human versions of the major

Histocompatability complex (MHC) genes that are found in most vertebrates (and thus are the most studied of the MHC genes).The proteins encoded by certain genes are also known as antigens, as a result of their historic discovery as factors in organ transplants. The major HLAs are essential elements for immune function.

Different classes have different functions:

- HLAs corresponding to MHC class I (A, B, and C) present peptides from inside the cell. For example, if the cell is infected by a virus, the HLA system brings fragments of the virus to the surface of the cell so that the cell can be destroyed by the immune system. These peptides are produced from digested proteins that are broken down in the Proteasomes. Foreign antigens presented by MHC class I attract killer T-cells (also called CD8 positive- or cytotoxic T-cells) that destroy cells.

- HLAs corresponding to MHC class II (DP, DM, DOA, DOB, DQ, and DR) present antigens from outside of the cell to T-lymphocytes. These particular antigens stimulate the multiplication of T-helper cells, which in turn stimulate antibody-producing B-cells to produce antibodies to that specific antigen. Self-antigens are suppressed by regulatory T cells.

- HLAs corresponding to MHC class III encode components of the complement system.

HLAs have other roles. They are important in disease defense. They are the major cause of organ transplant rejections. They may protect against or fail to protect (if down-regulated by an infection) against cancers. Mutations in HLA may be linked to autoimmune disease (examples: type I diabetes, coeliac disease). HLA may also be related to people's perception of the odor of other people, and may be involved in mate selection, as at least one study found a lower-than-expected rate of HLA similarity between spouses in an isolated community.

Aside from the genes encoding the six major antigen-presenting proteins, there are a large number of other genes, many involved in immune function, located on the HLA complex. Diversity of HLAs in the human population is one aspect of disease defense, and, as a result, the chance of two unrelated individuals with identical HLA molecules on all loci is very low. HLA genes have historically been identified as a result of the ability to successfully transplant organs between HLA-similar individuals.

In Infectious Disease

When a foreign pathogen enters the body, specific cells called antigen-presenting cells (APCs) engulf the pathogen through a process called phagocytosis. Proteins from the pathogen are digested into small pieces (peptides) and loaded onto HLA antigens (to be specific, MHC class II). They are then displayed by the antigen-presenting cells to T cells, which then produce a variety of effects to eliminate the pathogen.

Through a similar process, proteins (both native and foreign, such as the proteins of virus) produced inside most cells are displayed on HLAs (to be specific,

MHC class I) on the cell surface. Infected cells can be recognized and destroyed by CD8+ T cells.

Immune Tolerance

Immune tolerance – Autoimmunity, Criteria for autoimmunity, Classifications of autoimmune diseases in man, mechanism of autoimmunity

Occurs when an individual's immune system reacts against antigen on the tissue of other member of same species. There are two clinically relevant examples for this reactivity. Transplant rejection and transfusion reaction in which, immune system of the recipient of organ transplant or blood transfusion reacts against antigen on donor cell.

Because foetus is hybrid between mother and father it may express tissue specific antigen that are not found in mother. Occasionally these foetal antigens cross placenta and elicit immune response in mother. Maternal antibodies may be transported into foetal circulation to produce alloimmune disease in the foetus.

Maternal autoimmune diseases may cause transient neonatal disease. Mother may be producing Ig G autoantibodies specifically for her self-antigen. The foetus may also have same type of antigen. Therefore, symptoms of the same autoimmune disease may affect both mother and child even though autoantibodies are produced by mother's immune system.

Mechanism of this form of reaction is type II (tissue specific reaction). It does not occur by type I, III, or IV-because mediators of these reaction (viz: Ig E, immune complex, T-cells) do not readily cross placenta.

At birth, the source of antibody in foetal circulation is removed, although symptoms may be manifested immediately after birth. If successfully treated at birth will disappear as maternal antibodies are catabolised.

Child can be affected in following immunological disease:

- Graves's disease: An autoimmune disease, in which maternal antibody against the receptor for thyroid stimulating hormone cause neonatal hyperthyroidism.
- Myasthenia gravis: An autoimmune disease in which maternal antibody bind with acetylcholine receptor for neural transmitters on muscle cell, causing neonatal muscular weakness.
- Alloimmune neutropenia: Maternal antibody against neutrophils destroys neutrophils in foetus and neonates.
- Systemic Lupus Erythematosus: diverse maternal antibodies induce anomalies in the foetus. e.g.: congenital heart defect
- Rh and ABO alloimmunisation: Maternal antibody against erythrocyte antigen induces anaemia in child. e.g.: Erythroblastosis foetalis

Transplantation

Transplantation antigens [Histocompatibility molecule (Histocompatibility antigen)]: Histocompatibility molecules (antigens) are extremely important in induction and regulation of immune response and certain non-immunological function.

The principal physiological function of cell surface histocompatibility molecule (antigen) is to bind with peptide fragment of foreign proteins for presentation to appropriate antigen specific T cells. T-cells (in contrast to B cells) can recognise only membrane bound antigens. Hence histocompatibility antigens are critical to the induction of T-cell immunity.

Several genes code for histocompatibility antigens, but those that code for most important transplantation antigens are clustered on small segment of chromosome-6.This cluster constitutes the Major Histocompatibility Complex [MHC] also known Human Leukocyte Antigen Complex [HLA] because first identified in Leukocytes. MHC gene products are known as MHC antigens/HLA antigens.

MHC antigens are cell surface glycoproteins.HLA/MHC system is highly polymeric [variation between individuals]. Any two individuals express different HLA antigen. Based on the chemical structure, tissue distribution and function MHC gene products [MHC antigens] are classified into three categories:

1. *Class I MHC antigens:* Class I antigens are expressed on surface of all nucleated cell and platelets. They are encoded by three closely linked loci- HLA-A, HLA-B, HLA-C. Class I MHC antigens present foreign antigen to cytotoxic T-cells (CD8+ cells) in a groove present in the surface of the molecule [antigen binding cleft]. T -cell receptor [TCR] recognise MHC-peptide complex. CD8 molecule acts as co-receptor. Peptide antigen binds to MHC molecule in a complex process. Proteosomes in cytoplasm digest antigenic proteins to short peptides. They are transported to Endoplasmic reticulum. In ER peptide bind with newly synthesised class I molecule. It is then transported to cell surface for presentation to CD8+ cytotoxic T-lymphocytes. Class I antigens regulate the function of CD8+ cells. CD8+ cells carry receptor for class I MHC antigens. Class I antigens are important target in organ transplantation.

2. *Class II MHC antigens*: Class II antigens are coded by region called HLA-D in chromosome 6, which has three sub regions, HLA-DP, HLA-DQ, HLA-DR. Class II antigens are located on surface of macrophages, B-cells, activated T cells, endothelial cells and dendric cells (called as antigen presenting cells-APC). Class II MHC molecule have antigen binding cleft. Nature of the peptide that binds to class II molecule is different from that bind with class I molecule. Peptide-MHC complex is recognised by CD4+ cells (Helper T cells). CD4 molecule acts as co-receptor. Class II molecules regulate function of CD4+ (Helper T cells). CD4+ cells have receptor for class II molecules.

3. *Class III MHC antigens*: Class III antigens are components of complement system.

Role of MHC/HLA Complex

- Organ transplantation: The major importance of human histocompatibility antigen or HLA system lies in matching donor and recipient for organ transplantation. Recipient's immune system can recognise histocompatibility antigens on donor organ and accordingly accept or reject it. Both humoral and cell mediated immune response are involved in genetically non-identical transplant.

- Regulation of immune system: Class I antigens regulate function of cytotoxic T cells (CD8+). Class II antigens regulate function of helper T-cells (CD4+).

- Association of Disease with HLA: Several diseases have been found to be associated with some specific histocompatibility antigens, e.g. Inflammatory ankylosing spondylitis, Auto immune disorders, Rheumatoid arthritis – IDDM, Inherited disease of metabolism like Idiopathic Hemochromatosis.

Transplant Rejection

Allograft: Normal tissue that is transferred between genetically different individual of same species. Allogenic transplantation result in immune reaction. Two types of immune reaction:

- **HVG:** [Host versus Graft reaction]: Recipient's immune system recognise graft tissue as foreign and mount immune attack on graft.

- **GVH** [Graft versus Host reaction]: Immunocompetent graft attack immune compromised or eradicated host. e.g.: Bone marrow transplantation

Mechanism involved in rejection: Graft rejection depends on recognition of graft tissue as foreign by host. Graft rejection is a complex process which involves both cell mediated immunity (Type-IV) and antibody mediated immunity (Humoral) Type II and type III.

Antigen responsible for such rejection in human are, Major Histocompatibility Antigen system (HLA system/ MHC).HLA are produced by genes of MHC, which are set of membrane associated glycoproteins that are critical for recognition of self during cell-cell immunological reactions.HLA antigens are highly polymeric. Except identical twins' HLA of two individuals are different. Every individual recognise HLA molecule of another individual as foreign and react against it.

T-cell mediated reaction: It involve activation of CD8+ [cytotoxic T-cells] and delayed hyper sensitivity reaction triggered by activated CD4+ [helper cells]. T-cell mediated reaction initiated when recipient's lymphocytes encounter donor HLA antigens. (It is believed that interstitial dendric cells carried in donor organs are most important immunogens).

CD4+ helper T-cells activated to proliferation on encountering class II MHC antigens. CD8+ cells activated on encountering class I antigens. Mature CTLs (Cytotoxic T Cells/CD8+ cells) lyse the grafted tissue. In CD4+ activation, release cytokines IL-2, IL-4 and IL-5, etc. and cause increase vascular permeability, local accumulation of mono nuclear cells (Lymphocytes and Macrophages) Delayed hypersensitivity with microvascular injury, tissue ischemia, and destruction mediated by macrophages are the most important mechanism of graft destruction

Antibody mediated rejection: HLA antibodies are formed as part of host immune response against allograft. Hyper acute rejection occurs when preformed anti donor antibodies are present in the recipient. Such antibodies may be present in patient who already rejected a kidney transplant. Prior blood transfusion with HLA non-identical donors also lead to pre sensitisation because platelets and leukocytes are rich in HLA antigens.

In such cases rejection occur immediately after transplantation because circulating antibodies react with antigen and antigen antibody complex get deposited rapidly on vascular endothelium of grafted tissue. Complement fixation occurs and arthus type reaction follows. It mainly affects graft vasculature. Antibodies may cause injury by several mechanisms:

- Type I reaction
    - complement dependent cytotoxicity
    - antibody dependent cell mediated cytolysis
- Type III reaction
    - deposition of An-Ab complex

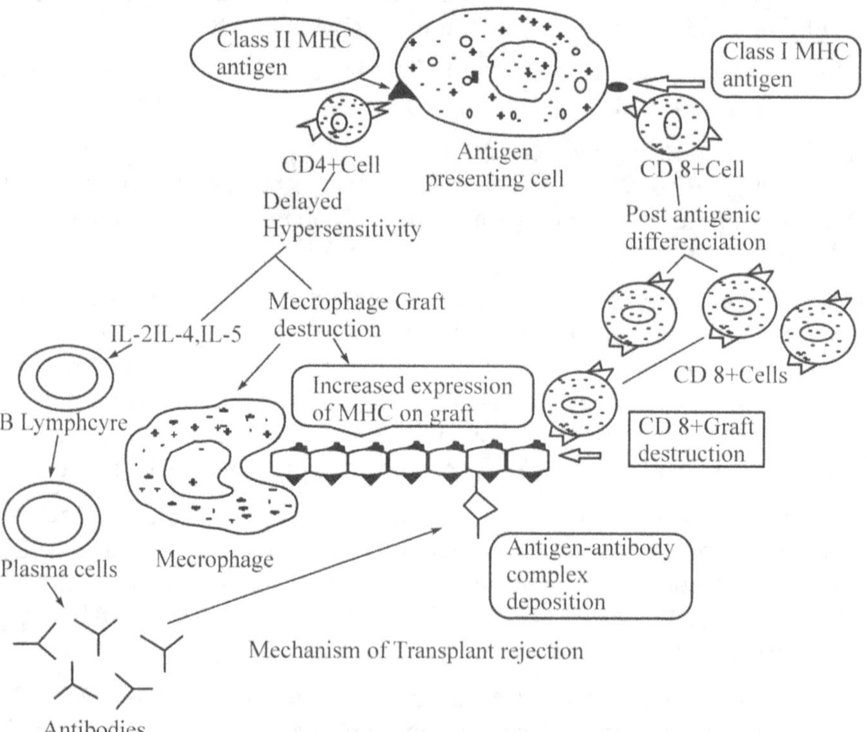

Fig. 4.7 Mechanism of transplant rejection.
(Source: emedicine.medscape.com/article/432209-overview)

Morphology of rejection reaction: On the basis of morphology and underlying mechanism rejection reaction are classified as:

- *Hyper acute rejection*: This form of rejection reaction occurs within minutes or hours after transplantation. Histological lesions are characterised by arthus reaction caused by antigen-antibody reaction at the level of vascular endothelium. Endothelial injury, thrombotic occlusion of capillaries and necrosis or arterial wall occurs. In kidney transplantation, a hyper acutely rejected kidney show rapid accumulation of neutrophils within arterioles, glomeruli and peritubular capillaries.

  Immunoglobulin and complements are deposited in vessel wall. These shows antigen-antibody reaction at vascular endothelium. Glomeruli undergo thrombotic occlusion; fibrinoid necrosis of arterial wall and such non-functional kidney are removed.

- *Acute rejection:* Occurs within days of transplantation in untreated recipient/even after months and years where immunosuppressants are employed. Acute graft rejection is a combined process in which both cell mediated and antibody mediated reactions are involved. Humoral rejection (antibody mediated) is associated with vasculitis. Cellular rejection is characterised by mononuclear infiltration, oedema, and interstitial haemorrhage in kidney. Acute graft rejection can be controlled by immunosuppressive therapy.

- *Chronic rejection* - Patient with chronic rejection have progressive rise in serum creatinine over a period of 4-6 months. Vascular changes consist of dense intimal fibrosis, resulting in renal ischemia, interstitial mononuclear cell infiltration.

Direct T-cell mediated rejection: T-cells of recipient recognise allogeneic (donor) MHC molecule on the surface of antigen presenting cells, in the graft, e.g. Dendric cells. CD8+ T-cell recognise class I HLA antigen and mature to cytotoxic T-cells (CTLs). CD4+ cells mature to T1 I effect or cells by class II antigen.

- Increase permeability
- Mononuclear accumulation
- Activate macrophage
- Graft injury

Indirect Pathway of T-cell mediated reaction: Peptide derived from donor tissue is presented by hostsown antigen presenting cells. According to genetic relationship transplantation tissue are classified into-

- *Autograft:* donor and recipient same individual.
- *Isograft:* same genotype.
- *Allograft:* same species but different genotype. Normal tissue that is transferred between genetically different individual of same species.
- *Xenograft:* different species.

Allogeneic transplantation result in immune reaction which is cell mediated (type IV), antibody mediated (type II, III).

Method of increasing graft survival: Because HLA antigens are major target in transplant rejection, minimising HLA disparity between donor and recipient would influence graft survival. In inter familial kidney transplant marked beneficial effect of matching class I antigen have been observed.

Additional matching of Class II antigen result in beneficial improvement in graft survival (CD4+ helper T-cells are not triggered if class II antigens are matched).Except in identical twins complete matching of cell histocompatibility antigens are not possible. Drugs like azathioprine, Steroids, Cyclosporine, anti-lymphocyte globulin, mono nuclear anti T-cell antibodies are employed. Immunosuppressive therapy may cause opportunistic fungal, viral and other infections. There is increased chance of developing lymphomas.

Hypersensitivity [Allergy, Autoimmunity, Alloimmunity]

Hypersensitivity, clinical significance and pathogenesis of hypersensitivity. Types I, II, III and IV. Biological significance Examples of clinically significant Hyper Sensitivity reactions are Allergy due to food, chemicals and drugs. Immunopathology is the study of derangement in immune system.

Hypersensitivity reactions [immunologic tissue injury]: Hypersensitivity is the altered immunological reaction to antigen that results in pathologic immune response after re-exposure. Hypersensitivity is defined as a state of exaggerated immune response to antigen. Hypersensitivity includes allergy, autoimmunity and alloimmunity. This classification is based on source of antigen against which the hypersensitivity response is directed.

- *Allergy:* It is the deleterious effect of hypersensitivity to environmental antigens (Allergen).

- *Autoimmunity:* it is the disturbance in immunological tolerance to self-antigen. In autoimmune disease, immune system reacts against self-antigen and destroys the host tissue. Antibodies against self-antigen are termed as autoantibodies.

- *Alloimmune reaction:* It occurs when immune system of one individual produces immunologic reaction against tissue of another individual. Alloimmunity can be observed during immunological reaction against transfusions, grafted tissue and foetus during pregnancy.

Mechanism of hypersensitivity reaction: Hypersensitivity reactions are divided into four distinct types:

- Type-I (Anaphylactic/Ig-E mediated)
- Type-II (Cytotoxic/Tissue specific reaction)
- Type-III (Immune complex mediated reaction)
- Type-IV (Cell mediated reaction)

Hypersensitivity reactions are immediate /delayed depending on time required for reaction to appear. Immediate hyper sensitivity reactions -in which immune reaction occur immediately (within seconds/minutes).Immediate type of hypersensitivity involves type-I, type-II and type-III. Immune response in these types is mediated by antibodies.

Delayed Hypersensitivity reaction -in which reaction slower in onset (develop within 24 to 48 hours) and effect is prolonged, e.g. Type-4.It is mainly mediated by cellular response.

Type I (Anaphylactic or atopic reaction): Anaphylaxis is a state of rapidly developing immune response to an antigen to which the individual is previously sensitised. Type I reaction/anaphylaxis is mediated by Ig-E antibodies. Most common allergic reactions are type I reactions. Type I reactions are characterised by production of antigen specific immunoglobulin-E (Ig-E) after exposure to antigen.

Most type I reactions are against environmental antigens (allergens). Most allergens are proteins that enter the host from environment. Allergens are environmental antigens that cause atypically exorbitant immunological response in genetically predisposed individual.

Typical allergens include:

- Pollen- Rag weed, timothy, mould and fungi: Penicillium notatum– Food-milk, egg, peanut, fish
- Animals-cat dander, dog dander – Cigarette smoke
- Component of house dust-faecal pellets of house mite
- Often allergens are contained in large particle or covered by non-allergic coat. Actual allergens are released after enzymatic break down.

Most allergens are either can react with protein or small molecular weight proteins. Role of Ig-E -exposure to an allergen causes Ig-E production by selected B cells. Ig-E binds to the crystalline fragment receptor (Fc receptor) on plasma membrane of mast cell. Now the individual is sensitised.

With further exposure to antigen (allergen), allergen's antigenic determinants bind to two molecules of mast cell bound Ig-E, initiating degranulation of mast cells and release of mast cell products-called anaphylactic mediators.[Sometimes Ig-E mediated response is beneficial, as in Ig-E mediated destruction of parasite].

Mechanism of Ig -E mediated hypersensitivity reaction: The product of mast cell degranulation can modulate almost all aspect of acute inflammatory response. The most potent mediator is histamine. Histamine act through H1 receptor and it contract bronchial smooth muscles, causing bronchoconstriction, increases vascular permeability causing oedema. Also causes vasodilation and increase in blood flow to affected area. Histamine increases gastric secretion through H2 receptor

Clinical manifestations of type I reactions are attributed mostly to histamine. Target tissue of type I reaction contain large number of mast cells and are sensitive to effect of histamine. These tissues are found primarily in git, skin, respiratory tract etc.

Symptoms include angioedema, oedema of larynx, urticaria, bronchospasm, hypotension, dysrhythmia, gastro intestinal cramps. Genetic predisposition [Atopic individuals]: certain individuals are prone to allergies called atopic individuals (10% of the total population).

Atopy means genetically determined allergy to inhaled or ingested allergens, e.g. Hay fever, bronchial asthma, food allergy, urticaria. Atopic individuals have high concentration of Ig-E and Fc receptor in their mast cell. Air way and skin of atopic individuals are more sensitive than normal.

Anaphylaxis: Most severe and immediate hypersensitivity reaction is anaphylaxis. Anaphylaxis is mediated by Ig-E antibodies. On re-exposure to specific antigen, Ig-E antibodies sensitise mast cells to release pharmacologically active mediators, called anaphylactic mediators.

These mediators are -Histamine, Serotonin, Chemotactic factor of Eosinophils, Neutrophils, Leukotrienes C4 and D4, Prostaglandin D2, Platelet activating factor, Cytokines, (TNFα, IL-1, IL-3etc.)

The effects of these agents are:

- increased vascular permeability
- smooth muscle contraction
- early vasoconstriction followed by vasodilation
- shock
- increased gastric secretion
- increased nasal, lachrymal secretion etc.,

Clinical manifestations of anaphylaxis include two types:

- *Systemic anaphylaxis:* Characterised by itching, erythema, contraction of respiratory bronchioles, pulmonary oedema, respiratory distress, shock and death, e.g.: administration of anti-sera (ATS), administration of drugs like penicillin, sting by wasp, bees etc.,

- *Localised anaphylaxis:* Characterised by urticaria, angioedema, allergic rhinitis, asthma etc.

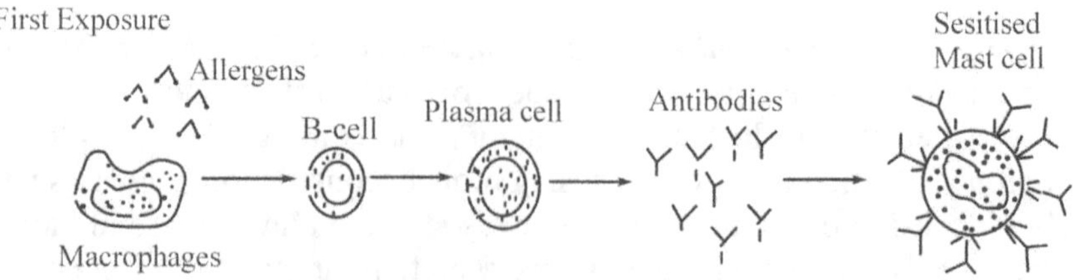

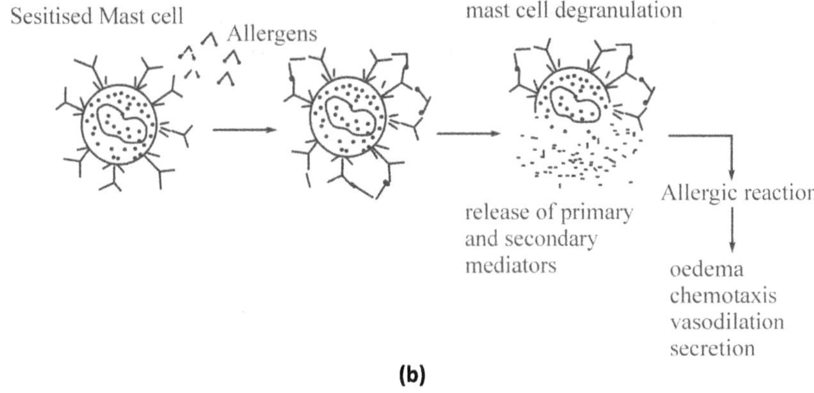

(b)

Fig. 4.8 (a) Second exposure (b) Diagram: Type I hypersensitivity reaction.

Test for Ig-E mediated hypersensitivity: allergic reaction can be life threatening, so allergic individuals must be made aware of specific allergen against which they are sensitised. Skin test with allergen -on injecting allergen intra-dermally or epicutaneously [prick test] of sensitized individual, local anaphylactic reaction occurs within few minutes. It consists of wheal and flare reaction. Radio-immunosorbant testing -measure the circulating level of total Ig-E. Radio allergosorbant testing -measure the circulating level of specific Ig-E antibodies.

Desensitisation: Minute quantities of allergens are injected over a prolonged period. This procedure reduces the severity of the allergic reaction in treated individuals. Desensitisation works by stimulating the production of blocking antibodies.

Type II Hypersensitivity Reaction [Tissue Specific Reaction]

Type II hypersensitivity reaction is generally characterised by destruction or altered function of target cell, through action of antibody against antigen present on the cell membrane of target cell. Most tissue have antigen expressed on their plasma membrane called tissue specific antigen. Type II reactions are limited to those tissue/organs that express the particular antigen. Environmental antigen [e.g. drugs, their metabolites etc.] may bind to plasma membrane of cells and function as target of type II reaction.

Certain drugs like penicillins, rifampicin etc., bind on surface of RBC and stimulate production of antibodies (haptens).Type II or tissue specific hypersensitivity reaction can alter cell/destroy it by four mechanisms. All begin with binding of antibody with tissue specific antigen.

(a) *Complement mediated lysis of cell:* Antibody (Ig-M, Ig-G); react with antigen present on surface of cell causing activation of complement system, which causes direct lysis of the cell.

(b) *Phagocytosis by macrophages:* antibodies make cell susceptible to phagocytosis by opsonisation. Macrophages recognise and bind to antibody on opsonised cells (subject of phagocytosis). It mainly affects blood cells. Examples., transfusion reaction, erythroblastosis foetalis, autoimmune haemolytic anaemia.

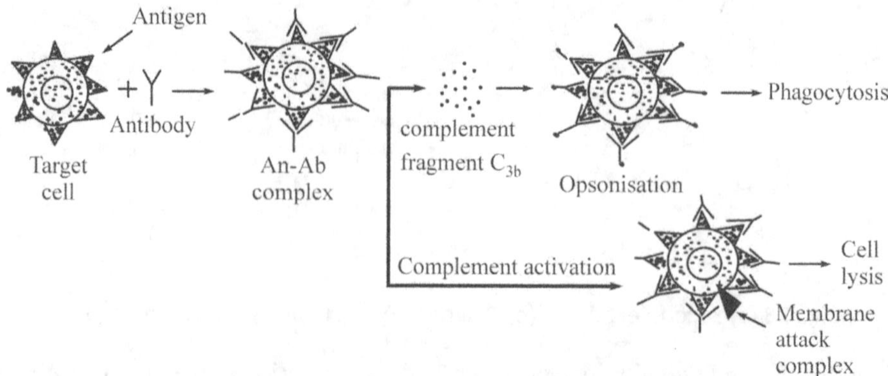

Fig. 4.9 Type-II Complement dependend reaction.

(c) *Antibody dependent cell mediated cytotoxicity:* leukocytes having Fc receptor bind with Fc fragmenton antibody (like Ig-G, Ig-M) and bring about lysis of the cell, e.g. Destruction of cell by cytotoxic Tcells [Tc cells]. Antibody on target cell gets bound to Fc receptor on Tc cells, which release toxic substance that destroy the cell. Other leukocytes like monocytes, neutrophils, eosinophils, NK cells etc., have Fc receptor, e.g. Destruction of parasites, tumour cells.

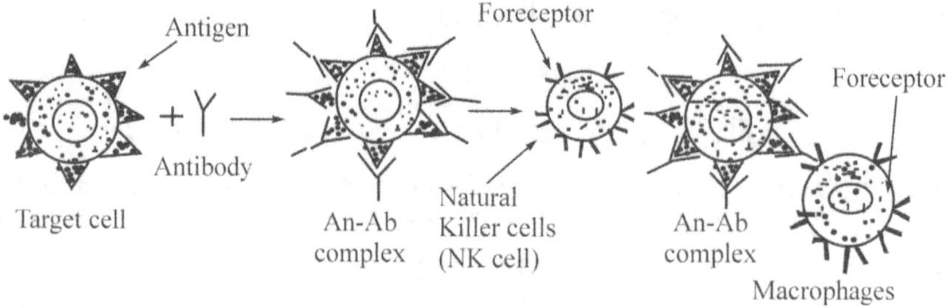

Fig. 4.10 Type II – Antibody dependent cell mediated cytotoxicity.

(d) *Modulation/blockade of receptor on target cell [Antibody dependent cellular dysfunction]:* In this case antibody do not destroy target cell but cause it to malfunction. Examples: Graves' disease - Thyroid autoantibodies stimulate TSH receptor and cause hyper function of thyroid gland [Hyperthyroidism]

Myasthenia Gravis: In myasthenia gravis auto-antibodies against acetyl choline receptor block neuromuscular transmission and cause muscle weakness

Anti-sperm antibody: Cause male sterility

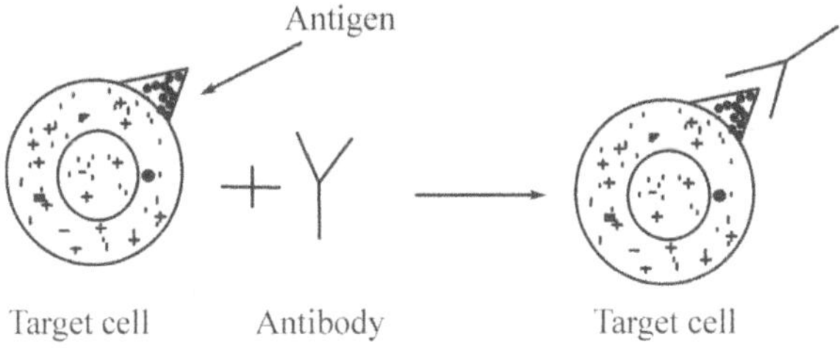

Fig. 4.11 Type III Immune complex mediated reaction.

Most of the type III hypersensitivity reactions are caused by antigen-antibody complexes (immune complexes) formed in circulation and later deposited in vessel wall or extra vascular tissue. Type III reactions are therefore not organ specific. Immune complexes have the capacity to activate a variety of serum mediators, principally complement system. Immune complex mediate diseases may be-

- Generalised (systemic), if immune complex formed in circulation and deposited in many organs, e.g. Serum sickness, Glomerulonephritis, Systemic lupus erythematosus (SLE)

- Localised (Arthus reaction) if immune complex are deposited in particular organ, e.g. Glomerulonephritis (kidney), Arthritis (joints), Local arthus reaction of skin

Regardless of whether immune complexes are formed in tissue or circulation their harmful effect is caused by complement activation; particularly generation of complement fragments that are chemotactic for neutrophils. Pathogenesis of immune complex disease can be classified into three phases-

- Phase I [Formation of antigen antibody complex in circulation]: When antigen is introduced into the circulation, it initiates the formation of antibodies (Ig-G, Ig-M), which react with antigen to from circulating antigen-antibody complexes.

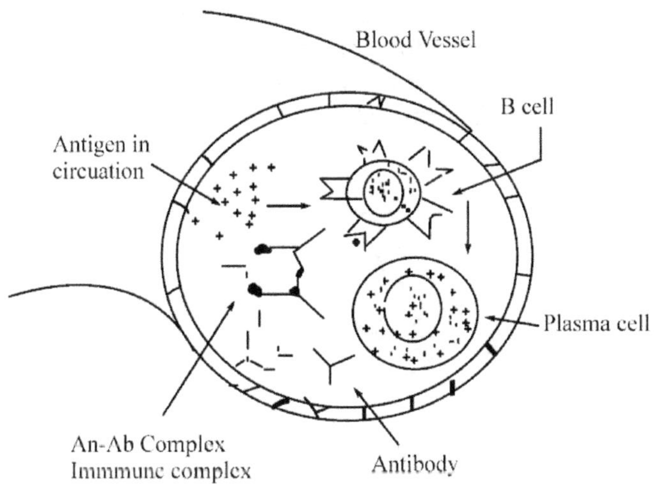

Fig. 4.12 Type III Phase-I immune complex formation.

- Phase II [Immune complex deposition]: Antigen-antibody complex formed in circulation are deposited invarious tissues like glomeruli, joints, skin, heart, small blood vessels etc.

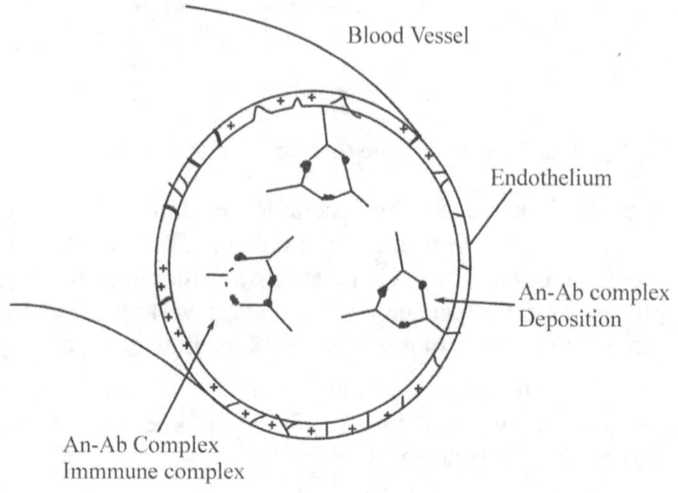

Fig. 4.13 Type-III [Phase-II immune complex deposition].

- Phase III [immune complex mediated acute inflammatory reaction]: Once complexes are deposited in tissues, they initiate acute inflammatory reaction and activation of complement system, with release of biologically active compounds like chemotactic factors, vasoactive amines, anaphylatoxins etc. Release of chemotactic factors attracts neutrophils and monocytes.

Neutrophils attempt to ingest immune complex, but often unsuccessful because immune complex are bound to tissue. During this process neutrophils release large quantity of lysosomal enzymes resulting in tissue damage (Fibrinoid necrosis). Immune complex also causes platelet aggregation and activation of Hageman factor which augment inflammatory process and microthrombi formation. The lesion may occur in blood vessels (vasculitis), renal glomeruli (glomerulonephritis), joints (arthritis) etc.

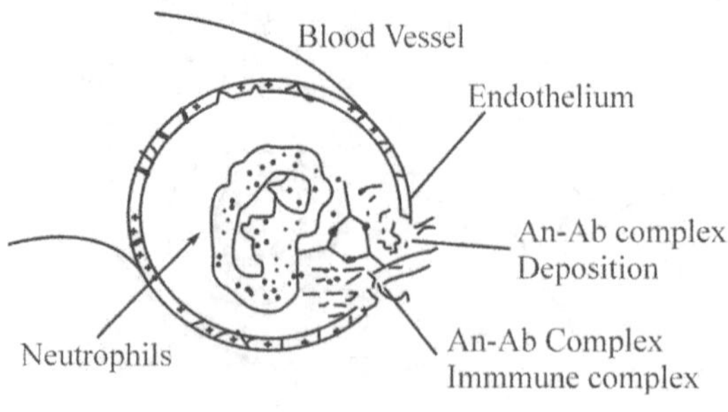

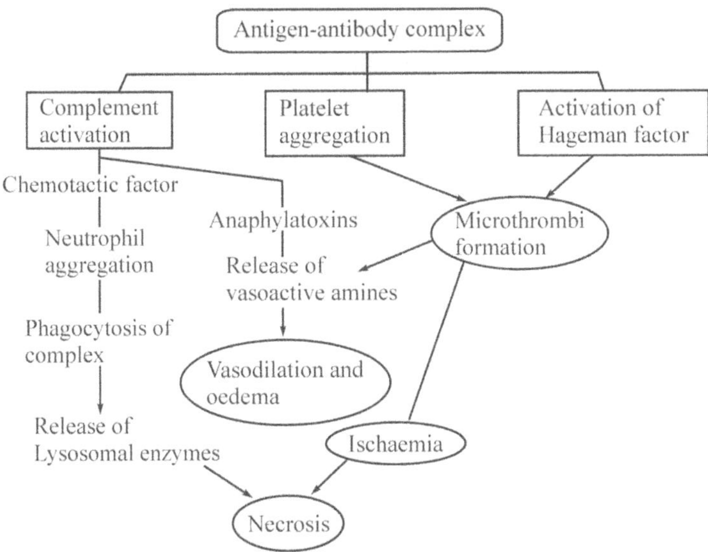

Fig. 4.14 (a) Type-III, Phase-III immune complex mediated acute inflammatory reaction. (b) Table: Effects of Aul-ab complex.

Antigen: Two types of antigens cause immune complex mediated reaction/injury

- *Exogenous antigens:* bacteria, virus, parasites, fungi etc.,
- *Endogenous antigens:* nuclear antigens, immunoglobulins, tumour antigens etc.

Type IV [Cell Mediated Tissue Reaction]

Type I, II, II l, hypersensitivity reactions are mediated by antibody. Type IV reaction are mediated by specifically sensitised T lymphocytes and do not involve antibody. Two types of lymphocytes are involved-

Cytotoxic T- lymphocytes (Tc cells) or CD8+ cells - Tissue destruction caused by direct killing of cells bytoxins from Tc cells (Toxic oxygen products), e.g. killing of virus infected cells, tumour cells, incompatible transplanted tissue etc.

Helper T cells or (CD4+ cells) - They produce lymphokines (IFN, IL-2, TNF- α etc.) that can recruit and activate phagocytic cells especially macro phages at inflammatory site. Classical delayed hypersensitivity reactions are mediated by these cells, e.g. tuberculin reaction.

Clinical examples for type IV reaction are graft rejection, tumour rejection, tuberculin reaction, allergic reaction due to contact with poison ivy, metals etc., (contact dermatitis).Type IV component also may be present in rheumatoid arthritis (self-antigen-type II collagen), autoimmune thyroiditis (self-antigen- protein on thyroid cell), (Hashimoto's disease), Insulin dependent diabetes mellitus (self-antigen - protein on β-cells of pancreas).

Diagnostic skin test for tuberculosis (tuberculin reaction) it is a best example for delayed hypersensitivity reaction (type IV hypersensitivity reaction in skin).The reaction produced in sensitised individuals on intra-dermal injection of the antigen (tuberculin) a component of mycobacteria.

It is called delayed hypersensitivity skin test because of its slow onset (it takes 24-72 hours to reach maximum intensity). In previously sensitised individuals, induration (hard white central area) and erythema (red dish surrounding area) occur within 24- 72 hours. The reaction site is infiltrated with T-lymphocyte and macrophages.

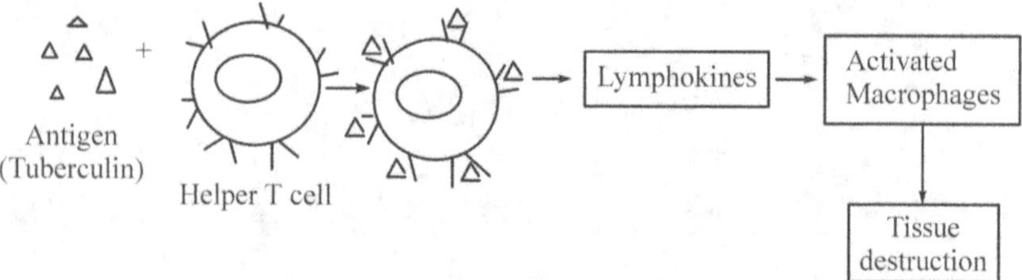

Fig. 4.15 Type -IV Tuberculin reaction.

Allergic contact dermatitis -allergic type IV reactions are elicited by some environmental antigens like industrial chemicals, cosmetics, food, metals, some topical medicines, poison ivy plant etc. Antigen with molecular weight less than 1000 Daltons usually do not induce an immune response directly but do so after binding with carrier protein in the host, such substances are called haptens. In allergic contact dermatitis, the carrier protein is in the skin of host. Example: Delayed reaction caused by contact with poison ivy -in poison ivy the antigen is plant catechol (Urushinol) that reacts with normal skin protein and evoke cell mediated immune response, characterised by lesion at site of contact.

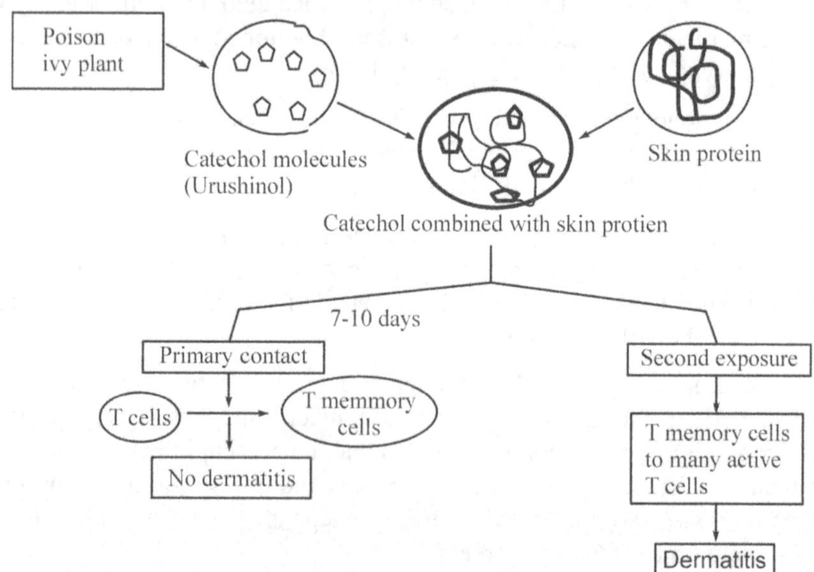

Fig. 4.16 Type-IV Delayed reaction caused by contact with poison ivy.

Skin reaction to industrial chemicals, cosmetics, detergents, clothing, food, metals, topical medicines are elicited by same mechanism.

Clinically Significant Hypersensitivity Reactions

Type I:

Systemic anaphylaxis

Local anaphylaxis - Hay fever, bronchial asthma, food allergy, angioedema.

Type II:

Autoimmune haemolytic anaemia, transfusion reaction, Erythroblastosis foetalis, Myasthenia gravis, Grave's disease, male sterility.

Type III:

Local arthus reaction -farmer's lung, injection of ATS.

Systemic reaction -glomerulonephritis, Good Pasture's syndrome, arthritis, uveitis, Systemic lupus erythematosus (SLE).

Type IV:

Tuberculin reaction, contact dermatitis, killing of virus infected cells, tumour cells, transplant rejection etc.

Auto Immunity

Auto immunity: Transplantation and immunologic tolerance, allograft rejections, transplantation antigens, mechanism of rejection of allograft.

Definition: Autoimmunity is the immune reaction against self-antigen. Autoimmunity is a state in which, body's immune system fails to distinguish between self and non-self and react by forming anti body against one's own tissue antigens (self-antigens).

Immunological tolerance: Immunological tolerance is a state in which individual is incapable of developing an immune response to a specific antigen.

Self-tolerance: Is norm al state of immunological non-responsiveness to self-antigen. Loss of tolerance to self-antigen is referred as autoimmunity. Self-tolerance is a normal phenomenon present since foetal life, and is defined as ability of individual to recognise self-tissue and antigen. So peripheral T-cell pool is lacking or deficient in self-reactive T-cells. Three important mechanisms involved in self-tolerance are-

(a) Clonal deletion

(b) Clonal anergy

(c) Peripheral suppression

Clonal Deletion

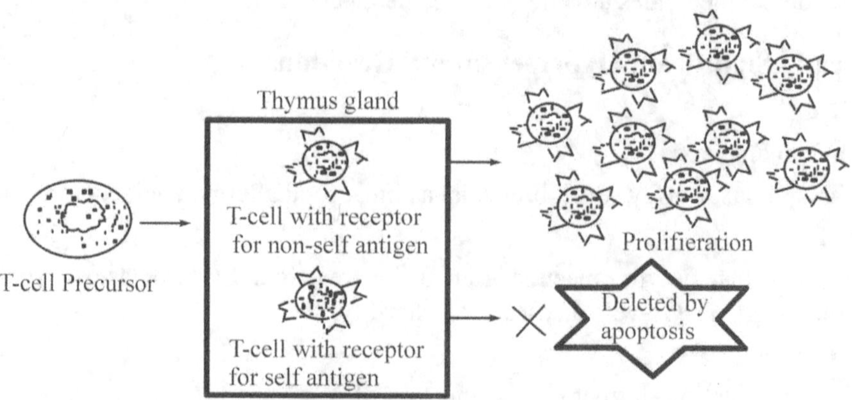

Fig. 4.17 Clonal deletion.

AIRE protein [Auto immune regulator protein]: A protein, which stimulates expression of peripheral self-antigens in thymus gland. It is critical for detection of self-reactive T cells.

Slippage: Clonal deletion is far from perfect. Many self-antigens are not expressed in thymus. T-cells bearing receptor for such antigens escape to periphery. Clonal deletion by activation induced cell death -CD4+ cells that recognise self-antigen receive signal that promote their death by apoptosis.

Fas-Fas ligand system: Fas - lymphocytes and many other cells express Fas (CD9 5), [a member of TNF receptor family]. FasL - a membrane protein (similar to TNF) expressed on activated T lymphocytes. Fas-FasL binding induces apoptosis of activated T-lymphocytes [peripheral deletion of auto reactive T-cells].

Self-antigens are abundant in peripheral tissues and cause repeated and persistent stimulation of self-antigen specific T cells, leading eventually to their elimination via apoptosis. Mutation in Fas gene cause autoimmune lymphoproliferative syndrome.

Clonal anergy: Prolonged or irreversible functional inactivation of lymphocytes, induced by encounter of antigen under certain conditions. Normally activation of helper T-cells (CD4+) requires two signals.

- First – An encounter of peptide antigen with class II MHC molecules on surface of antigen presenting cells[APC e.g. macrophages, dendric cells etc.].

- Second - A co-stimulatory signal provided by the antigen presenting cells [B7-1, B7-2].

To stimulate second signal, certain T-cell associated molecule like CD28 must bind to the ligand on APC. If antigen is presented by cell that does not bear CD 28 ligand, a negative signal is delivered and the cell becomes anergic. Clonal anergy of T-cells may occur during their development in thymus or in peripheral tissue.

Since co-stimulatory signal not expressed/weakly expressed by most of the normal cells, encounter between auto reactive T-cell with a specific antigen on the normal cell, (in the absence of co-stimulatory signal) lead to anergy. A special form of peripheral unresponsiveness occurs if a T-cell that bear self-antigen receptor encounter the antigen on cell that do not express MHC class II molecule.

- *B cell anergy:* Clonal anergy affect B-cells also, and is the major mechanism of B-cell tolerance to self-antigen. It is believed that B-cells which encounter antigen, before they are fully mature; the antigen receptor complex is endocytosed and never re-appears. Anergic cell cannot be activated by a relevant APC with co-stimulatory signal. If B-cell encounter antigen in the absence of specific helper T-cell stimulation B-cell become anergic.

- *Regulatory T-cells:* These prevent immune reaction against self antigen, e. g. CD4+ with CD25+ (mechanism not clear). They are produced in thymus and periphery. They secrete cytokines-IL-10, TGF-β, it inhibits lymphocyte activation and receptor function.

- *Foxp3 - transcription factor:* This is required for development and function of CD4+ regulatory T-cells. Mutation of Foxp3 results in severe autoimmunity in human, e.g. IpEx- immune dysregulation, poly-endocrinopathy, enteropathy, x linked.

- *Peripheral suppression by suppressor T-cells:* Suppressor T cells [CD8+ sub type] do not allow autoreactive lymphocytes [T or B] to proliferate and differentiate [activation]. Suppressor T cells inhibit auto reactivity by secreting cytokines [e.g. TGF-β], which down regulate many immune responses. IL 10, TGF β inhibit lymphocyte activation and receptor function.

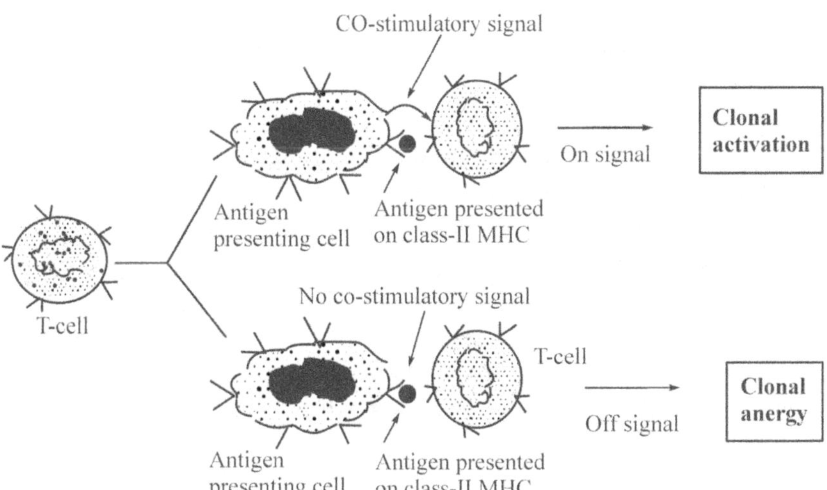

Fig. 4.18 Clonal anergy.

Mechanism of Autoimmune Diseases

(https://www.ncbi.nlm.nih.gov/pmc/articles/PMC3266166/)

HLA types are inherited, and some of them are connected with autoimmune disorders and other diseases. People with certain HLA antigens are more likely to develop certain autoimmune diseases, such as type I diabetes, ankylosing spondylitis, celiac disease, SLE (systemic lupus erythematosus), myasthenia gravis, inclusion body myositis, Sjögren syndrome, and narcolepsy. HLA typing has led to some improvement and acceleration in the diagnosis of celiac disease and type 1 diabetes; current serotyping can resolve, in one step, DQ8. HLA typing in autoimmunity is being increasingly used as a tool in diagnosis. In celiac disease, it is the only effective means of discriminating between first-degree relatives that are at risk from those that are not at risk, prior to the appearance of sometimes-irreversible symptoms such as allergies and secondary autoimmune disease.

Autoimmunity is the breakdown of immunological tolerance in which the body's immune system begins to recognise self-antigen as foreign. The mechanisms by which immune tolerance of the body broken, causing autoimmunity may be immunological, genetic or microbial factors.

Immunological Factors

- Bye pass of the helper T-cell tolerance - Complex formation of self-antigen with drugs or microorganism can stimulate production of auto antibodies, e.g. auto immune haemolytic anaemia, caused by methyldopa binding on red cell surface. Partial degradation of self-antigen can expose new antigenic determinants.

- Polyclonal (antigen non-specific) activation of B cells - Self-reactive B cells can be activated by some microorganism and their products, e.g. Bacterial lipopolysaccharide (endotoxin) − Epstein Barr virus [EBV]

- Imbalance of suppressor/helper T-cell function - Decreased suppressor T-cell increased helper T-cell activity.

- Sequestered antigen release from tissue (Hidden antigen) - Some antigens are hidden from immune system [sequestered antigen]. They do not communicate with blood or lymph.

Any self-antigen that is completely sequestered during development is likely to be viewed as foreign if introduced into circulation. If antigen of this tissue released in to blood/lymph result in immune response. Due to trauma or infection antigen from testis, brain, eyes etc., are released into blood, lead to prolonged tissue inflammation or injury. e.g. Post traumatic orchitis, uveitis, Autoantibody against lens crystals, Anti-sperm antibodies in trauma to testis.

Genetic Factors

Role of susceptibility genes - Autoimmune diseases show strong genetic predisposition. Most human autoimmune disorders have complex multi-genetic pattern of susceptibility and are not attributed to single gene mutation. Eg:. HLA gene mutation, Fas-FasL gene mutation, AIRE gene mutation [AIRE-autoimmune regulatory protein], CTLA-4 gene etc.

Many autoimmune diseases have familial incidence (origin), e.g. SLE, Auto immune thyroiditis etc. Tissue involved in auto immunity show increased expression of class II HLA antigen.

Microbial Factors

Microbial infection - virus (EBV infection), bacterial- (streptococci, klebsiella), microplasma, have been implicated in pathogenesis of autoimmune diseases. Microbes trigger autoimmune reaction in several ways:

1. Viral antigen and auto-antigen [self-antigen] become associated to form immunogenic unit

2. Some virus [EBV] causes polyclonal activation of B cells

3. Viral infection can cause loss of suppressor T-cell function

4. Cross reactivity between autologous antigen [self-antigen] and microbial antigen

5. Infection may up regulate the expression of co-stimulators on antigen presenting cells. If these cells are presenting self-antigen, the result may be break down of clonal anergy and activation of T-cells specific for self-antigen.

6. Molecular mimicry -some microbial antigens have same amino acid sequence as self-antigen. Immune response against microbial antigen result in self-reactive lymphocytes, e.g. Rheumatic heart disease; Anti body against streptococcal protein cross-react with myocardial proteins and cause myocarditis.

7. Tissue injury, that is common in infection may release self-antigen or structurally alter self-antigen so that they are able to activate T-cells.

8. Epitope spreading -important mechanism of persistence and evolution of autoimmune disease. Infection/initial autoimmune response may release and damage self-antigen and expose the epitopes of antigen that are normally concealed from immune system (Cryptic antigen)

Autoimmune Diseases

Definition: To call a disease as autoimmune disease, these pre-requisites are needed:

1. Presence of autoantibodies

2. Presence of autoimmune reaction

3. Evidence that such reaction is not due to tissue destruction caused by another disease

4. Absence of any other well-defined cause for the disease

5. Proved by experimental model (if any)

A. **Organ specific (Localised):** Auto immune response directed to a single organ/tissue.

- *Endocrine gland:* Hashimoto's thyroiditis, Graves' disease, Insulin dependent diabetes mellitus, Idiopathic Addison's disease
- *Alimentary tract:* Ulcerative colitis, Crohn's disease, Autoimmune atrophic gastritis, Autoimmune pernicious anaemia.
- *Blood:* Autoimmune haemolytic anaemia, Autoimmune thrombocytopenia
- *Others:* Myasthenia gravis, Autoimmune orchitis, Autoimmune encephalomyelitis, Good pasture's syndrome [antibody against basement membrane of lungs, kidney], Primary biliary cirrhosis, Membranous glomerulonephritis, Autoimmune hepatitis, Multiple sclerosis [auto reactive T-cells react against CNS myelin)

B. **Systemic [Non-organ specific]:** Autoimmune reaction against wide spread antigen.

- Systemic lupus erythematosus
- Rheumatoid arthritis
- Scleroderma (Progressive systemic sclerosis)
- Poly arthritis nodosa (PAN)
- Sjogren's syndrome
- Mixed connective tissue disease
- Reiter's syndrome
- Inflammatory myopathies

Systemic Lupus Erythematosus [SLE]: SLE is a classic example for systemic autoimmune disease. It is characterised by acute and chronic inflammatory lesions widely scattered in the body. There is presence of various nuclear and cytoplasmic autoantibodies in plasma. Antibodies identified against nuclear and cytoplasmic components of the cell, e.g. antibody against cell surface antigen of blood cells, anti-nuclear antibodies, antibody to DNA, antibody to histone, antibody to non-histone protein of RNA Antibody to double stranded DNA is diagnostic of SLE. It is predominantly a disease of women. It occurs in any age group.

Etiology: The exact etiology is not known. The limitless number of autoantibodies to self-constituents indicate that fundamental defect in SLE is failure of regulatory mechanism that sustain self-tolerance. No single cause has been identified but environmental, genetic and immunological influences are suspected.

- Genetic factors - Family members of SLE patients have increased risk of developing the disease. Concordance in monozygotic twins show same pattern of SLE. Some lupus patients have inherited deficiency of complement C2 and C4. Inherited deficiency of complement C2 and C4 which impair removal of immune complex by mononuclear phagocyte system and favour tissue deposition of immune complex. Defect in MHC gene.

- Environmental factors- Certain drugs like -D-penicillamine, procainamide, hydralazine etc., – viral infection, e.g. EBV infection
- Certain hormones, e.g. Oestrogen – ultra violet light
- Toxins-Inherited defect in B-cells, stimulation of B-cells by microorganism, T-helper cell hyper activity, T-suppressor cell defect
- Hormone factors -Lupus occurs primarily in women, of child bearing age. Hence role of hormones aresuspected.

Pathogenesis [SLE]: Autoantibodies -antibodies against various nuclear and cytoplasmic antigens are found, e.g. antinuclear antibodies (ANA).Immune complexes are formed by autoantibodies, e.g.- DNA-anti DNA antibody complex, Immunoglobulin-anti-immunoglobulin antibody complex.

These immune complexes get deposited in various site like small blood vessels, renal glomeruli etc. They produce lesion (injury) by type III hypersensitivity. Autoantibody against red cells, white cells, platelets etc., cause lesion by type II hypersensitivity. Lymphocyte dysfunction -defect in suppressor T cell function and prolonged polyclonal B cell activation causes increased antibody response.

Clinical features: It is a multi-system disease with variable presentation. Butter fly like erythematous rash on skin, painful joints [synovitis, arthritis], chest pain [pleuritis], renal impairment [glomerulonephritis], hematologic derangement (haemolytic anaemia, thrombocytopenia), neurological disorders [seizure, Psychosis], fever, weight loss, fatigue

Pathology: LE cells -are phagocytic leucocytes (neutrophils, macrophages etc.) that engulfed the denaturednucleus of injured cell. Antibody against double stranded DNA (smith antigen).

- *Skin:* Immune complex deposited in skin stimulate inflammatory reaction leading to liquefactive degeneration of dermis of skin.
- *Joints:* acute lupus arthritis
- *Kidney:* produce glomerular changes– Heart - fibrinoid necrosis of valves
- *Vessels:* vasculitis, inflammatory lesion in blood vessels

Other changes: Hyperplasia of lymph node, spleen, inflammatory reaction of lungs, liver etc. Cytopenia, leukopenia, haemolytic anaemia, thrombocytopenia etc.

Scleroderma [Progressive systemic sclerosis]: It is characterised by small vessel destruction and fibrosis of skin and multiple internal organs. Vascular endothelial cell damage triggers connective tissue over growth and excessive fibrosis throughout the body. Skin is most commonly affected but git, kidney, heart, muscle, lungs are frequently involved.

Clinical features: Include fibrosis of multiple organs. On Skin, sclerotic atrophy of skin is observed. Marked increase in compact collagen in dermis and thinning of epidermis. Claw like deformity of hands.

CREST syndrome involves:

- Calcinosis [abnormal deposition of calcium in tissue]
- Raynaud's phenomenon [spasm of digital arteries, sensitivity of hand and finger to cold]
- Oesophageal dismotility
- Sclerodactylyl [scleroderma of digits (Hardening and thickening of skin)]
- Telangiectasia [lesion caused by dilation of small group of blood vessels]
- Oesophageal fibrosis causing dysphagia, hypomotility
- Malabsorption syndrome
- Respiratory distress
- Malignant hypertension
- Pulmonary hypertension
- Biliary cirrhosis

Etiology and Pathogenesis: Systemic sclerosis is a disease of unknown cause. Excessive deposition of collagen is the hall mark of systemic sclerosis.

- *Immunologic hypothesis*: Fibrosis is secondary to abnormal activation of immune system. A variety autoantibodies found in scleroderma patients like antibody to smooth muscles, rheumatoid factor, ANA (anti-nuclear antibody) etc. High level of ANA [antinuclear antibodies] detected in systemic sclerosis patients. Activated T-cells release cytokines [IL-1, TNF-α, TGF-β], which enhance fibroblast growth and increase collagen synthesis.

- *Vascular hypothesis:* Endothelial cell injury is due to autoantibodies or antigen-antibody complex resulting in aggregation and activation of platelet which increase vascular permeability and fibroblast proliferation. The endothelial injury may be due to serum cytotoxic factors, cellular/ humoral autoimmunity or toxins. T-cell sensitisation to collagen and humoral hypersensitivity (antibody mediated) also postulated. A variety of autoantibodies are found in scleroderma patients like antibody to smooth muscles, rheumatoid factor, ANA (anti-nuclear antibodies) etc. Antinuclear antibodies (ANA) are specific in scleroderma patients, e.g. Antibody to centromere.

Pathology: Involves vascular fibrosis and fibrinoid necrosis.

- *Skin:* Oedema, degenerative changes in dermal collagen, later dermal sclerosis, atrophy of epidermis and skin tightness is characteristic of clinical scleroderma.

- *GIT:* Lower 2/3rdof oesophagus develops fibrosis and motility dysfunction. Fibrosis in small bowel etc, Kidney -renal arterial intimal proliferation and acute collapse of renal blood flow. Which cause renalcortical ischaemia, malignant hypertension, and acute renal failure. Lungs -Idiopathic pulmonary fibrosis, progressive dyspnoea on exertion.

- *Musculoskeletal system:* Inflammatory synovitis in joints. Skeletal muscle oedema and perivascular mononuclear inflammation.

Sjögren's syndrome: It is an idiopathic (self-generated/without known cause) autoimmune disorder which affects organs and exocrine glands [especially lachrymal and salivary glands]. Sjögren's syndrome is characterised by dry eyes [keratoconjunctivitis scicca], dry mouth (xerostomia), resulting from immunologically mediated destruction of lachrymal glands and salivary glands. It is also known as scicca syndrome. It is often associated with other autoimmune disease like, rheumatoid arthritis, SLE, polymyositis, scleroderma, vasculitis, mixed connective tissue disease or thyroiditis.

Clinical features: 90% of the patients are women between 40-60 years. Symptoms result from inflammatory destruction of exocrine glands. Keratoconjunctivitis (dry eyes) produce blurred vision, burning, itching, thick secretion accumulates in conjunctival sac. Xerostomia (dry mouth) result in difficulty in swallowing, cracks and fissures in mouth, dryness of buccal mucosa. Enlarged and inflamed lachrimal gland, parotid gland. Bronchitis, Pneumonitis in lungs is observed. Concurrent autoimmune disease like rheumatoid arthritis. High risk of developing lymphoid malignancies.

Etiology and pathogenesis: Sjögren's syndrome involve both type II (antibody mediated) and type IV (cell mediated), hypersensitivity reactions. The lesion in salivary and lacrimal gland is mediated by T-lymphocyte, B-cells and plasma cells. There is lymphocytic infiltration and fibrosis of lacrimal and salivary glands. Auto antibodies like antinuclear antibodies (ANA) found in 90% of the cases. Antibody to salivary duct cells, rheumatoid factor also identified.

Pathology: Dense, periductual lymphocytic infiltrate composed of large and small lymphocytes and plasma cells. Duct destruction is seen. Later atrophy, fibrosis and fatty replacement may occur.

Inflammatory myopathies: Inflammation and injury to skeletal muscle mediated immunologically, e.g.-Dermatomyositis, Polymyositis, Inclusion body myositis.

- *Dermatomyositis:* Inflammatory disease of skin as well as skeletal muscle. Distinct skin rash that accompany or precedes muscle disease. Discolouration of eyelids, periorbital oedema, dusky red patches on finger joints, elbow, and knees. Muscle weakness, myalgia, dysphagia (difficulty to swallow).Interstitial lung disease, vasculitis, myocarditis etc. Development of visceral cancer.

- *Polymyositis:* Polymyositis is an idiopathic disease characterised by prominent muscle weakness andchronic inflammatory myopathy. It differs from dermatomyositis by lack of cutancous involvement.

Pathogenesis: Lymphocyte mediated muscle cell damage is thought to be the underlying mechanism. Auto antibodies to extractable nuclear antigens PM1, JO-1 are most specific for these diseases. Dermatomyositis -capillaries are principal target in dermatomyositis. Microvasculature attacked by antibodies and complements. B cells and CD4+ T cells mediate muscle destruction. Polymyositis is caused by CD8+ T cells and macrophages. They mediate damage of muscle cells.ANA and increased expression of class I and class II HLA antigen also seen.

Clinicopathologic features: Symmetrical proximal upper and lower extremity muscle weakness is characteristic. E.g.., Erythematous scaling rash on skin and Grave's disease [Primary hyperthyroidism], [Diffuse toxic goitre] It is associated with production of autoantibodies to TSH receptor. These antibodies bind to TSH receptor and stimulate thyroid growth and hyper secretion.

Pathogenesis: Over activity of thyroid caused by excessive stimulation of gland by thyroid stimulating immunoglobulins.[Cross reactivity with infectious antigen similar to TSH, recognition of neoantigen, alteration in anti-idiopathic antibody network]

Pathology: Symmetrical enlargement of thyroid gland to two/four times its normal size. Severe hyperplasia of follicular epithelium. Follicles are small and contain little colloid. Other diseases: Mixed connective tissue disease, Bullons disease of skin.

Rheumatoid arthritis: Chronic inflammatory disease that affect primarily the joints. It is an autoimmune disease. Activation of helper T-cells and other lymphocytes, release inflammatory mediators that cause destruction of joints. Cytokines play important role [TNF, IL-1]. T-cells stimulate other cells [macrophages, endothelial cells to produce cytokines. Metalloproteinases [collagenase, stromelysin, elastase, etc.] contributes to cartilage destruction. Pannusinflammatory exudates in joints.

Auto Immuno Defficiency Syndrome

HIV Infection

The best example of the importance of CD4+ T cells is demonstrated with human immunodeficiency virus (HIV) infection. HIV targets cells that express CD4, and can infect macrophages, dendritic cells (both groups express CD4 at low levels) and CD4+ T cells.

It has been proposed that during the non-symptomatic phase of HIV infection, the virus has a relatively low affinity towards T cells (and has a higher affinity for macrophages), resulting in a slow kill rate of CD4+ T cells by the immune system. This is initially compensated for via the production of new helper T cells from the thymus (originally from the bone marrow). Once the virus becomes lymphotropic (or T-tropic) however, it begins to infect CD4+ T cells far more efficiently (likely due to a change in the co-receptors it binds to during infection), and the immune system is overwhelmed.

At this point, functional CD4+ T cell levels begin to decrease, eventually to a point where the CD4+ T cell population is too small to recognize the full range of antigens that could potentially be detected. The lack of full antigen cover results in the core symptoms of acquired immune deficiency syndrome (AIDS). CD4 T cell depletion during AIDS allows various pathogens to escape T cell recognition, thus allowing opportunistic infections that would normally elicit a helper T cell response to bypass the immune system. While these complete bypass situations only occur when the helper T cell response is necessary for infection clearance, most infections increase in severity and/or duration because the immune system's helper T cells provide a weaker contribution to a less efficient immune response.

Two components of the immune system are particularly affected in AIDS, due to its CD4+ T cell dependency:

1. CD8+ T cells are not stimulated as effectively during the AIDS stage of HIV infection, making AIDS patients very susceptible to most viruses, including HIV itself. This decline in killing of CD4+ T cells results in the virus being produced for a longer period (the infected CD4+ T cells are not killed as quickly), increasing the proliferation of the virus, and accelerating the development of the disease.

2. Antibody class switching declines significantly once helper T cell function fails. The immune system loses its ability to improve the affinity of their antibodies, and is unable to generate B cells that can produce antibody groups such as IgG and IgA. These effects are primarily due to the loss of any helper T cell that can interact with the B lymphocyte correctly. Another symptom of AIDS is the reduction in antibody levels due to a decrease in Th2 cytokines (and less interactions by helper T cells). All of these complications result in an increased susceptibility to aggressive bacterial infections, especially in areas of the body not accessible by IgM antibodies.

If the patient does not respond to (or does not receive) HIV treatment they will succumb usually to either cancers or infections; the immune system finally reaches a point where it is no longer coordinated or stimulated enough to deal with the disease.

Inhibition of CD4 T-cell expansion during HIV infection is also due to microbial translocation in an IL-10-dependent way. Indeed, triggering PD-1, expressed on monocytes and up-regulated upon monocytes activation, by its ligand PD-L1 induces IL-10 production which inhibits CD4 T-cell function.

T helper cells (Th cells) are a type of T cell that play an important role in the immune system, particularly in the adaptive immune system. They help the activity of other immune cells by releasing T cell cytokines. These cells help suppress or regulate immune responses. They are essential in B cell antibody class switching, in the activation and growth of cytotoxic T cells and in maximizing bactericidal activity of phagocytes such as macrophages.

Mature Th cells express the surface protein CD4 and are referred to as CD4+T cells. CD4+ T cells are generally treated as having a pre-defined role as helper T cells within the immune system. For example, when an antigen-presenting cell expresses an antigen on MHC class II, a CD4+ cell will aid those cells through a combination of cell to cell interactions and through cytokines. Nevertheless, there are rare exceptions; for example, sub-groups of regulatory T cells, natural killer cells, and cytotoxic Tcells express CD4. All the latter CD4+ T cell groups are not considered T helper cells.

T helper 17 cells (Th17) are a subset of T helper cells producing interleukin 17 (IL-17). They are developmentally distinct from Th1 and Th2 cells. They create inflammation and tissue injury in autoimmune disease such as multiple sclerosis (which was previously thought to be caused by Th1 cells), psoriasis, autoimmune uveitis, juvenile diabetes, rheumatoid arthritis, and Crohn's disease. Th17 has also been suspected to play a role in allergen-induced airway responses.

Their normal role is to provide anti-microbial immunity at epithelial / mucosal barriers. They produce cytokines (such as interleukin 22) which stimulates epithelial cells to produce anti-microbial proteins to clear out certain types of microbe (such as Candida and Staphylococcus). Thus, a lack of Th17 cells leaves the host susceptible to opportunistic infections.

The original function of Th17 cells is to protect the body against bacteria and fungi. Though Th17 cells are implicated in anti-fungal immunity, it is thought to be limited to particular sites with detrimental effects observed.Th17 cells produce two main members of the IL-17 family, IL-17A and IL-17F, which cause recruitment, activation and migration of neutrophils. They also secrete IL-21 and IL-22. Th17 cells mediate the regression of tumors in mice. Th17 may contribute to the development of late phase asthmatic response due to its increases in gene expression relative to Treg cells.

The importance of helper T cells can be seen from HIV, a virus that infects CD4+ cells. Towards the end of an HIV infection the number of functional CD4+ T cells falls, which leads to the symptomatic stage of infection known as the acquired immunodeficiency syndrome (AIDS). There are also some rare disorders that result in the absence or dysfunction of CD4+ T cells. These disorders produce similar symptoms, and many of these are fatal.

The pathophysiology of AIDS is complex. Ultimately, HIV causes AIDS by depleting CD4+ T helper lymphocytes. This weakens the immune system and allows opportunistic infections. T lymphocytes are essential to the immune response and without them; the body cannot fight infections or kill cancerous cells. The mechanism of CD4+T cell depletion differs in the acute and chronic phases.

After the virus enters the body there is a period of rapid viral replication, leading to an abundance of virus in the peripheral blood. During primary infection, the level of HIV may reach several million virus particles per milliliter of blood.

This response is accompanied by a marked drop in the numbers of circulating CD4+ T cells. This acute viremia is associated in virtually all people with the activation of CD8+ T cells, which kill HIV-infected cells, and subsequently with antibody production, or seroconversion. The CD8+ T cell response is thought to be important in controlling virus levels, which peak and then decline, as the CD4+ T cell counts rebound. A good CD8+ T cell response has been linked to slower disease progression and a better prognosis, though it does not eliminate the virus.

Although the symptoms of immune deficiency characteristic of AIDS do not appear for years after a person is infected, the bulk of CD4+ T cell loss occurs during the first weeks of infection, especially in the intestinal mucosa, which harbors the majority of the lymphocytes found in the body. The reason for the preferential loss of mucosal CD4+ T cells is that a majority of mucosal CD4+ T cells express the CCR5 co-receptor, whereas a small fraction of CD4+ T cells in the bloodstream do so.

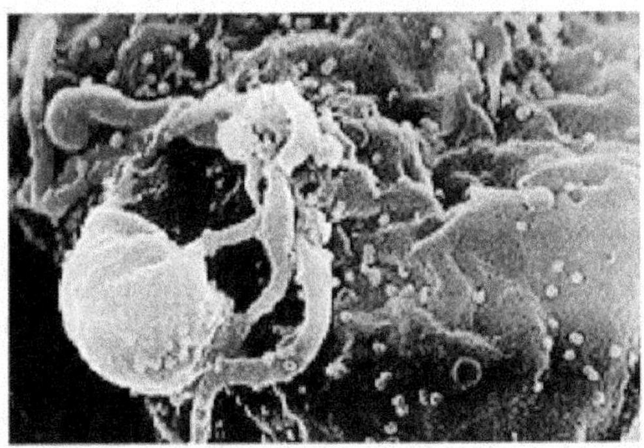

Fig. 4.19 Scanning electron micrograph of HIV-1, colored green,
budding from a cultured lymphocyte.
(Source: https://en.wikipedia.org/wiki/HIV)

HIV attaches to and penetrates host T cells via CD4+ molecules and chemokine receptors. After attachment, HIV RNA and several HIV-encoded enzymes are released into the host cell. Viral replication requires that reverse transcriptase (an RNA-dependent DNA polymerase) copy HIV RNA, producing proviral DNA; this copying mechanism is prone to errors, resulting in frequent mutations. These mutations facilitate the generation of HIV that can resist control by the host's immune system and by antiretroviral drugs. Proviral DNA enters the host cell's nucleus and is integrated into the host DNA in a process that involves integrase, another HIV enzyme. With each cell division, the integrated proviral DNA is duplicated along with the host DNA. Subsequently, the proviral HIV DNA can be transcribed to HIV RNA and translated to HIV proteins, such as the envelope glycoproteins 41 and 120. These HIV proteins are assembled into HIV virions at the host cell inner membrane and budded from the cell surface within an envelope of modified human cell membrane. Each host cell may produce thousands of virions. After budding, protease, another HIV enzyme, cleaves viral proteins, converting the immature virion into a mature, infectious virion.

Virions have a plasma half-life of about 6h. The high volume of HIV replication and high frequency of transcription errors by HIV reverse transcriptase result in many mutations, increasing the chance of producing strains resistant to host immunity and drugs.

During the acute phase, HIV-induced cell lysis and killing of infected cells by cytotoxic T cells accounts for CD4+ T cell depletion, although apoptosis may also be a factor. During the chronic phase, the consequences of generalized immune activation coupled with the gradual loss of the ability of the immune system to generate new T cells appear to account for the slow decline in CD4+ T cell numbers.

A vigorous immune response eventually controls the infection and initiates the clinically latent phase. However, CD4+ T cells in mucosal tissues remain depleted throughout the infection, although enough remain to initially ward off life-threatening infections.

Continuous HIV replication results in a state of generalized immune activation persisting throughout the chronic phase. Immune activation, which is reflected by the increased activation state of immune cells and release of proinflammatory cytokines, results from the activity of several HIV gene products and the immune response to ongoing HIV replication. Another cause is the breakdown of the immune surveillance system of the mucosal barrier caused by the depletion of mucosal CD4+ T cells during the acute phase of disease. This results in the systemic exposure of the immune system to microbial components of the gut's normal flora, which in a healthy person is kept in check by the mucosal immune system. The activation and proliferation of T cells that results from immune activation provides fresh targets for HIV infection.

A major cause of CD4+ T cell loss appears to result from their heightened susceptibility to apoptosis when the immune system remains activated. Although new T cells are continuously produced by the thymus to replace the ones lost, the regenerative capacity of the thymus is slowly destroyed by direct infection of its thymocytes by HIV. Eventually, the minimal number of CD4+ T cells necessary to maintain a sufficient immune response is lost, leading to AIDS.

The virus, entering through which ever route, acts primarily on the following cells:

- Lymphoreticular system
  - CD4+ T-Helper cells
  - Macrophages
  - Monocytes
  - B-lymphocytes
  - Certain endothelial cells
- Central nervous system:
  - Microglia of the nervous system

- Astrocytes
- Oligodendrocytes
- Neurones – indirectly by the action of cytokines and the gp-120

The virus has cytopathic effects but how it does it is still not quite clear. It can remain inactive in these cells for long periods, though. This effect is hypothesized to be due to the CD4-gp120 interaction.

- The most prominent effect of HIV is its T-helper cell suppression and lysis. The cell is simply killed off or deranged to the point of being function-leapses leading to the familiar AIDS complications, like infections and neoplasms (vide supra).

- Infection of the cells of the CNS causes acute aseptic meningitis, subacute encephalitis, vacuolar myelopathy and peripheral neuropathy. Later it leads to even AIDS dementia complex.

- The CD4-gp120 interaction (see above) is also permissive to other viruseslike Cytomegalovirus, Hepatitis virus, Herpes simplex virus, etc. These viruses lead to further cell damage i.e. cytopathy.

Acquired immune deficiency syndrome (AIDS) is caused by the HIV or human immunodeficiency virus. The infection causes progressive destruction of the cell-mediated immune (CMI) system, primarily by eliminating CD4+ T-helper lymphocytes.

Pathology of AIDS: HIV infection passes through a series of steps or stages before it turns into AIDS. These stages of infection as outlined in 1993 by the Centers for Disease Control and prevention are:

1. Seroconversion illness – this occurs in 1 to 6 weeks after acquiring the infection. The feeling is like a bout of flu.

2. Asymptomatic infection – After seroconversion, virus levels are low and replication continues slowly. CD4 and CD8 lymphocyte levels are normal. This stage has no symptoms and may persist for years together.

3. Persistent generalised lymphadenopathy (PGL) – The lymph nodes in these patients are swollen for three months or longer and not due to any other cause.

4. Symptomatic infection – This stage manifests with symptoms. In addition, there may be opportunistic infections. This collection of symptoms and signs is referred to as the AIDS-related complex (ARC) and is regarded as a prodrome or precursor to AIDS.

5. AIDS – this stage is characterized by severe immunodeficiency. There are signs of life-threatening infections and unusual tumours. This stage is characterized by CD4 T-cell count below 200 cells/mm^3.

6. There is a small group of patients who develop AIDS very slowly, or never at all. These patients are called non-progressors.

Geographical pathology of HIV/AIDS: Genetics and geographical location has a role in the pattern of opportunistic infections. A second determinant is the speed of decline in the immune system. Many of the opportunistic infections are of low virulence and are only encountered if patients survive with low CMI.

Genetics and earlier site of stay also plays a role. For example, African HIV-infected patients reside in the UK have high rates of tuberculosis and this is usually a reactivation of latent infection acquired in the country of origin.

Decreased immunity leads to opportunistic infections and certain cancers. Opportunistic infections are caused by organisms that do not cause infections in healthy individuals. HIV also directly damages certain organs like the brain. Some opportunistic infections include:

Viral infections:

- Cytomegalovirus (CMV)
- Herpes simplex
- Molluscum contagiosum
- Herpes zoster
- Measles
- Human papilloma virus (HPV)
- Human herpes virus 8 (HV8)
- Epstein-Barr virus (EBV)

Bacterial infections:

- Recurrent bacterial pneumonia (commonly *Streptococcus pneumoniae*)
- *Mycobacterium tuberculosis*
- Non-tuberculosis mycobacteriosis (particularly *M. avium*-intracellulare complex)
- Systemic non-typhoid Salmonella infections (notably *S. enteritidis and S. typhimurium*)
- Pseudomonas spp. *septicaemia* and *vasculitis*
- Bartonella spp. (causing bacillary angiomatosis)
- Rhodococcus equi
- Nocardia spp.

Fungal infections:

- Candida severe infection
- Pneumocystis jiroveci pneumonia
- Cryptococcus neoformans
- Histoplasma capsulatum
- Coccidioides immitis
- Aspergillus spp.
- Penicillium marneffei

- Protozoal infections
- Toxoplasma gondii
- Cryptosporidium parvum
- Isospora belli
- Leishmania spp.
- Microsporidia spp. (commonly Encephalitozoon intestinalis, Enterocytozoon bieneusi)
- Acanthamoeba spp.
- Trypanosoma cruzi

Tumours:

- Kaposi's sarcoma
- Primary cerebral lymphoma
- High-grade non-Hodgkin lymphoma
- Carcinoma (invasive) of the cervix
- Carcinoma of the conjunctiva
- Carcinoma of the anus
- T-cell lymphoma
- Hodgkin's disease
- Lymphoproliferative disease, pre-lymphomatous

Other conditions:

- HIV-wasting syndrome (fever, weight loss, diarrhoea)
- HIV-associated dementia or memory loss
- Various dermatitis patterns (e.g. pruritic rash, eosinophilic folliculitis)
- Skeletal myopathy
- Peripheral and autonomic neuropathy
- Cardiomyopathy
- Pulmonary hypertension
- Vasculitis
- HIV-associated nephropathy (HIVAN)
- Haemolytic uraemic syndrome (HUS) and thrombotic thrombocytopaenic purpura (TTP)
- Oral and oesophageal ulcers
- Dyshaemopoiesis and marrow serous atrophy

Worldwide infections:

- Candidiasis

- Pneumocystosis in infants
- Cryptococcosis
- Progressive multifocal leukoencephalopathy (PML)
- CMV infection in children
- Bacteraemia

Diseases those are geographically restricted:

- Leishmaniasis or Kalazar (Mediterranean, Central & South America)
- Penicilliosis (Far East)
- Histoplasmosis (USA, Africa, Caribbean, South America)
- Coccidioidomycosis (USA)
- Trypanosomiasis cruzi (South America)
- Conjunctival carcinoma or cancer (sub-Saharan Africa)

Diseases that vary greatly in prevalence according to socio-economic circumstances, medical facilities and route of HIV infection:

- Tuberculosis
- Non-tuberculosis mycobacterioses
- Toxoplasmosis
- Pneumocystosis in adults
- CMV
- Lymphoma
- HIV multinucleate giant cell encephalitis
- Kaposi's sarcoma
- Disease that is ethnically restricted
- HIV-associated nephropathy (in blacks)

Many opportunistic infections that complicate HIV are reactivations of latent infections. Thus, epidemiologic factors that determine the prevalence of latent infections also influence risk of specific opportunistic infections. In many developing countries, prevalence of latent TB and toxoplasmosis in the general population is higher than that in developed countries. Dramatic increases in reactivated TB and toxoplasmic encephalitis have followed the epidemic of HIV-induced immunosuppression in these countries.

Other Tissues

HIV also infects nonlymphoid monocytic cells (eg, dendritic cells in the skin, macrophages, brain microglia) and cells of the brain, genital tract, heart, and kidneys, causing disease in the corresponding organ systems. HIV strains in several compartments, such as the nervous system (brain and CSF) and genital tract (semen), can be genetically distinct from those in plasma, suggesting that they have been selected by or have adapted to these anatomic compartments.

Some patients present with cancers (eg, Kaposi sarcoma, B-cell lymphomas) that occur more frequently, are unusually severe, or have unique features in patients with HIV infection. In other patients, neurologic dysfunction may occur.

Hematologic disorders (eg, cytopenias, lymphomas, cancers) are common and may be usefullyevaluated with bone marrow aspiration and biopsy. This procedure can also help diagnose disseminated infections with MAC, M. tuberculosis, Cryptococcus, Histoplasma, human parvovirus B19, P. jirovecii, and Leishmania. Most patients have normocellular or hypercellular marrow despite peripheral cytopenia, reflecting peripheral destruction. Iron stores are usually normal or increased, reflecting anemia of chronic disease (an iron-reutilization defect). Mild to moderate plasmacytosis, lymphoid aggregates, increased numbers of histiocytes, and dysplastic changes in hematopoietic cells are common.

Combinations of 3 or 4 drugs from different classes are usually necessary to fully suppress replication of wild-type HIV. Nucleoside reverse transcriptase inhibitors (NRTIs) are phosphorylated to active metabolites that compete for incorporation into viral DNA. They inhibit the HIV reverse transcriptase enzyme competitively and terminate synthesis of DNA chains.

- Nucleotide reverse transcriptase inhibitors (nRTIs) competitively inhibit the HIV reverse transcriptase enzyme, as do NRTIs, but do not require initial phosphorylation.

- Non-nucleoside reverse transcriptase inhibitors (NNRTIs) bind directly to the reverse transcriptase enzyme.

- Protease inhibitors (PIs) inhibit the viral protease enzyme that is crucial to maturation of immature HIV virions after they bud from host cells.

- Entry inhibitors (EIs), sometimes called fusion inhibitors, interfere with the binding of HIV to CD4+receptors and chemokine co-receptors; this binding is required for HIV to enter cells. For example, CCR-5 inhibitors block the CCR-5 receptor.

- Integrase inhibitors prevent HIV DNA from being integrated into human DNA.

Combining drugs often increases the risk that either drug will have an adverse effect. Possible mechanisms include the following:

- Hepatic metabolism of PIs by cytochrome P-450: The result is decreased metabolism (and increased levels) of other drugs.

- Additive toxicities: For example, combining NRTIs, such as d4T and didanosine (ddI), increases the chance of adverse metabolic effects and peripheral neuropathy.

- Bone complications of ART include asymptomatic osteopenia and osteoporosis, which are common. Uncommonly, osteonecrosis of large joints such as the hip and shoulder causes severe joint pain and dysfunction. Mechanisms of bone complications are poorly understood.

Amyloidosis

Amyloidosis is a rare disease that results from accumulation of inappropriately folded proteins. These misfolded proteins are called amyloids. When normally soluble proteins fold to become amyloids, they become insoluble and deposit in organs or tissues, disrupting normal function. The type of protein that is misfolded and the organ or tissue in which the misfolded proteins are deposited determines the clinical manifestations of amyloidosis.

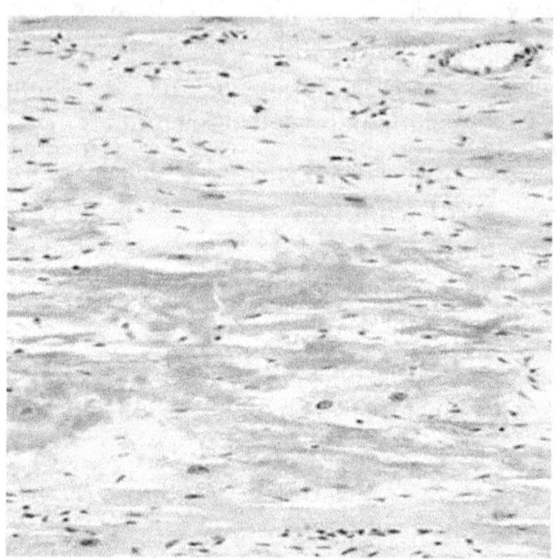

Fig. 4.20 Micrograph showing amyloid deposition (red fluffy material) in the heart (cardiacamyloidosis). Congo red stain.
(Source: https://en.wikipedia.org/wiki/Amyloidosis)

Classification

Various descriptive classification systems were proposed based on the organ distribution of amyloid deposits and clinical findings. There are different types of amyloidosis, including:

Primary (systemic AL) amyloidosis: This occurs without a known cause, but it has been seen in people with a blood cancer called multiple myeloma. This is the most common type of amyloidosis. Systemic means it affects the entire body. The most commonly affected body parts are the kidney, heart, liver, intestines, and certain nerves. AL stands for "amyloid light chains," which is the type of protein responsible for this type of amyloidosis.

Secondary (systemic AA) amyloidosis: This is the result of another chronic inflammatory disease, such as lupus, arthritis, tuberculosis, inflammatory bowel disease (Crohn's disease and ulcerative colitis), and certain cancers. It most commonly affects the spleen, kidneys, liver, adrenal gland, and lymph nodes. AA means the amyloid type A protein causes this type of amyloidosis.

Dialysis-related amyloidosis (DRA): This is more common in older adults and people who have beenon dialysis for more than five years. This form of amyloidosis is caused by deposits of beta-2 microglobulin that build up in the blood. Deposits can occur in many different tissues, but most commonly affects bones, joints, and tendons.

Familial, or hereditary, amyloidosis (AF): This is a rare form that is passed down through families. It is caused by an abnormal amyloid transthyretin (TTR) protein, which is made in the liver. This protein is responsible for the most common forms of hereditary amyloidosis.

Senile systemic amyloidosis (SSA): This is caused deposits of normal TTR in the heart and other tissues. It occurs most commonly in older men.

Organ-specific amyloidosis: This is cause deposits of amyloid protein in single organs, including the skin (cutaneous amyloidosis).

Another classification is primary or secondary:

Primary (i.e., idiopathic) amyloidosis: Primary amyloidoses arise from a disease with disordered immune cell function, such as multiple myeloma or other immunocyte dyscrasias. In which no associated clinical condition was identified.

Secondary amyloidosis (i.e., secondary to chronic inflammatory conditions): Secondary (reactive) amyloidoses occur as a complication of some other chronic inflammatory or tissue-destroying disease. Examples are reactive systemic amyloidosis and secondary cutaneous amyloidosis.[15]

Another system classified amyloidosis as

- Myeloma-associated amyloidosis
- Familial amyloidosis
- Localized amyloidosis.

Additionally, based on the tissues in which it is deposited, it is divided into mesenchymal (organs derived from mesoderm) or parenchymal (organs derived from ectoderm or endoderm).

An older clinical method of classification refers to amyloidoses as systemic or localised

- Systemic amyloidoses affect more than one body organ or system. Examples are AL, AA and Aβ2m.
- Localised amyloidoses affect only one body organ or tissue type. Examples are Aβ, IAPP, Atrialnatriuretic factor (in isolated atrial amyloidosis), and Calcitonin (in medullary carcinoma of the thyroid)

Causes and Types of Amyloidosis

Many different proteins can lead to the formation of amyloid deposits, but only a few have been linked to significant health problems. The type of protein and where it collects determines the type of amyloidosis you have. Amyloid deposits may collect throughout your body or in just one area.

The modern classification of amyloid disease tends to use an abbreviation of the protein that makes the majority of deposits, prefixed with the letter A. For example, amyloidosis caused by transthyretin is termed "ATTR". Deposition patterns vary between patients but are almost always composed of just one amyloidogenic protein. Deposition can be systemic (affecting many different organ systems) or organ-specific. Many amyloidoses are inherited, due to mutations in the precursor protein.

Other forms are due to different diseases causing overabundant or abnormal protein production - such as with overproduction of immunoglobulin light chains (termed AL amyloidosis), or with continuous overproduction of acute phase proteins in chronic inflammation (which can lead to AA amyloidosis).

Symptoms of Amyloidosis

Symptoms of amyloidosis are often subtle. They can also vary greatly depending on where the amyloid protein is collecting in the body. It is important to note that the symptoms described below may be due to a variety of different health problems. General symptoms of amyloidosis may include:

- Changes in skin colour
- Clay-colored stools
- Fatigue
- Feeling of fullness
- Joint pain
- Low red blood cell count (anaemia)
- Shortness of breath
- Swelling of the tongue
- Tingling and numbness in legs and feet
- Weak hand grip
- Weakness
- Weight loss

Cardiac (Heart) Amyloidosis

Amyloid deposits in the heart can make the walls of the heart muscle stiff. They can also make the heart muscle weaker and affect the electrical rhythm of the heart. This condition can cause less blood to flow to your heart. Eventually, your heart will no longer be able to pump. If amyloidosis affects your heart, you may have:

- Shortness of breath with light activity

- An irregular heartbeat
- Signs of heart failure, including swelling of the feet and ankles, weakness, fatigue, and nausea, among others

Renal (Kidney) Amyloidosis

Your kidneys filter waste and toxins from your blood. Amyloid deposits in the kidneys make it hard for them to do this job. When your kidneys do not work properly, water and dangerous toxins build up in your body. If amyloidosis affects the kidneys, you may have:

- Signs of kidney failure, including swelling of the feet and ankles and puffiness around the eyes.
- High levels of protein in your urine.

Gastrointestinal Amyloidosis

Amyloid deposits along your gastrointestinal (GI) tract slow down the muscle contractions that help move food through your intestines. This interferes with digestion. If amyloidosis affects your GI tract, you may have:

- Decreased appetite
- Diarrhoea
- Nausea
- Stomach pain
- Weight loss

Liver Amyloidosis

Liver involvement can cause:

- Liver enlargement,
- Fluid build-up in the body,
- Abnormal liver function tests.

Amyloid Neuropathy

Amyloid deposits can damage the nerves outside your brain and spinal cord called the peripheral nerves. The peripheral nerves carry information between your brain and spinal cord (central nervous system) and the rest of your body. For example, they make your brain perceive pain if you burn your hand or stub your toes. If amyloidosis affects your nerves, you may have:

- Balance problems
- Problems controlling your bladder and bowel
- Sweating problems
- Tingling and weakness

- Light-headedness when standing due to a problem with your body's ability to control blood pressure

Amyloidosis can also involve other organs including the lungs, skin, and spleen. Amyloidosis comprises of a heterogeneous group of diseases in which normally soluble plasma proteins are deposited in the extracellular space in an abnormal, insoluble, fibrillar form.

Amyloid A (AA) amyloidosis is the most common form of systemic amyloidosis worldwide. It is characterized by extracellular tissue deposition of fibrils that are composed of fragments of serum amyloid A (SAA) protein, a major acute-phase reactant protein, produced predominantly by hepatocytes. AA amyloidosis occurs in the course of a chronic inflammatory disease of either infectious or noninfectious etiology, hereditary periodic fevers, and with certain neoplasms such as Hodgkin disease and renal cell carcinoma.

In developing countries, the most common instigator of AA amyloidosis is chronic infection; in industrialized societies, rheumatic diseases, such as rheumatoid arthritis (RA), are the usual stimuli. The United States is a major exception to this in that immunoglobulin-related amyloid light chain type (AL) of amyloidosis is more frequent than AA as the cause of systemic amyloid deposition.

In AA amyloidosis, the kidney, liver and spleen are the major sites of involvement. It becomes clinically overt mainly when renal damage occurs, manifesting either as proteinuria, nephrotic syndrome, or derangement in renal function.

The tissue fibril consists of a 7500-dalton cleavage product of the SAA protein, which is an acute phase reactant, and like C-reactive protein, is synthesized by hepatocytes under the transcriptional regulation of cytokines including interleukin (IL)-1, IL-6 and tumor necrosis factor (TNF). Under the influence of the inflammatory cytokine IL-6, hepatic transcription of the messenger ribonucleic acid (mRNA) for SAA may increase 1000-fold when exposed to an inflammatory stimulus.

Intact circulating SAA (molecular weight 12,500 Dalton) is complexed with high-density lipoproteins (HDL). During the course of inflammation, the apolipoprotein SAA (apoSAA) apparently displaces apolipoprotein A1 (apoA1) from the HDL particles and facilitates HDL-cholesterol uptake by macrophages.

The conversion of SAA into amyloid fibrils occurs through its specific interaction with heparan sulphate, a ubiquitously expressed glycosaminoglycan component of the extracellular matrix. SAA specifically binds to heparan sulfate (HS) glycosaminoglycan, a common constituent of all types of amyloid deposits that has been shown to facilitate conformational transition of a precursor to beta-pleated sheet structure. The protein has also been shown to be chemotactic for neutrophils, and it stimulates degranulation, phagocytosis, and cytokine release in these cells.

Until relatively recently, the erythrocyte sedimentation rate (ESR) and the serum C-reactive protein (CRP) level were used to monitor inflammation clinically. Increases in both CRP and SAA have been associated with active atherosclerotic coronary artery disease and cited as evidence for the inflammatory nature of that disease process. SAA also has been used to monitor the dissemination of malignancy.

Pathogenesis: Native cells have two different ways of making different proteins. Some cells make proteins in one piece; others, cells make only protein fragments and the fragments come and join together to form the whole protein. But such a protein can sometimes fall apart into the original protein fragments. This process of "flip flopping" happens frequently for certain protein types, especially the ones that cause amyloidosis. The fragments or actual proteins are at risk of misfolding as they are synthesized, to make a poorly functioning protein. This causes proteolysis, which is the directed breakdown of proteins by cellular enzymes called proteases or by intramolecular digestion; proteases come and digest the misfolded fragments and proteins. The problem occurs when the proteins do not dissolve in proteolysis. This happens because the misfolded proteins sometimes become robust enough that they are not dissolved by normal proteolysis.

The stabilized balls of protein fragments are called oligomers. When the fragments do not dissolve, they get spit out of proteolysis and when these fragments are exposed to water, these hydrophobic pieces tend to aggregate with other hydrophobic pieces to form oligomers. The reason they aggregate is that the parts of the protein that do not dissolve in proteolysis are the β-pleated sheets, which areextremely hydrophobic. This ball of fragments gets stabilized by GAGs (glycosaminoglycans) and SAP (serum amyloid P), a component found in amyloid aggregations that is thought to stabilize them and prevent proteolytic cleavage.The oligomers can aggregate together and further stabilize to make amyloid fibrils. Both the oligomers and amyloid fibrils are toxic to cells and can interfere with proper organ function. Chronic or acute, recurrent, substantial elevations of SAA are necessary but not sufficient for the development of amyloidosis. The median plasma concentration of SAA in healthy persons is 3 mg/L, but the concentration can increase to more than 2000 mg/L during the acute-phase response.

Many individuals with long-standing inflammatory disease, although severely compromised by their primary condition, clearly do not develop tissue amyloid deposition. What determines any patient's risk for the development of this complication of inflammation is not known. Therapy, genetic factors, and environmental factors have all been proposed as possible contributors to the response of the primary disease.

1. **Primary amyloidosis (AL)**
   - Patients with AL produce light chains that are inherently prone to misfolding from a native alpha-helical state into an insoluble beta-pleated sheet configuration.

- The development of amyloidosis is linked both to the quantity of light chain that is produced, as well as a qualitative thermodynamic tendency for the immunoglobulin light chain fragment to misfold into the amyloid configuration.

- Significant differences in gene usage are found in AL. Patients with clones derived from the 6aV lambda VI germline gene usage is more likely to present with dominant renal involvement. Those with clones derived from 1c, 2a2, and 3r V lambda genes are more likely to present with cardiac and multisystem disease.

- The kidney is the primary target organ in AL. The monoclonal light chain assembles and deposits extracellularly, resulting in disruption of the glomerular basement membrane. The light chains interact with mesangial cells, which catabolise them into fragments that form amyloid fibrils.

- Cardiac amyloidosis resembles idiopathic restrictive cardiomyopathy, but ventricular long axis function is depressed in all patients with cardiac amyloidosis compared with only 36% of patients with idiopathic restrictive cardiomyopathy. The 2 disorders have distinct pathophysiological profiles with impairment in longitudinal function even if left ventricular filling isnormal. Amyloid infiltration of the heart also results in conduction abnormalities. Clinical evidence of cardiac involvement is seen in 22% to 34% of AL patients. Death is due to a cardiac cause in over half of patients.

- Amyloid deposits in the vasa nervorum results in clinical findings similar to ischaemic neuropathy and lead to a mixed axonal demyelinating picture. Carpal tunnel syndrome is associated in half of patients.

2. Secondary amyloidosis (AA)

- Secondary amyloidosis results from the improper processing of serum amyloid A protein (AA), which instead of being broken down to constituent amino acids cannot be broken down beyond an 8.5-kDa fragment labelled amyloid A protein. This protein is common to all forms of amyloidosis related to long-standing infections such as bronchiectasis (cystic fibrosis), osteomyelitis, chronic mycobacterial infections, inflammatory bowel disease, familial periodic fever syndrome and Castleman's disease.

- The most common organs involved are the kidney, GI tract and thyroid. Patients who are long-term survivors of non-familial secondary amyloidosis can develop cardiac amyloidosis, but with a frequency much lower than that seen in familial and light chain forms. The most common late sequelae of sustained production of AA amyloid is dialysis-dependent renal failure.

3. Inherited amyloidosis (AF)

- Most forms of inherited amyloidosis are a consequence of misfolding of an inherited mutant transthyretin (TTR) molecule. There are other rarer forms of inherited amyloidosis due to mutations of apolipoprotein A1, apolipoprotein A2, fibrinogen and lysozyme.
- This usually presents as either familial cardiomyopathy or familial peripheral and autonomic neuropathy.

4. Senile amyloidosis (SSA)

- There is a form of amyloidosis associated with an unmutated (native) TTR. This occurs in the elderly and is referred to as senile systemic amyloidosis; it was formerly known as senile cardiac amyloidosis.

Cellular and Extracellular Tissue Factors

Mononuclear phagocytes might play a role in degradation of SAA and initiation of development of AA amyloidosis. The factors responsible for determining the site of deposition in any form of amyloidosis have not been identified. AA fibrils have been generated in tissue cultures by incubating SAA with macrophages. Deposits are frequently found in tissues with large numbers of phagocytic cells, notably the liver and spleen, but other affected organs, such as the kidneys, do not have the same cellular composition.

5

Neoplasia – Cancer

Syllabus: Differences between benign and malignant tumors, Histological diagnosis of malignancy, invasions and metastasis, patterns of spread, spread of malignant tumors, disturbances of growth of cells, classification of tumors, general biology of tumors, etiology and pathogenesis of cancer.

Definition: The term 'neoplasia' means new growth and the mass of tissue formed is called 'neoplasm'. All new growths are not neoplasm. e.g.: embryogenesis, regeneration, repair, hyperplasia, hormonal stimulation etc.

Neoplasm or tumour is mass of tissue formed as a result of abnormal, excessive, uncontrolled, autonomous, purposeless proliferation of cells. Proliferation and maturation of cells in normal adult is controlled. Neoplastic cells lose control and regulation of replication and form abnormal mass of tissue. Branch of science which deals with study of neoplasm or tumour is called oncology. Neoplasm (Tumour) may be benign or malignant.

Types of Neoplasms

- *Benign neoplasms:* are slow growing, localised, do not invade into local surrounding tissue, or spread to other sites and do not cause much difficulty to host.

- *Malignant neoplasm [cancer]:* proliferate rapidly, invade into local tissue (invasiveness) and can disseminate (metastasis) to other tissue and organs, and may eventually cause death of the host. The common term used for all malignant tumours is cancer.

All tumours (benign and malignant) have two components-Parenchyma and supportive stroma. Parenchyma consists of proliferating tumour cells. Parenchyma determines the nature and evolution of tumour. Supportive stroma composed of fibrous connective tissue and blood vessels. Stromal connective tissue provides a frame work for parenchyma on which parenchymal tumour cell grow. Tumour derives their nomenclature on the basis of parenchymal component comprising them.

Characters of Malignant Neoplasm

1. Variation from normal histological characters is known as cellular atypia or dysplasia. Loss of uniformity and architectural orientation (architectural anarchy): e.g.: encountered in epithelia. Do not necessarily progress to cancer. (Pre-invasive neoplasia or carcinoma *in situ*).

2. *Pleomorphism:* It is variation in cell size, shape, and staining characters of cytoplasm, nucleus, nucleolus.

3. *Anaplasia:* (complete loss of differentiation): It is the hall mark of malignant neoplasm. Anaplasiarefers to complete loss of specialised histological features such that tissue of origin cannot be predicted. Differentiation is the extent to which parenchymal cell resemble normal cell structurally and functionally. Benign tumours are well differentiated whereas anaplasia is found in many malignant tumours.

4. *Invasiveness (Local invasion):* Growth of cancer is accompanied by infiltration, invasion and destruction of surrounding tissue. Invasiveness is the ability to transgress normal boundaries. Invasiveness of cancer permits them topenetrate into blood vessels, lymphatics, and body cavities (provide opportunity for spread). Benign tumours have no invasiveness. They remain localised to their site of origin Benign tumour have fibrous capsule.

   Biochemical basis for invasiveness:
   - Malignant cells are less tightly adherent than normal cell.
   - Calcium content of malignant cells is less than normal cell.
   - Cancer cells may repel each other due to their high negative charge on their surface.
   - Some neoplasms release its enzymes like Hyaluronidase, collagenase, etc. which disrupt the basement membrane allowing the tumour cell to enter the matrix of surrounding tissue or to migrate through the tissues (Invasiveness).

5. *Metastasis:* It is the ability to spread to distant site. The ability to transgress (break) normal tissue boundaries and to invade locally (invasiveness) or to penetrate lymphatics and blood vessels and to spread distant sites (metastasis) is the major criteria of malignancy. Benign tumour does not metastasis.

6. *Clonality:* cancer cell population develop from a single cell.

7. **Autonomy:** Normally inhibitory influences control cell growth and proliferation. Neoplastic cells exhibit uncontrolled proliferation. Cancer cells do not follow normal control in cell cycle.

8. **Rate of growth:** rate of growth of tumour depends on proportion of cell undergoing mitosis, duration of cell cycle, rate of cell loss. Benign tumour grows slowly. Cancer grows rapidly. Emergence of aggressive sub clones of transformed cells cause explosive growth of malignant cell. Growth rate correlate with rate of differentiation. The proliferation and maturation of cells

in normal adult is controlled, as a result of which some cells proliferate throughout life (labile) some have limited proliferation (stable cells) while other do not replicate (permanent cells).

9. **Aneuploidy:** Majority of the malignant neoplasm show abnormal DNA content.

10. **Blood supply:** Tumour angiogenesis factor stimulate the endothelial cell mitosis and new blood vessel growth in tumour.

11. Loss of orientation: Large mass of tumour cells grow in disorganised, anarchic fashion (pleomorphism). Encountered in epithelia. Mitoses appear in abnormal location in epithelium.

Comparison between benign and Malignant Tumour

Benign	Malignant
Differentiation and anaplasia: Well differentiated. [Cells resemble tissue of origin]	Lack of differentiation with anaplasia. [Poor resemblance to tissue of origin] Malignant tumour ranges from well differentiated to undifferentiated.
Boundaries: Encapsulated	Irregular
Local invasion: Do not invade or infiltrate to surrounding normal tissue (surrounding tissue normally compressed)	Infiltrate to surrounding normal tissue
Metastasis: Absent	Frequently present
Rate of growth: Grow slowly Rate of growth of tumour depends on proportion of cell undergoing mitosis, duration of cell cycle, and rate of cell loss.	Grow rapidly Malignant tumour cells have increased metabolic rate. Cancer cells (malignant cells) do not follow normal control in cell cycle. Growth persists even after cessation of stimuli which evoked it.
Mitoses: Few, Normal	Numerous, Abnormal.
Nuclei: Little altered	Enlarged, Often irregular
Prognosis: Local complication	Death by local and metastatic complications
Cytoplasmic basophilia: slight	Marked
Haemorrhage and Necrosis: Inconspicuous	Often extensive

Benign Tumour Classification and Nomenclature

Tumour nomenclature includes indication of tumour's derivation and its possible behaviour. Benign tumour has suffix -oma which is preceded by cell origin. e.g.: Adenoma, fibroma

Malignant Tumour use Suffix

- Carcinoma if the tumour derived from epithelial origin.
- Sarcoma if derived from mesenchyme e.g. Adenocarcinoma, fibrosarcoma (tumour of connective tissue)

Unfortunately, many tumours do not confirm the above rules. e.g.: Lymphoma not benign proliferation of lymphoid cells but malignant tumour.

Benign Epithelial Tumours: Papilloma, adenoma, cystadenoma

Malignant Epithelial Tumour: Squamous carcinoma, adenocarcinoma, transition cell carcinoma, basalcell carcinoma.

Benign Connective Tissue Tumours

- *Uterine leiomyoma:* consists of inter weaving bundles of smooth muscle cells.
- *Lipoma:* It consists of lobulated mass of adipose tissue usually in subcutaneous tissue. They may be present in other sites like small intestine.
- *Chondromas (enchondromas):* These are benign cartilage tumour usually arising in the small bones of hands and feet. e.g.: Ollier's disease, Maffucci's syndrome
- *Osteomas:* These are benign bone forming tumours.
- *Fibroma:* benign tumour of fibrous tissue.

Malignant Connective Tissue Tumour (Sarcoma)
Classification and Nomenclature

They are less common than carcinomas. But often highly aggressive in their behaviour. [Sar- means fleshy].

- *Osteosarcoma:* Usually a tumour of children and young adult.
- *Chondrosarcoma:* Old age group.
- *Leiomyosarcoma:* Smooth muscle of uterus or wall of alimentary canal.
- *Rhabdomyosarcoma (skeletal muscle):* Commonest soft tissue tumour of children and adolescent.
- *Liposarcoma:* Arise in deep sub cutaneous tissue of trunk, proximal limbs and retroperitoneum.
- *Malignant fibrous histiocytoma:* Commonest soft tissue sarcoma of adult arising in the deep soft tissueof limps and retroperitoneum (posterior to peritoneum). This is highly malignant tumour with poor prognosis.
- *Neuroectodermal tumours:* Portion of ectoderm of early embryo which give rise to central andperipheral nervous system.
- *Gliomas:* They are derived from astrocytes (neuroglial cell of ectodermal origin), oligodendrocytes (nonneuronal cells of ectodermal origin) and ependymal cells (ependymal membrane lining the cerebral ventricles and central canal of spinal cord). Relatively rare but second commonest tumour of children. They may cause Jacksonian epilepsy, hemiparesis (incomplete paralysis of one side) hemi anopiaby virtue of their position.
- *Astrocytoma:* Tumour composed of astrocytes. Most common type of primary brain tumour and also found throughout central nervous system.

- *Haemopoietic tumours:* These are derived from blood cells and are called leukaemia. There are many different types arising from various stages of maturation of lymphocytes/myeloid cells. It occurs in children and adult. There are chronic and acute. They are highly sensitive to chemotherapy.

- *Acute leukaemia:* It involves proliferation of immature (blast) cells. There are two main types:
    - *Acute lymphoblastic leukaemia (ALL):* found predominantly in children.
    - *Acute non-lymphoblastic leukaemia (ANLL):* Myeloid, monocytes, erythroid, mega karyocytic etc.

Clinically these patients (ALL and ANLL) have recurrent infections, anaemia, bleeding.

- *Chronic leukaemia:* Chronic lymphatic leukaemia (CLL); chronic granulocytic leukaemia (CGL)

- *Lymphoreticular tumours:* These are derived from lymphoid cells of lymph node. There are two majorcategories. Hodgkin's disease, Non-Hodgkin's lymphoma. Etiology involves Viral infection, immunosuppression. Hodgkin's disease: This is primary disease of young adult involving lymph node but extend into extranodular tissue. It is characterised by presence of Reed Stenberg cells [a binucleated cell with mirror image nuclei].

- *Non Hodgkin's lymphoma:* These are tumours derived from B or T lymphocytes.

- *Germ cell tumours:* derived from cells of the embryonic germ cell layers. In males there are two main types:
    - *Seminoma:* Non seminomatous germ cell tumours
    - *Teratoma:* Tissue derived from germ cell and contains more than one type of tissue arranged in totally disorganised fashion.
    - *Dysgerminoma:* Undifferentiated germ cell tumour of ovary.

Ovarian cystic teratoma:

Choriocarcinoma: a rise from placental tissue and secrete chorionic gonadotropin.

Seminoma: Testicular tumour occurs in men in their 5th decade. It arises from testicular tubules.

Testicular teratoma:

Hepatoma: carcinoma of hepatocytes.

- *Mixed tumours:* Occasional tumours contain mixture of tissue type. Arise from single germ layer. This occurs due to collision between two tumours arising in adjacent tissue. Metaplastic change in tumour.

- *Adenosquamous carcinoma:* Carcino sarcoma: Combination of malignant tumour of epithelium (carcinoma) and that of mesenchymal tissue (sarcoma) such as in thyroid. Teratoma: Most common site ovaries and testis (Gonadal teratomas) also occur at extra gonadal site-head, neck, mediastinum etc. (Arise from totipotent cells).

- ***Blastoma:*** Hamartoma: Endocrine tumours: These tumours regularly produce hormones and often have clinical effect of overproduction of hormone. Carcinoma of epidermis elaborates keratin. Hepatocellular carcinoma elaborates bile. Tumour markers: Some tumour produce substance which may be detected biochemically in blood orurine which may be used in diagnosis, follow up of tumour.

- ***Carcino embryonic antigen (CEA):*** in colonic cancer. If CEA level rises, it indicates recurrence of metastasis.

- ***Human chorionic gonadotropin (HCG):*** Alpha protein is used similarly in teratomas.

- ***Prostatic acid phosphate (PAP), Prostate specific antigen (PSA):*** can be used in diagnosis of prostate carcinoama. It is possible to localise substance such as HCG or PSA in histological tissue secretions using immunological techniques (immunocytochemistry).

Special Categories of Tumour

- ***Teratoma:*** Tissue derived from germ cell and contains more than one type of tissue arranged in totally disorganised fashion. e. g.: Ovarian cystic teratoma.

- ***Blastoma [embryoma]:*** are group of malignant tumours which arise from embryonal or partially differentiated cells which would normally from blastema of the organ and tissue during embryogenesis. These tumours occur frequently in infants and children. e.g.: Neuroblastoma, Nephroblastoma.

- ***Hamartoma:*** Benign tumour made of mature but disorganised cells of tissue indigenous to particular organ. e.g.: Lung hamartoma. Hamartoma of lungs consist of mature cartilage, mature smooth muscle and epithelium. Thus, all mature differentiated tissue elements which comprise bronchus are present in it but are jumbled up as a mass.

- ***Choristoma:*** ectopic islands of normal tissue. e.g.: Adrenal cells under kidney capsule.

Mechanism of Carcinogenesis (Spread of Tumour)

Carcinogenesis or oncogenesis or tumorigenesis is the formation of a cancer, whereby normal cells are transformed into cancer cells. The process is characterized by changes at the cellular, genetic, and epigenetic levels and abnormal cell division, in some cancers forming a malignant mass.

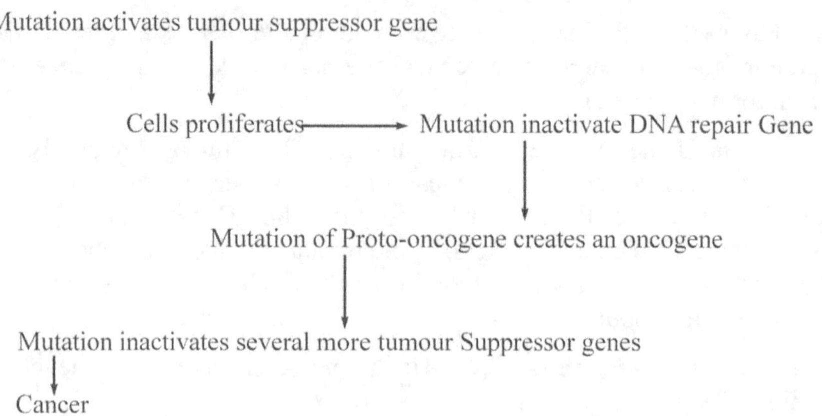

Fig. 5.1. Schematic diagram of mechanism of carcinogenesis.

Tumour may Spread by Following Methods

- *Spread by infiltration:* Spread of cancer cell through tissue space is one of the chief characteristic of malignant tumour. Cancer cells are amoeboid and motile. Cells of benign tumour and normal cells are incapable of movement because they are firmly anchored to one another by cell adhesiveness. Loss of adhesiveness in cancer cell is due to deficiency of calcium.

- *Lymphatic spread:* Tumour cells can rapidly enter the lymphatic channels. Spread by blood [Haematogenous]: Cancer cells may reach blood either by thoracic duct or by direct invasion of blood vessels. Portal system of veins is invaded by tumour of GIT pancreas and can produce secondary tumour in liver. Pulmonary veins are invaded by primary bronchogenic carcinoma.

- *Spread by natural passage:* Tumour cells are carried along bronchus, bowel, ureter etc. e.g.: simultaneous occurrence of tumour in renal pelvis, and bladder.

- *Spread through serous cavities:* It explains the frequent transfer of tumour cells from stomach to ovaries (through peritoneal cavity).

- *Spread by inoculation:* Tumour cells may be inoculated into surrounding tissue in an operation.

Etiologic Agents [Known Factors Causing Cancer]

(i) *Chemical carcinogens*

  (a) *Direct acing carcinogens:* They can induce cancer without undergoing any prior metabolic activation). They directly interact with DNA and damage it.

   - Alkylating agents: e.g.:
     - Cyclophosphamide
     - Chlorambucil

- Busulfan
- Melphalan

- Acylating agents: e.g.:
  - Dimethyl carbamyl chloride
  - 1-acetyl imidazole

(b) *Indirect acting carcinogens (Procarcinogens):* They require metabolic activation in the body to become ultimate carcinogen:

- Polycyclic aromatic hydrocarbons e.g.:
  - Bezanthracene
  - Dibenzanthrazene
  - 3-methyl cholanthrene
  - benzopyrene etc. (produced in combustion of tobacco).

- Aromatic amines and azo dyes: e.g.:
  - 2-naphthyl amine
  - Benzidine
  - 2-acetyl aminofluorene
  - dimethyl amino azobenzene etc. (activated by cytochrome P450 oxygenase system).

- Azo dyes: e.g.:
  - butter yellow
  - scarlet red

(ii) *Physical carcinogens:* e.g.: Ultra violet light, ionizing radiation (α, β, , and x rays etc.) asbestos, plastic glass etc.

(iii) *Viral carcinogens:*

- DNA oncogenic virus: e.g.:
  - Human papilloma virus
  - Epstein Barr virus
  - Hepatitis B virus

- RNA oncogenic virus: e.g.:
  - Human T cell Lymphotrophic virus
  - Hepatitis C virus

(iv) *Hormones:* e.g.: Oestrogen, contraceptive hormones anabolic steroids

(v) *Promoters:* e.g.: Dietary fat (colon cancer) hormones, diethylstilbesterol (endometrial carcinoma) saccharine, cyclamate (bladder cancer)

(vi) *Miscellaneous:* e.g.: Chromium, nickel arsenic (skin cancer), asbestos, cigarette smoke (bronchogenic carcinoma, mesothelioma, gastro intestinal cancer) vinyl chloride.

Pathogenesis of Cancer
[Carcinogenic Agents and their Cellular Interaction]

Mutation hypothesis: Neoplasia involves multi factorial, multistage process of progressive mutation in the genetic makeup of the cell. Transformation of normal cell to a neoplastic cell involves change within the genetic makeup of the cell. Hereditary, chemicals, physical agents, radiation, virus may be the factor in this change.

Monoclonality of tumour: Most of the human cancer arise from single cell by genetic transformation/mutation or 'the first step occurs in single cell'. Cancer cells display a type of clonal evolution that enables insidious selection of most aggressive, rapidly growing, invasive clones. This selection process gives rise to sub clones that are fiercely resistant to all known mode of therapy that ultimately prove lethal.

Genetic theory of cancer: Cell growth in normal as well as abnormal cell type is under genetic control. In cancer, there is abnormality in genes of cell/normal genes with abnormal function. Abnormality in genetic composition may be from inherited or induced mutation. Mutated cell transmit their characters to next progeny of cells and result in cancer. In normal cell, there are four regulatory genes:

- Proto-onchogenes: Growth promoting genes
- Anti-onchogenes: Growth suppressor genes
- Apoptosis regulatory genes: Control programmed cell death
- DNA repair genes: They regulate the repair of DNA damage that occurred during mitosis also control the damage to proto-onchogenes and anti-onchogenes

Genetic damage to these normal controlling genes produce transformed cell with abnormal cell growth.

In cancer, there is:

(a) Activation of growth promoting onchogenes (Produce excessive and autonomous growth)

(b) Inactivation of cancer suppressor genes (permitting cellular proliferation of transformed cell)

(c) Abnormal apoptosis regulatory genes cause escaping the cell death by apoptosis

(d) Failure of DNA repair genes cause inability to repair the DNA damage resulting in mutation.

Addition of p53 gene to breast cell culture can suppress their growth. Agents causing genetic damage and neoplastic transformation of cell:

(a) ***Chemical carcinogenesis:*** Induction of cancer by chemical carcinogens occur after a delay-often several years in man. Factors which influence the induction of cancer are dose, mode of administration, susceptibility of the individual and various predisposing factors. Basic mechanism of chemical carcinogenesis is by induction of mutation in proto-onchogenes and anti-onchogenes.

Chemical carcinogenesis is progressive process involving two stages: Initiation and Promotion.

- *Initiation:* Initiation result from exposure of cell to an appropriate dose of carcinogenic agent. Initiation cause permanent DNA damage. Initiator alone is not sufficient for tumour formation.

- *Promotion:* Promoters can induce tumour in initiated cell. Promoters are non tumourogenic by themselves. Cellular changes produced by promoter do not affect DNA directly and are reversible. Promoter applied before cannot induce tumour.

(b) ***Reactive electrophile:*** Direct acting carcinogens are intrinsically electrophilic while indirect acting carcinogens become electrophilic (electron deficient) after metabolic activation. Highly reactive electrophile binds to electron rich portion of other molecule of the cell such as DNA, RNA, other proteins etc. (covalent bond)

- *Target molecule:* The primary target of electrophile is DNA producing mutagenesis. Any gene in DNA may be the target of chemical carcinogen. Change in DNA produce initiated cell. Mutation of cancer suppresser genes, oncogenes and genes regulation apoptosis result in malignant transformation e.g.: Mutation of Gene P53

- *Initiated Cell [mutated cell]:* Unrepaired alterations in DNA are essential first step in process of initiation. Unrepaired damage produced in DNA become permanent and fixed when that cell undergoes a least one cycle of proliferation. This result in transferring changes to the next progeny of cell (heritable change).

Promotion of Carcinogenesis

Promotion is the next sequential stage in chemical carcinogenesis. Tumour promoters act by further clonal proliferation and expansion of initiated cell (Mutated cell).They do not damage DNA, hence not mutagenic but instead enhance the effect of direct acting carcinogens and pro carcinogens.

They differ from initiator in following respect:

- They do not produce sudden change

- They require application or administration, following initiator exposure for sufficient time, sufficient dose
- They do not damage DNA hence not mutagenic. e. g.: Phorbol esters, Phenols, Hormones, Artificial sweeteners, Drugs like phenobarbital.

Examples: Dietary fat: colon cancer, Diethyl stilbesterol - endometrial cancer, Saccharine, Cyclamate - Bladder cancer. Urathane when applied to skin of mouse will not produce evident neoplasia, but when it is followed by repeated application of croton oil a neoplasm develops. Croton oil is harmless unless the process is initiated by urathane.

Ames test: to test/screen mutagenic potential of a chemical. Use salmonella typhimurium bacteria.

Physical carcinogenesis: Physical agents in carcinogenesis are divided into two:
   (a)   Radiation: both UV and ionising radiation
   (b)   Non radiation physical agents

Radiation carcinogenesis: UV and ionising radiation show long period of latency between initial exposure (mutation) and cancer. They have sequential stage of initiation and promotion in their evolution like chemical carcinogens.

Ultra Violet light (UV): the main source of UV radiation is sun light, welder's arch, UV lamb etc. UV light penetrates the skin only few mm so its effect is limited to the skin. In human exposure to UV-light cause various form of skin cancer-squamous cell carcinoma, basal cell carcinoma, malignant melanoma, etc. There is high incidence of cancer in fair skinned Europeans, albinos, New Zealand, Australia (close to equator) and in farmers and outdoor workers. UV light inhibits cell division, induce mutation and inactivate enzymes:

- UVA (320-400nm)
- UVB (280-320nm)
- UVC (200-280nm)

UVB cause mutation in oncogenes and tumour suppressor genes. The most important biochemical effect UV radiation is formation of pyrimidine dimer in DNA. Pyrimidine dimer causes transcription errors. UV induced DNA damage is repaired in normal individual but persons excessively exposed to UV radiation such damage are unrepaired. Hereditary defect in DNA repair mechanism is with high incidence of cancer. UV radiation also induces mutation in proto oncogenes and anti oncogenes.

Ionising radiation: Ionising radiation of all kind, x rays, alpha, beta, gamma rays, radio activeisotopes, protons, neutrons, can cause cancer in experimental animals. Radiation induced cancer are, all form of leukaemias, cancer of thyroid, skin, breast, ovary, uterus, lung myeloma, salivary gland etc. The risk is increased by higher dose and with high LET [linear energy transfer]: Neutrons> α rays> x rays> rays. High incidence of osteosarcoma, malignant tumour of skin observed in X-ray workers and radio therapist. Miners in reactive element have high incidence of cancer. Xeroderma pigmentosum, Bloom's disease: Japanese atom bomb survivors after World War II have increased frequency of malignant tumours: e.g.:chronic myeloid leukaemia.

Radiation damage the DNA of the cell by two possible mechanisms:

(a) It may dislodge ion from water and other molecules of the cell and result in formation of highly reactive free radicles, which bring about the damage.

(b) It may directly alter the cellular DNA.

Damage to DNA resulting in mutagenesis is the most important action of ionising radiation. It may cause chromosomal breakage, translocation, point mutation etc. The effect depends on type of radiation, dose, frequency, individual susceptibility, immune competence etc. Non-radiation physical carcinogens: The tumerogenesis by these materials in human is rare.

Viral carcinogenesis: Virus of either DNA or RNA type can cause genetic transformation. The neoplastic change involves the integration of new genetic information from virus- in the form of DNA nucleotide sequence –into host's cellular genome.

Retrovirus and oncogenes: Retroviruses are RNA viruses. RNA virus or Retroviruses have two identical strands of RNA and enzyme reverse transcriptase. Reverse transcriptase is RNA dependent DNA synthase –a single stranded viral DNA is formed. DNA dependent DNA synthase from another strand of complimentary DNA resulting in double stranded viral DNA or pro virus. Pro virus then integrates into DNA of the host cell genome. The integrated provirus act just like host cell genes, transmitting genetic information to the cell progeny.

Some retroviruses contain onc or more nucleotide sequence capable of inducing malignant transformation-these sequences are called viral onchogenes. Several viral onchogenes have been proved to induce cancer in experimental system.

- Human T cell leukaemia virus (Type-I) [HTLV-I]: RNA oncogenic virus associated with T-cell leukaemia/ lymphoma. Transmission: Sexual, Blood products, breast feeding. CD4+ is the major target (like AIDS). Infection stimulates prolipheration of T-cells.

- Hepatitis C virus: DNA onchogenic viruses: DNA oncogenic viruses have direct access to the host cell nucleus and are incorporated into genome of host cell.

DNA viruses are classified into papova viruses, Herpes virus, Adeno virus, Pox virus, Hepadna virus etc.

- *Human papilloma virus:* Benign squamous papilloma (wart), Squamous cell carcinoma of cervix, anogenital region.

- *Ebstein Barr virus:* Nasopharyngeal carcinoma, Hodgkin's disease, B-cell lymphoma, Burkitt's lymphoma

- *Hepatitis B virus [Hepadna virus]:* Hepatocellular carcinoma (Liver cancer).

Concepts Related to Cancer Vaccines
(https://en.wikipedia.org/wiki/cancer_vaccine)

A cancer vaccine is a vaccine that either treats existing cancer or prevents development of a cancer. Vaccines that treat existing cancer are known as therapeutic cancer vaccines. Some types of cancer, such as cervical cancer and some liver cancers, are caused by viruses (oncoviruses). Traditional vaccines against those viruses, such as HPV vaccine and hepatitis B vaccine, prevent those types of cancer. Oncophage was approved in Russia in 2008 for kidney cancer. Sipuleucel-T, Provenge, was approved by the FDA in April 2010 for metastatic hormone-refractory prostate cancer.

CancerVax (Canvaxin), Genitope Corp (MyVax personalized immunotherapy), and FavId (Favrille Inc) are examples of cancer vaccine projects that have been terminated, both due to poor phase III results. Cancer vaccines seek to target a tumor-specific antigen and distinct from self-proteins. Selection of the appropriate adjuvant to activate antigen-presenting cells to stimulate immune responses, is required. An effective vaccine also should seek to stimulate long term memory to prevent tumor recurrence. Some scientists claim both the innate and adaptive immune systems must be activated to achieve total tumor elimination.

6

Shock

Definition: Shock commonly called circulatory collapse (cardio vascular collapse) may develop following any serious assault on body's homeostasis-such as profuse haemorrhage, severe trauma, extensive burn, large myocardial infarction, massive pulmonary embolism or bacterial sepsis.

Shock constitute wide spread hypo-perfusion of tissue (systemic hypo-perfusion) due to reduction in blood volume, cardiac output, re-distribution of blood resulting in inadequate effective circulation. Perfusion deficit cause insufficient delivery of oxygen (hypoxia) and nutrients and inadequate clearance of metabolite.

Cellular hypoxia cause shift of aerobic metabolism to anaerobic metabolism, resulting in increased lactate production and lactic acidosis and hypotension. Shock is reversible initially. Persistence or worsening of shock leads to irreversible injury and death of the cell and finally the individual.

Classification of Shock

Shock is commonly divided in to five major types:

1. *Cardiogenic shock:* It is caused by failure of myocardial pump. Myocardial infarction, arrhythmia, extrinsic pressure [cardiac tamponade, out flow obstruction (pulmonary embolism)] may be the cause.

2. *Hypo-volemic/haemorrhagic shock:* This type of shock is due to inadequate blood/plasma volume caused by haemorrhage, fluid loss, from severe burns, trauma, diarrhoea etc.

3. *Septic shock (endotoxic shock):* This is caused by severe bacteraemic infections (systemic microbial infection). Most commonly by gram negative bacteria (endotoxic shock), gram positive organism and fungi.

4. *Neurogenic shock:* Happens due to an aesthetic accidents or spinal cord injury. Cause loss of vascular tone and peripheral pooling of blood.

5. *Anaphylactic shock:* It is caused by Ig-E mediated type-I hypersensitivity reaction. Systemic vasodilation, hypotension, increased vascular permeability, decreased tissue perfusion, cellular anoxia etc.

Pathogenesis of septic shock: It results from spread of microbes from severe localised infection into bloodstream, e.g. Abscess, Peritonitis, Pneumonia, etc. Majority of causes are produced by endotoxin producing g(-) ve bacilli, e.g. E. coli, Klebsiella pneumoniae, Proteus species, Pseudomonas aeruginosa, Seratia, Bacterioides etc., hence called endotoxic shock.

Endotoxins are bacterial cell wall lipo-polysaccharides (LPS). It has toxic fatty core and complex polysaccharide coat. It is released when cell walls are degraded, e.g. as in inflammation. LPS form complex with LPS-binding protein in serum.LPS directly cause injury or alteration of function of cell.

LPS indirectly initiate synthesis and release of mediators. These mediators affect number of organ systems, e.g.-Heart -myocardial dysfunction, Vascular system -vasodilation and hypotension, Leukocyte activation and aggregation, Endothelial cell activation/injury, Disseminated intravascular coagulation, Lungs -acute respiratory distress syndrome (ARDS), Liver -liver failure, Kidney -acute renal failure, CNS -culminating coma

Mediators of inflammation include:

- Cytokines -INF, Tumour Necrosis factor (TNF), Interleukin (1, 2, 6, 8 etc.)
- Nitric oxide
- Complement C5a, C3a
- Prostaglandins
- Leukotrienes
- Kinin system
- Oxygen metabolites
- Catecholamines
- Endorphin
- Myocardial depressant factor etc.,

Endotoxin [LPS] mediated activation of mononuclear phagocyte system and consequent release of IL-1 and TNF-α is the key event in pathogenesis of septic shock. Cytokines cause endothelial activation, leukocyte adhesion and aggregation and capillary thrombosis. They also stimulate secondary mediators like prostaglandins, platelet activating factor, nitric oxide etc. Antibody against TNF, IL-1 receptor antagonist, decreased TNF receptor etc., protect against septic shock in animals and humans.

Suppression of secondary mediators (induced by cytokines) - ameliorate haemodynamic complications of septic shock in some experimental models.LPS is unique for each bacterial species. 'LPS-LPS binding protein' complex bind to TLR-4 (mammalian tall like receptor protein-4)-a signal transduction protein, which activate endothelial cells and cytokines mediators. TLR-4 (Mammalian tall like receptor protein-4) participates in innate (natural) immune response to microbial components.

TLR-4 (activated by LPS) activates vascular wall cells, cytokine mediators, complements, leukocytes.TLR-4 eradicates invading microorganism.LPS in low dose cause activation of complement system, monocyte and macrophage and cause bacterial eradication. LPS-in moderate dose causes cytokine induced secondary effect-fever, leucocytosis, increased synthesis of acute phase reactants.

LPS in high level cause syndrome of septic shock:

- Systemic vasodilation and hypotension
- Diminished myocardial contractility
- Acute respiratory distress syndrome (ARDS)
- Hypo-perfusion
- Wide spread endothelial injury and activation
- Activation of coagulation system (DIC-disseminated intravascular coagulation)
- Vasodilation, myocardial pump failure, DIC, cause hypo-perfusion, multi-organ system failure (liver, kidney, CNS etc.).
- Antibody to LPS binding protein
- Antibody/antagonist to TNF, IL-1
- Inhibitors to secondary mediators like no, prostaglandin etc.

Stages of Shock

Shock is a progressive disorder that if uncorrected may lead to death. Usually shock evolves through three stages:

(a) *Non-progressive phase:* During this stage, reflex compensatory mechanisms are activated and perfusion of vital organs preserved.

(b) *Progressive stage:* It is characterised by tissue hypo-perfusion and onset of ever widening circulatory and metabolic disorder.

(c) *Irreversible stage:* this stage occurs if cellular and tissue injury is so severe that even if therapy correct haemodynamic defect, survival is not possible.

(a) *Non-progressive phase:* During this stage, reflex compensatory mechanisms are activated and perfusion of vital organs preserved. During early shock, a variety of neurohumoral mechanisms come into play to maintain cardiac output and blood pressure. Peripheral vasoconstriction is responsible for coolness and pallor of skin seen in cardiac and hypovolemic shock.

These include

- Baroreceptor reflex
- Release of catecholamines
- Activation of renin angiotensin axis

- Anti-diuretic hormone
- Generalised sympathetic stimulation etc.,

The effect of all these is to produce:

- Tachycardia
- Peripheral vasoconstriction
- Conservation of fluid by kidney

(b) ***Progressive phase:*** It is characterised by tissue hypo-perfusion and onset of ever widening circulatory and metabolic disorder. Uncorrected shock passes to progressive phase during which vital organs experience significant hypoxia. With persistent oxygen deficit, there is anaerobic glycolysis with excessive production of lactate (lactic acid), which induce metabolic lactic acidosis. Lowering of pH dilate microcirculation, cause pooling of blood, worsen cardiac output, cause anoxic injury to endothelial cells and cause disseminated intravascular coagulation (DIC). Function of vital organs begins to deteriorate (fail).Patient is confused, urinary output fall.

(c) ***Irreversible stage:*** This stage occurs if cellular and tissue injury is so severe that even if therapy correct haemodynamic defect, survival is not possible. In irreversible stage, wide spread cell injury allows leakage of lysosomal enzymes which further aggravate the shock stage. Myocardial depressant factor (NO) worsen already poor cardiac performance. At this stage patient have complete renal shut down due to acute tubular necrosis.

Morphological Changes

Morphological changers are similar to hypoxic injury. Failure of multiple organ system

Brain	:	Ischaemic encephalopathy
Heart	:	Sub endocardial haemorrhage and necrosis (zonal lesion)
Kidney	:	Acute tubular necrosis
Liver	:	Haemorrhagic necrosis
Lungs	:	Diffuse alveolar damage

Clinical Manifestation

(a) Hypovolemic/cardiogenic shock: hypotension, a sheen grey pallor (paleness), cool clammy (wet) cyanotic skin, threaddy pulse, rapid cardiac and respiratory rate, renal insufficiency.

(b) Septic shock -skin warm/flushed due to peripheral vasodilation.

7
Biological Effects of Radiation

Acute radiation syndrome (ARS), also known as radiation poisoning, radiation sickness or radiation toxicity, is the compilation of health effects which present within 24 hours of exposure to high amounts of ionizing radiation.

Effects of Radiation on Cells

The mechanism by which radiation causes damage to human tissue, or any other material, is by ionization of atoms in the material. Ionizing radiation absorbed by human tissue has enough energy to remove electrons from the atoms that make up molecules of the tissue. When the electron that was shared by the two atoms to form a molecular bond is dislodged by ionizing radiation, the bond is broken and thus, the molecule falls apart. When ionizing radiation interacts with cells, it may or may not strike a critical part of the cell.

Chromosomes are considered as the most critical part of the cell since they contain the genetic information and instructions required for the cell to perform its function and to make copies of itself for reproduction purposes. Cellular degradation due to damage to DNA and other key molecular structures within the cells in various tissues. This destruction, particularly as it affects ability of cells to divide normally, causes the symptoms. The symptoms can begin within one or two hours and may last for several months.

Skin Changes

Cutaneous radiation syndrome (CRS) refers to the skin symptoms of radiation exposure. Within a few hours after irradiation, a transient and inconsistent redness (associated with itching) can occur. Then, a latent phase may occur and last from a few days up to several weeks, after which, intense reddening, blistering and ulceration of the irradiated site are visible.

Healing occurs by regenerative means: however, very large skin doses can cause permanent hair loss, damaged sebaceous and sweat glands, atrophy, fibrosis (mostly Keloids), decreased or increased skin pigmentation, and ulceration or necrosis of the exposed tissue.

Cells are undamaged by the dose: Ionization may form chemically active substances which in some cases alter the structure of the cells. These alterations may be the same as those changes that occur naturally in the cell and may have no negative effect.

Cells are damaged: Repair the damage and operate normally some ionizing events produce substances not normally found in the cell. These can lead to a breakdown of the cell structure and its components. Cells can repair the damage if it is limited. Even damage to the chromosomes is usually repaired. Many thousands of chromosome aberrations (changes) occur constantly in our bodies. We have effective mechanisms to repair these changes.

Cells die as a result of the damage: If a cell is extensively damaged by radiation, or damaged in such a way that reproduction is affected, the cell may die. Radiation damage to cells may depend on how sensitive the cells are to radiation.

All cells are not equally sensitive to radiation damage cells which divide rapidly and/or are relatively non-specialized tend to show effects at lower doses of radiation then those which are less rapidly dividing and more specialized. e.g. - more sensitive cells are those which produce blood.

This system (called the hemopoietic system) is the most sensitive biological indicator of radiation exposure. The relative sensitivity of different human tissues to radiation can be seen by examining the progression of the Acute Radiation Syndrome.

Cancer

If a damaged cell needs to perform a function before it has had time to repair itself, it will either be unable to perform the repair function or perform the function incorrectly or incompletely. The result may be cells that cannot perform their normal functions or that now are damaging to other cells. These altered cells may be unable to reproduce themselves or may reproduce at an uncontrolled rate. Such cells can be the underlying causes of cancers.

According to the linear no-threshold model, any exposure to ionizing radiation, even at doses too low to produce any symptoms of radiation sickness can induce cancer due to cellular and genetic damage. The probability of developing cancer is a linear function with respect to the effective radiation dose.

In radiation-induced cancer, the speed at which the condition advances, the prognosis, the degree of pain, and every other feature of the disease are not believed to be functions of the radiation dosage.

Alpha and beta radiation have low penetrating power and are unlikely to affect vital internal organs from outside the body. During spaceflight, particularly flights beyond low Earth orbit, astronauts are exposed to both galactic cosmic radiation (GCR) and solar particle event (SPE) radiation. Evidence indicates past SPE radiation levels which would have been lethal for unprotected astronauts. GCR levels which might lead to acute radiation poisoning are less well understood.

Radiotherapy treatments are typically prescribed in terms of the local absorbed dose, which might be 60 Gy or higher. The dose is fractionated (about 2 Gy per day for curative treatment), which allows for the normal tissues to undergo repair, allowing it to tolerate a higher dose than would otherwise be expected. The dose to the targeted tissue mass must be averaged over the entire body mass, most of which receives negligible radiation, to arrive at a whole-body absorbed dose that can be compared to the table above.

Cell Phone Radiation and Oxidative Stress

Free radicals are a group of highly reactive molecules consisting of unpaired electrons in the outer orbit. Free radicals that are derived from oxygen metabolism are known as reactive oxygen species (ROS).

DNA strand break and apoptosis: DNA damage in cells may have an important implication as it is cumulative. Normally, DNA is capable of repairing itself. Through a homeostatic mechanism, cells maintain a delicate balance between DNA damage and repair. DNA damage accumulates if this balance is altered. Most cells can repair single-strand DNA breaks. However, DNA double strand breaks, if not properly repaired, are known to lead to cell death or apoptosis.

Effect on male reproductive system: A number of recent reports have suggested a possible link between cell phone use and male infertility men undergoing infertility evaluations and reported that the duration of possession and the daily. Pathophysiological effects of radiation are also observed on atherosclerosis development and progression, and the incidence of cardiovascular complications.

Radiation therapy while important in the management of several diseases is implicated in the causation of atherosclerosis and other cardiovascular complications. Subsequently, it was discovered that the heart is sensitive to radiation and many cardiac structures may be damaged by radiation exposure. A significantly higher risk of death due to ischemic heart disease has been reported for patients treated with radiation for Hodgkin's disease and breast cancer.

Certain cytokines and growth factors, such as TGF-β1 and IL-1 β, may stimulate radiation-induced endothelial proliferation, fibroblast proliferation, collagen deposition, and fibrosis leading to advanced lesions of atherosclerosis. The treatment for radiation-induced ischemic heart disease includes conventional pharmacological therapy, balloon angioplasty, and bypass surgery.

Endovascular irradiation has been shown to be effective in reducing restenosis-like response to balloon-catheter injury in animal models. Caution must be exercised when radiation therapy is combined with doxorubicin because there appears to be a synergistic toxic effect on the myocardium.

Damage to endothelial cells is a central event in the pathogenesis of damage to the coronary arteries. Certain growth factors that interfere with the apoptotic pathway may provide new therapeutic strategies for reducing the risk of radiation-induced damage to the heart. Somatic effects Somatic effects may be divided into two classes based on the rate at which the dose was received.

- Prompt somatic effects are those that occur soon after an acute dose (typically 10 rad or greater to the whole body in a short period of time).A prompt effect is the temporary hair loss which occurs about three weeks after a dose of 400 rad to the scalp. New hair is expected to grow within two months after the dose, although the color and texture may be different.

- Delayed somatic effects are those that may occur years after radiation doses are received. E.g. an increased potential for the development of cancer and cataracts. Since some forms of cancer are among the most probable delayed effects, the established dose limits were formulated with this risk in mind.

Genetic or heritable effects: appear in the future generations of the exposed person as a result of radiation damage to the reproductive cells. Genetic effects are abnormalities that may occur in the future generations of exposed individuals. Potential biological effects depend on how much and how fast a radiation dose is received. Radiation doses can be grouped into two categories acute and chronic radiation dose. Relatively smaller doses result in gastrointestinal effects, such as nausea and vomiting, and symptoms related to falling blood counts, such as infection and bleeding.

Relatively larger doses can result in neurological effects and rapid death. Treatment of acute radiation syndrome is generally supportive with blood transfusions and antibiotics, with some more exotic treatments, such as bone marrow transfusions, being required in extreme cases. Similar symptoms may appear months to years after exposure as chronic radiation syndrome when the dose rate is too low to cause the acute form. Radiation exposure can also increase the probability of developing some other diseases, mainly different types of cancers. These diseases are sometimes referred to as radiation sickness, but they are never included in the term acute radiation syndrome.

Acute Dose

An acute radiation dose is defined as a large dose (10 rad or greater, to the whole body) delivered during a short period of time (on the order of a few days at the most). If large enough, it may result in effects which are observable within a period of hours to weeks.

Acute doses can cause a pattern of clearly identifiable symptoms (syndromes). These conditions are referred to in general as Acute Radiation Syndrome. Radiation sickness symptoms are apparent following acute doses >100 rad.

Blood-forming organ (Bone marrow) syndrome (>100 rad) is characterized by damage to cells that divide at the most rapid pace (such as bone marrow, the spleen and lymphatic tissue). Symptoms include internal bleeding, fatigue, bacterial infections, and fever.

Gastrointestinal tract syndrome (>1000 rad) is characterized by damage to cells that divide less rapidly (such as the linings of the stomach and intestines). Symptoms include nausea, vomiting, diarrhea, dehydration, electrolytic imbalance, loss of digestion ability, bleeding ulcers, and the symptoms of blood-forming organ syndrome.

Central nervous system syndrome (>5000 rad) is characterized by damage to cells that do not reproduce such as nerve cells. Symptoms include loss of coordination, confusion, coma, convulsions, shock, and the symptoms of the blood forming organ and gastrointestinal tract syndromes. Scientists now have evidence that death under these conditions is not caused by actual radiation damage to the nervous system, but rather from complications caused by internal bleeding, and fluid and pressure build-up on the brain. Other effects from an acute dose include:

- 200 to 300 rad to the skin can result in the reddening of the skin (erythema), similar to mild sunburn and may result in hair loss due to damage to hair follicles.
- 125 to 200 rad to the ovaries can result in prolonged or permanent suppression of menstruation in about fifty percent (50%) of women.
- 600 rad to the ovaries or testicles can result in permanent sterilization.
- 50 rad to the thyroid gland can result in benign (non-cancerous) tumors.

As a group, the effects caused by acute doses are called deterministic. Broadly speaking, this means that severity of the effect is determined by the amount of dose received. Deterministic effects usually have some threshold level - below which, the effect will probably not occur, but above which the effect is expected. When the dose is above the threshold, the severity of the effect increases as the dose increases.

Chronic Dose

A chronic dose is a relatively small amount of radiation received over a long period of time. The body is better equipped to tolerate a chronic dose than an acute dose. The body has time to repair damage because a smaller percentage of the cells need repair at any given time. The body also has time to replace dead or non-functioning cells with new, healthy cells. This is the type of dose received as occupational exposure. These effects include some forms of cancer and genetic effects.

Prenatal radiation exposure: Since an embryo/fetus is especially sensitive to radiation (embryo/fetus cells are rapidly dividing) special considerations are given to pregnant workers. Protection of the embryo/fetus is important because the embryo/fetus is considered to be at the most radiosensitive stage of human development, particularly in the first 20 weeks of pregnancy. Potential effects associated with prenatal radiation doses include:

- Growth retardation
- Small head/brain size
- Mental retardation
- Childhood cancer

8

Environmental and Nutritional Diseases

The health consequences of climate change will depend on its extent and rapidity, the severity of the ensuing consequences, and humankind's ability to mitigate the damaging effects. Even in the best case scenario, however, climate change is expected to have a serious negative impact on human health by increasing the incidence of a number of diseases, including

- Cardiovascular, cerebrovascular, and respiratory diseases, all of which will be exacerbated by heat waves and air pollution.

- Gastroenteritis, cholera, and other food- and water-borne infectious diseases, caused by contamination as a consequence of floods and disruption of clean water supplies and sewage treatment, after heavy rains and other environmental disasters.

- Vector-borne infectious diseases, such as malaria and dengue fever, due to changes in vector number and geographic distribution related to increased temperatures, crop failures and more extreme weather variation (e.g., more frequent and severe El Niño events).

- Malnutrition, caused by changes in local climate that disrupt crop production. Such changes are anticipated to be most severe in tropical locations, in which average temperatures may already be near or above crop tolerance levels. It is estimated that by 2080, agricultural productivity may decline by 10% to 25% in some developing countries as a consequence of climate change.

Toxicity of Chemical and Physical Agents

Toxicology is defined as the science of poisons. It studies the distribution, effects, and mechanisms of action of toxic agents. More broadly, it also includes the study of the effects of physical agents such as radiation and heat. We now consider some basic principles regarding the toxicity of exogenous chemicals and drugs.

- The definition of a poison is basically a quantitative concept strictly dependent on dosage. Pollutants contained in air, water, and soil is absorbed through. Xenobiotics are exogenous chemicals in the environment that may be absorbed by the body through inhalation, ingestion, or skin contact.

- Chemicals may be excreted in urine or feces or eliminated in expired air, or they may accumulate in bone, fat, brain, or other tissues.

- Chemicals may act at the site of entry, or they may be transported to other sites. Some agents are not modified upon entry in the body, but most solvents and drugs are metabolized to form water-soluble products (detoxification) or are activated to form toxic metabolites.

- Most solvents and drugs are lipophilic, which facilitates their transport in the blood by lipoproteins and penetration through lipid components of cell membranes.

- Xenobiotic metabolism. Xenobiotics can be metabolized to nontoxic metabolites and eliminated. The reactions that metabolize xenobiotics into nontoxic products, or activate xenobiotics to generate toxic compounds, occur in two phases. In phase I reactions, chemicals can undergo hydrolysis, oxidation, or reduction. Products of phase I reactions often are metabolized into water-soluble compounds through Phase II reactions of glucuronidation, sulfation, methylation, and conjugation with glutathione (GSH). Water-soluble compounds are readily excreted.

- The most important cellular enzyme system involved in phase I reactions is the cytochrome P-450 system, located primarily in the endoplasmic reticulum (ER) of the liver but also present in skin, lungs, and gastrointestinal (GI) mucosa and in practically every organ. The system catalyzes reactions that either detoxify xenobiotics or activate xenobiotics into active compounds that cause cellular injury. Both types of reactions may produce, as a byproduct, reactive oxygen species (ROS), which can cause cellular damage. Examples of metabolic activation of chemicals through the P-450 system are the conversion of carbon tetrachloride to the toxic trichloromethyl free radical and the generation of a DNA-binding metabolite from benzo [a] pyrene (BaP), a carcinogen present in cigarette smoke. The cytochrome P-450 system also participates in the metabolism of a large number of common therapeutic drugs such as acetaminophen, barbiturates, and anticonvulsants, and in alcohol metabolism.

- P-450 enzymes vary widely in activity among different people, owing to both polymorphisms in the genes encoding the enzymes and interactions with drugs that are metabolized through the system. The activity of the enzymes also may be decreased by fasting or starvation, and increased by alcohol consumption and smoking.

Nutritional Diseases

Not only in 3rd world countries! - even developed ones - poor social classes (namely children), homeless persons, lonely aged people, chronic alcoholics, patients with psychiatric disorders (anorexia nervosa, bulimia nervosa)

- Primary (shortage of nutrition)

- Secondary (metabolic disorders, increased requirements - growth, pregnancy, increased losses (chronic diseases)

Protein-Energy Malnutrition

- Most frequent and most important
- Dimension of epidemy (Africa - Ethiopia - up to 25% of children; 50% of all deaths are children <5y)
- Range of clinical syndromes, 2 main forms - marasmus & kwashiorkor
- Deficiency of proteins, mainly animal.
- Most common in Africa. Children, who have been weaned too early (arrival of another child) and fed by exclusively carbohydrate diet.
- Kwashiorkor is more severe than marasmus - loss of visceral proteins - hypoalbuminemia - generalized edema, ascites
- Skin lesions, hair changes, fatty liver, defects of immunity, secondary infections, anemia

Marasmus

- Deficiency of energy (calories) - due to starving – growth retardation - arrest, loss of muscle mass, serum albumin is normal, subcutaneous fat is used as a fuel - extremities are emaciated
- Anemia, immune deficiency (namely cellular immunity)

Vitamin Deficiencies

- For healthy body 45-50 compounds are necessary (9 amino acids, 2 fatty acids, several trace elements and 13 vitamins).Vitamin deficiency are of two types, primary (diet) or secondary (malabsorption, metabolic disorders, liver diseases)

Deficiency state

- *Eyes:* xerophtalmia, small corneal opaque (squamous keratinizing) plaques (Bitot's spots), keratomalacia > total blindness
- *Respiratory tract:* squamous metaplasia, pulmonary infections
- *Urinary tract:* pelvic keratinization > stones
- *Skin:* hyperkeratosis

Vitamin D

Maintenance of normal plasma Ca and P levels, important for normal development and mineralization of bones. Two sources are involved. They are:

- Endogenous synthesis in the skin (UV light) from 7-dehydrocholesterol - 80% of needed amount
- Exogenous - dietary sources (deep-sea fish, plants, grains)

Causes of hypo-vitaminosis

- Decreased endogenous synthesis (inadequate exposure to sunlight)
- Decreased absorption (dietary lack, malabsorption syndrome)
- Enhanced degradation (drugs)
- Impaired synthesis of metabolites (liver diseases, renal disorders)
- Target resistance (congenital lack of receptors)
- Phosphate depletion (renal tubular disorders, long-term use of antacids)

Deficiency state

- Children - before closing of epiphyses - rickets (rachitic rosary, pigeon breast deformity, lumbar lordosis, bowing of the legs)
- Adults - after closing of epiphyses - osteomalacia (impaired remodelation of bone mass, no mineralization of osteoid - microfractures (vertebral bodies, femoral necks)
- HypervitaminosisD - hypercalcaemia - metastatic calcification, urolithiasis

Vitamin K

- Required cofactor for synthesis of clotting factors VII, IX, X Causes of hypovitaminosis:
- Fat malabsorption syndromes
- Destruction of endogenous vitamin K synthesizing flora (broad spectrum ATB)
- Neonatal period (low reserve, no bacterial flora)
- Diffuse liver disease
- Iatrogenic decrease (warfarin)

Deficiency state

- Bleeding diathesis (e.g. Hemorrhagic disease of the newborn - intracranial bleeding, any site - skin, umbilicus, viscera)
- Adults - hematomas, hematuria, melena, ecchymoses, bleeding from the gums

Vitamins B

- Coenzymes
- Major source - grains, rice, vegetables, fish, meat, yeast, seed oils
- In deficiency - involved mainly highly metabolic active tissues with short cell-turnover period (skin, oral mucosa, stomach, bone marrow, neural system)

Vitamin B1 (Thiamine)

- Widely available in the diet – non polished rice, grains
- Avitaminosis in 3rd world - in severe malnutrition

- Avitaminosis in developed countries - in chronic alcoholics (25%!) (malnutrition, decreased absorption from the gut)
- Affected peripheral nerves, heart, brain
- Dry beri-beri (polyneuropathy) - degeneration of myelin sheaths and axons (motoric, sensoric and vegetative)
- Wet beri-beri (cardiovascular syndrome) - dilatation, right heart failure, peripheral edema
- Wernicke-korsakoff syndrome - ophthalmoplegia, nystagmus, ataxia of gait and stance, confusion, apathy, amnesia, psychosis

Vitamin B2 (Riboflavin)

- Avitaminosis associated with changes at the angles of the mouth (cheilosis or cheilitis), glossitis, ocular (keratitis) and skin changes (nasolabial dermatitis), bone marrow (erythroid hypoplasia - anemia)

Niacin (Nicotinic acid)

Deficiency state:

- Pellagra (rough skin) - 3 Ds
- Dermatitis - neck - chronic inflammation, fissures, depigmentation, hyperpigmentation
- Diarrhea - atrophy of columnar epithelium of GIT mucosa, inflammation and subsequent ulceration
- Dementia - degeneration of the neurons of the brain

Vitamin B12 (Cyanocobalamine)

- Deficiency in strict vegetarians or in chronic atrophic gastritis - pernicious anemia (lack of synthesis of intrinsic factor in gastric mucosa due to autoimmune inflammation with severe destruction of corporal glands)
- In deficiency - megaloblastic anemia (decreased number of RBC, increased size; hyper-segmentation of neutrophilic leucocytes) and demyelinization of spinal cord and peripheral nerves, which is a neuroanemic syndrome

Vitamin C (Ascorbic acid)

- Fruits and vegetables - not synthesized endogenously
- Involved in metabolism of collagen and basic intercellular matrix - involvement of vessel walls - increased fragility - bleeding
- Deficiency in adults - scurvy
- Deficiency in children - möller-barlow disease - subperiostal hematomas

Scurvy
- Sailors, travelers, today elderly persons, homeless people, etc.
- petechial skin bleeding, ecchymoses, epistaxis, melena, intraarticular bleeding
- gingival swelling, hemorrhages, secondary bacterial infection - periodontitis
- hyperkeratotic papular rash
- impaired wound healing, defective osteoid - pathologic fractures
- anemia

Hypervitaminosis C
- Mega doses of vitamin C (several grams/day) - no effect in prevention or in treatment
- Excretion into urine - urolithiasis
- Hyperacidity in stomach - mucosal erosions

Trace Elements
- 14 inorganic elements - Fe, Cu, Co, I, Zn, Se, Mn, Mo, Cr, F, Si, Ni, Sn (tin), Va
- activity in enzymes
- primary deficiency - only I (thyroid gland - goiter)
- secondary deficiency:
- Zn - skin lesions, neurological and psychiatric syndromes, growth retardation, hypogonadism in males
- Cu - ancmia, impaired synthesis of connective tissue matrix
- Se - China - Keshan disease - dilated cardiomyopathy

Obesity
- Disorder of energetic balance - food derived energy chronically exceeds energy expenditure, excess calories are stored as fat
- Some genetic predispositions (multifactorial disease)

Diet and Cancer
- Not completely clear - no clear evidence, that diet can cause or prevent from ca
- Most frequently accused: Red meat, animal fat, cholesterol, refined sugar, chemical additives
- Assumption of WHO - 1/3 of all cancers are due to improper nutrition
- Oral cavity, pharynx, esophagus - alcohol, smoking of cigarettes
- Colorectal cancer - increased intake of fat, reduced intake of fibers
- Liver cancer - aphlatoxin (nuts, grains) - cirrhosis - hepatocellular ca
- Breast cancer - fat intake (in USA 10% of females - increasing incidence)

Pathogenesis of Starvation

The terms malnutrition and starvation are used interchangeably, when in reality, there are specific definitions for each. Malnutrition is the inadequate intake of any of the required nutrients. This can even occur in animal receiving large amounts of food, but is not able to ingest, digest, absorb, or utilize this food. Causes for this inability are injuries, poor teeth, parasitism, disease, foreign bodies in the digestive tract, tumors, or an increased motility of the digestive tract. Malnutrition can also occur if the food is inadequate in one or more of the required nutrients. If an animal is not able to obtain food for an extended period of time either for the above reasons or due to an unavailability of food or insufficient energy intake, this is defined as starvation. Malnutrition and starvation can be caused by diseases, injuries, the range the animal lives on, or the environmental conditions it must live in. Starvation and malnutrition occur in several wildlife species and routinely eliminates the young, old, weak, and sick animals. Winter is when mortality usually occurs due to the negative energy balance brought about by the cold weather, deep snow, increased energy demands, snow covered food, and human and predator induced stress.

Pathophysiology

If an animal is forced into an inadequate plane of nutrition, there are many physiological changes as the animal attempts to satisfy its energy requirements. At the cellular level, catabolism (the breaking down in the body of complex chemical compounds into simpler ones) continues to supply the substances required for anabolism (the usage of nutritive matter and its conversion into living substance) and to continue vital functions. Reserve stores of nutrients contained in the individual are utilized to compensate for the lack of nutritional intake. Energy is generated from the utilization of proteins, fats, and carbohydrates.

The most readily usable material, the carbohydrate glycogen, is utilized first. This is derived from glycogen stored in the liver and is exhausted within a few hours. This is followed by stored fat from the various subcutaneous deposits, around the kidney, and in the mesentery and omentum tissue.

Fat deposits in the parenchymatous organs are utilized next. The last area of the body to lose its fat deposits is the marrow of the bones. The final source of energy available is the protein comprising the cytoplasm of the cells. It is at this time that ketosis and an increase in nitrogen excretion may occur.

Ketosis (a condition in which ketone substances appear in the blood and urine) is commonly seen in malnourished animals. This is because it is necessary for the animal to derive its energy from the stored fat and protein. After all the fat reserves have been exhausted, nitrogen excretion rises due to the protein catabolism which occurs just prior to death.

The animal will eventually reach a point where the cells of the body are unable to perform the functions necessary for life. Death results from lack of sufficient blood glucose to provide the energy needs of the brain and hypoglycemic shock occurs.

Cachexia causes weight loss and increased mortality. Other causes of weight loss include anorexia, sarcopenia, and dehydration. The pathophysiology of cachexia appears to be cytokine excess. Other potential mediators include testosterone and insulin-like growth factor I deficiency, excess myostatin, and excess glucocorticoids. Numerous diseases can result in cachexia, each by a slightly different mechanism. Both nutritional support and orexigenic agents play a role in the management of cachexia.

Cytokines in the Pathogenesis of Cachexia

Cytokines are cell-associated proteins produced by inflammatory cells that function as paracrine intercellular mediators. Systemic inflammation mediated through cell injury or activation of the immune system triggers an acute inflammatory response that causes excess cytokine elaboration. Cytokines play a major role in immunomodulation and have been implicated in the etiology of anorexia, weight loss, cognitive dysfunction, anemia, and frailty. Excessive elaboration of proinflammatory cytokines such as interleukin IL-1, IL-2, interferon γ, and tumor necrosis factor α (TNF-α) is probably the most common cause of cachexia observed in acutely ill patients.

Cytokines activate nuclear transcription factor κB (NF-κB), which results in decreased muscle protein synthesis. Cytokine activation is also responsible for the reduction of MyoD protein, a transcription factor that modulates signaling pathways involved in muscle development. MyoD binding to myosin heavy chain IIb promoter region is necessary for myosin expression in fast twitch muscles.

TNF-α and interferon γ act synergistically to inhibit the activation of messenger RNA for myosin heavy chain synthesis. TNF-α and interferon γ are highly specific for stimulating the proteolysis of myosin heavy chains.

Starvation Ketosis: When hepatic glycogen stores are exhausted (after 12-24 hours of total fasting), the liver produces ketones to provide an energy substrate for peripheral tissues. Ketoacidosis can appear after an overnight fast but it typically requires 3 to 14 days of starvation to reach maximal severity.

Typical ketoanion levels are only 1 to 2 mmol/l and this will not much alter the anion gap. The acidosis even with quite prolonged fasting is only ever of mild to moderate severity with ketoanion levels up to a maximum of 3 to 5 mmol/l and plasma pH down to 7.3. This is probably due to the insulin level, which though lower, is still enough to keep the FFA levels less than 1mM. This limits substrate delivery to the liver restraining hepatic ketogenesis. Ketone bodies also stimulate some insulin release from the islets. The anion gap will usually not be much elevated.

9
Pathophysiology of Common Diseases

Degenerative Diseases of Brain (Parkinsonism, Alzheimer's Disease)

Degenerative Diseases of Brain

These are diseases of grey matter characterised principally by progressive loss of neurons with associated secondary changes in white matter. Pattern of neurological loss is selective affecting one/more neurons while leaving others intact. Disease arises without any previous neurological deficit. In some diseases, there is intra cellular abnormalities (like lewy bodies, neurofibrillatory tangles). In others, there is only loss of affected neuron.

Degenerative diseases are classified according to anatomical regions of the brain that are primarily affected:

- ***Degenerative disease affecting cerebral cortex:*** Their principal clinical manifestation is dementia that is progressive loss of cognitive function independent of state of attention. E.g., Alzheimer's disease (AD) – Picks disease.

- ***Degenerative disease of basal ganglia and brain stem:*** Disease affecting these regions of brain is frequently associated with movement disorders like rigidity, abnormal posturing and chorea (involuntary, purposeless, rapid motion). They manifest either as reduction in voluntary movement/abundance of involuntary movement. E.g., Idiopathic Parkinson disease – Shy drager's syndrome, Progressive supranuclear palsy – Striatonigral degeneration

(i) Parkinsonism (Idiopathic Parkinson disease)

Definition: Parkinsonism is a clinical syndrome characterised by diminished facial expression, stooped posture (bend posture), slowness of voluntary movement, festinating giat (style of walking-progressively shortened and accelerated steps), rigidity and pill rolling tremor. This type of motor disturbances seen in number of conditions that have in common damage to nigrostriatal dopaminergic system. Parkinsonism may be induced by drugs that affect this system particularly dopamine antagonist and toxins.

Pathophysiology: The disease seen with increasing frequency in old age. Few patients with idiopathic Parkinson disease present with dementia clinically similar to that of Alzheimer's disease. Epidemiological data shows genetic, viral and environmental toxins as possible cause. It is a commonly occurring degenerative disorder of basal ganglia caused by failure/damage of nigrostriatal dopaminergic system.

Dopaminergic neurons of substantia nigra project to the striatum and their degeneration in Parkinson disease is associated with reduction in striatal dopamine content. Nigral and basal ganglial loss of neurons with depletion of dopamine (an inhibitory neurotransmitter) is the principal biochemical alteration in Parkinson's disease.

There is imbalance in the dopaminergic (inhibitory) and cholinergic (excitatory) in caudate and putamen of basal ganglia. This is manifested by hypertonia (tremor and rigidity) and akinasia (immobility). Severity of the motor syndrome is proportional to dopamine deficiency. Involvement of other receptor may contribute to dementia.

Parkinson's disease can be induced by drugs that affect this system like dopamine antagonist, toxins (MPTP), neuroleptics, anti-emetics etc. [MPTP: 1-methyl, 4-phnyl, 1, 2, 3, 4,-tetra hydro pyridine].

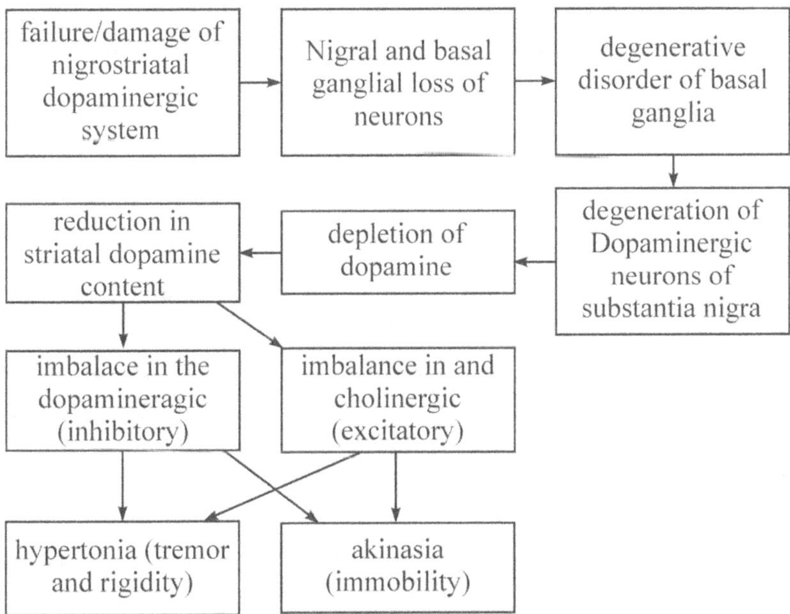

Fig. 9.1 Pathophysiology of parkinson's disease.

Clinical manifestations: Parkinson's disease begins at the age of 40. Clinical manifestations include:

- Diminished facial expressions, stooped posture, slowness of voluntary movement, festinating giat (progressively shortened accelerated steps), rigidity, pill rolling tremor, slurred speech, etc.,
- Autonomic effects: inappropriate diaphoresis, orthostatic hypotension, gastric retention, constipation, urinary retention etc.,
- Dementia, depression

Pathology: Typical gross finding is pallor of substantia nigra/locus ceruleus. Microscopically there is loss pigmented -catecholaminergic neurons in the region associated with gliosis [an excess astroglia] (neuroglial cells) in damaged area of CNS. Lewy bodies may be found in some remaining neurons-they are intra cytoplasmic eosinophilic round elongated inclusions that have dense core surrounded by pallor rim.

Treatment: Treatment of Parkinson disease is symptomatic. Dopamine deficiency is corrected by replacement therapy with L-dopa (precursor of dopamine). Recent development in IPD is neural transplantation, stereotactic implants of foetal mesenchymal tissue in to striatum

(ii) Alzheimer's Disease

Definition: Dementia of all etiologies is one of the most commonly encountered organic mental syndromes. Alzheimer's disease-is primary degenerative dementia (PDD).Dementia of Alzheimer's type is a severe cognitive dysfunction (understanding disability) in older person which selectively affects neurons in basal forebrain, amygdala, hippocampus and cerebral cortex.

Pathophysiology: The major morphologic CNS alterations in PDD include– cortical atrophy, neuronal loss, neuro-fibrillatory tangles, and neuritic plaques. Deterioration in neuronal cytoskeletal structure can also occur. These structures are important for supporting neuronal metabolism, surface membrane components and cellular transport of neurotransmitters. These changes can disturb neurotransmission resulting in alteration in receptor function in specific brain regions.

PDD (primary degenerative dementia) selectively affect neurons in basal forebrain, amygdala, hippocampus, and cerebral cortex. Hippocampus, entorhinal cortex (in temporal lobe), amygdala are required for normal memory function. Cholinergic dysfunction is a common finding in memory and cognitive defect.

PDD affect the cholinergic neurons of cerebral cortex, hippocampus and amygdala [decrease choline acyl transferase activity and decreased cholinergic transmission]. Nucleus basilis is the principal source of extrinsic cholinergic innervation of cortex. Degeneration of this nucleus in PDD results in reduction of cholinergic transmission to cortex and other neuronal system.

Attention has been focused on Aβ and its precursor protein- APP (amyloid precursor protein) as possible etiologic agent. Normal processing of APP includes cleavage of peptide bond in middle of Aβ sequence-this prevents the formation of insoluble aggregates of Aβ. Mutation in gene coding for amyloid precursor protein cause a deposition of amyloid (A, β-4,3,-amino acid peptide).

The development of amyloid deposits occurs from abnormal processing of precursor molecule-in such a way that increased amount of this peptide accumulates. Increased rate of generation of amyloidogenic Aβ have been found in cells expressing some of the mutations associated with FAD (familial Alzheimer's disease). In PDD post mortem specimens shows high density of neuro-fibrillatory tangles and neuritic plaques in cortex and hippocampus.

Morphology: Gross examination of brain shows variable degree of cortical atrophy with widening of cerebral sulci that is most pronounced in frontal, temporal and parietal lobes. There is compensatory ventricular enlargement secondary to loss parenchyma. Microscopic abnormalities of AD are neurofibrillatory tangles, senile (neuritic) plaques and amyloid angiopathy (blood vessel).

- *Neurofibrillatory tangles:* are abnormal neurons in which cytoplasm filled with sub-microscopic filamentous structure that displace/ encircle the nucleus. Ultra structurally-they are composed of paired helical filaments (PHF).

- *Neuritic plaques (senile plaques):* are formed from degenerated neurons-and has an amyloid core. Neuritic plaques are focal spherical collection of dilated, tortuous, silver-staining neuritc process (dystrophic neuritis)-surrounding a central amyloid core. Plaques can be formed in hippocampus, amygdala, and neocortex. The dominant component of plaque core is -Aβ 4, 3, amino acid peptide-derived from amyloid precursor protein-(APP).

Clinical manifestation: Usually occur above 50years.The disease becomes clinically apparent as insidious impairment of higher intellectual functions with alterations in mood and behaviour. Later progressive disorientation, memory loss, aphasia [defect/loss of the power of expression by speech writing or signs or of comprehending spoken/written language due toinjury/disease of the brain centres]-indicating severe cortical dysfunction-eventually over 5-10 years patient become profoundly disabled, mute and immobile.

Individual become progressively more forgetful over time-particularly in relation to recent events. Memory loss increase as disease advances- and person become disoriented, confused and loss the ability to concentrate. Abstraction, problem solving and judgement skills gradually deteriorate. Failure of mathematical calculation ability, language, visual and spacial perception. Dyspraxia [partial loss of ability to perform co-ordinated acts]. Deterioration of cognition [include all aspects of thinking, perceiving, remembering].

Behavioural changes: Behavioural reaction caused by patient's awareness of their deterioration. Irritability, agitation, restlessness, anxiety, depression. Motor changes may also occur like hand eye incoordination, imbalance etc. With continued deterioration patient become totally dependent on environment for orienting cues (continuation of speech).

Evaluation and treatment: From history, mental status evaluation, course of illness, biopsy, or autopsy. Use of memory aid. Maintaining unimpaired cognitive functions. Maintain/improving general state of hygiene, nutrition and health.

(iii) Schizophrenia

Definition: Schizophrenia is a mental disorder characterized by a disintegration of the processes of thinking and of emotional responsiveness, is complex. A number of theories attempt to explain the link between altered brain function and schizophrenia.

Pathophysiology: *Hypothesis:*

1. The dopamine hypothesis of schizophrenia. This attributes psychosis to the faulty distribution, regulation, and function of dopaminergic neurons. Dopamine is involved in the advancement and reinforcement of the abnormal thought patterns inschizophrenia. Dopamine facilitates abnormal long-term potentiation within the striatum, basal ganglia, cingulate cortex (specifically the cingulate gyrus), and prefrontal cortex, among other limbic system structures. The "dopamine hypothesis of schizophrenia" proposes that a malfunction involving dopamine pathways is the cause of (the positive symptoms of) schizophrenia. High levels of D2 receptors intensify brain signals and can exacerbate positive symptoms (i.e. hallucinations and paranoia) in schizophrenia. It is still thought that dopamine mesolimbic pathways may be hyperactive, resulting in hyperstimulation of D2 receptors and positive symptoms.

2. Glutamate hypothesis of schizophrenia Interest has also focused on the neurotransmitter glutamate and the reduced function of the NMDA glutamate receptor in schizophrenia. The glutamate blocking drugs such as phencyclidine and ketamine can mimic the symptoms and cognitive problems associated with the condition. Reduced glutamate function is linked to poor performance by frontal lobe and hippocampal function. Glutamate affect dopamine function thereby ensuring the role of glutamate pathways in schizophrenia. ErbB4 protein abnormalities are also associated with neuro-pathophysiology of the schizophrenic brain.

A reduction of cAMP levels in these glutaminergic neurons lowers the activity of the NMDA receptor, a receptor crucial for the phenomena of LTP. This then leads to altered K+, Na+, and Ca 2+ levels within the cell. Protein reelin, is a crucial modulator of NMDA function in the hippocampus. It is in lowered concentrations in both schizophrenic and psychotic bipolar disorder patients.

This protein enhances Long Term Potentiation (LTP) activity. The risk for psychotic disorders is associated with alterations in the expression and distribution of a wide variety of G protein coupled receptors. The presynaptic metabotropic receptors are of specific interest in this disorder. They act as auto receptors, regulating glycine and glutamate receptors, also known as NMDA receptors. NMDA receptors are unique in that they are voltage dependent and are blocked by Mg2+ ions. Only when there is a depolarization do these Ca2+ channels open. This is the primary reason for the phenomena of LTP.

The NMDA component has largely been suggested by abnormally low levels of glutamate receptors found in postmortem brains of people previously diagnosed with schizophrenia. It involves a complex interplay between 5-HT1A, 5-HT2A, 5-HT1B, 5-HT2C, 5-HT6, and 5-HT7, D2, D1, the endocannabinoid system, including CB2, which regulates glial cell NT release.

3. ***Serotonin hypothesis of schizophrenia:*** Serotonin has been implicated in a variety of behaviors and somatic functions that are disturbed in schizophrenia: cognition, including memory; perception and attention; sensory gating; mood; aggression; sexual drive; appetite; energy level; pain sensitivity; endocrine function; and sleep. The biochemical and anatomical complexity and diversity of the serotonergic system and its extensive interactions with multiple neurotransmitters provide the physiological substrate for the ability of 5-HT to influence all these behaviors.

4. Another hypothesis of schizophrenia formulated included abnormal immune system development which explains roles of prenatal hazards, post-pubertal onset, stress, genes, climate, infections, and brain dysfunction. The immune hypothesis is supported by findings of high levels of immune markers in the blood of schizophrenia patients. High levels of immune markers have also been associated with having more severe psychotic symptoms.

Neurological:

Those with a diagnosis of schizophrenia have both changes in brain structure and brain chemistry, including dopamine. That differences seem to most commonly occur in the frontal lobes, hippocampus and temporal lobes. Due to the alteration in neural circuits some feel schizophrenia should be viewed as a collection of neuro developmental disorders. These differences have been linked to the neurocognitive deficits often associated with schizophrenia.

Abnormal findings in the prefrontal cortex, temporal cortex and anterior cingulate cortex are found before the first onset of schizophrenia symptoms. These regions are the regions of structural deficits found in schizophrenia and first-episode patients. Positive symptoms, such as thoughts of being persecuted, were found to be related to the medial prefrontal cortex, amygdala, and hippocampus region. Negative symptoms were found to be related to the ventrolateral prefrontal cortex and ventral striatum.

Psychological:

Many psychological mechanisms have been implicated in the development and maintenance of schizophrenia. Cognitive biases have been identified in those with the diagnosis or those at risk, especially when under stress or in confusing situations. Some cognitive features may reflect global neurocognitive deficits such as memory loss, while others may be related to particular issues and experiences.

Despite a demonstrated appearance of blunted effect, recent findings indicate that many individuals diagnosed with schizophrenia are emotionally responsive, particularly to stressful or negative stimuli, and that such sensitivity may cause vulnerability to symptoms or to the disorder. Evidence for the role of psychological mechanisms comes from the effects of psychotherapies on symptoms of schizophrenia.

Early hypotheses linking hallucinogens and schizophrenia:

The first hypotheses were concerning the involvement of 5-HT in schizophrenia by Wooley and Shaw and Gaddum based on the attribution of the psychotomimetic effects of lysergic acid diethylamide (LSD, which is structurally related to 5-HT and its antagonists at brain 5-HT receptors. These investigators proposed that serotonergic activity might be decreased in schizophrenia. The major problems with this hypothesis was that the primary effect of LSD was to produce visual hallucinations, which are relatively rare in schizophrenia, not auditory hallucinations, which are the most common perceptual disturbance in schizophrenia. Additionally, paranoid delusions, conceptual disorganization, and the wide range of cognitive impairments characteristic of schizophrenia: disturbances in working memory, semantic memory, and executive function, are generally absent during LSD intoxication. Another problem with the LSD hypothesis was that LSD is a full or partial agonist rather than antagonists at many 5-HT receptors.

The 5-HT deficiency hypothesis was superseded by the proposal that the production of endogenous methylated indoleamines with psychotomimetic properties (e.g., N, N-dimethyl tryptamines) might be important to the etiopathology of schizophrenia. However, no consistent differences were found in the amounts of the N-methyl-transferase enzyme which synthesizes this type of compound in the brain, the level of methylated indoleamines, or their metabolites in plasma or urine of schizophrenic patients and normal controls.

The serotonin hypothesis of schizophrenia:

A relatively small group of biochemical and psychopharmacologic studies constituted the main effort in this regard. Biochemical studies of the density of specific types of 5-HT receptors in brain generally produced intriguing findings that supported the hypothesis of some type of serotonergic dysfunction in schizophrenia. The major breakthrough restoring interest in the role of 5-HT in schizophrenia was the identification of numerous 5-HT receptor subtypes and their extensive impact on multiple neurotransmitters and behaviors. In addition, it was thought that at least some of the extraordinary ability of clozapine to improve schizophrenic symptoms more effectively and with fewer side effects than typical neuroleptics could be attributed to its ability to block 5-HT 2 A receptors.

Etiology of schizophrenia Serotonin has been implicated in a variety of behaviors and somatic functions that are disturbed in schizophrenia: cognition, including memory; perception and attention; sensory gating; mood; aggression; sexual drive; appetite; energy level; pain sensitivity; endocrine function; and sleep.

The biochemical and anatomical complexity and diversity of the serotonergic system provide the physiological substrate for the ability of 5-HT to influence all these behaviors. There might be enhanced dopaminergic and serotonergic neurotransmission in subcortical areas in schizophrenia, leading to positive symptoms, and decreased dopaminergic and serotonergic activity, perhaps in the prefrontal cortex, which led to negative symptoms. Functional alterations in the serotonergic system (including both pre-and postsynaptic function) affect multiple neurotransmitter systems (e.g., glutamate, GABA, norepinephrine [NE], acetylcholine, and DA) and cause the various behavioral disturbances in schizophrenia. Pharmacologic manipulation of the serotonergic system can reduce or exacerbate positive, negative or disorganization symptoms and cognitive function, as well as modulate extrapyramidal function (e.g., extrapyramidal symptoms [EPS] and tardive dyskinesia or dystonia [TD]).

Taken together, these findings support the role of brain 5-HT dysfunction in schizophrenia. However, CSF 5-HIAA levels, at best, provide an integrated measure of serotonergic activity in multiple brain regions. They cannot distinguish between selective changes in different regions or provide any index of the necessary integration between serotonergic activity and that of other neurotransmitters.

(iv)   Depression and Mania

Definition: Scientific studies have found that numerous brain areas show altered activity in patients suffering from depression, and this has encouraged advocates of various theories that seek to identify a biochemical origin of the disease, as opposed to theories that emphasize psychological or situational causes. Among the theories of a biologically based cause of depression are those involving genetics and circadian rhythms, but the most prominent and widely researched is the monoamine hypothesis.

Circadian rhythm: Depression may be related to the same brain mechanisms that control the cycles of sleep and wakefulness and therefore may be related to abnormalities in the circadian rhythm, or biological clock. F or example, rapid eye movement (REM) sleep— the stage in which dreaming occurs—may be quick to arrive and intense in depressed people. REM sleep depends on decreased serotonin levels in the brain stem. Overall, the serotonergic system is least active during sleep and most active during wakefulness. Prolonged wakefulness due to sleep deprivation activates serotonergic neurons, leading to processes similar to the therapeutic effect of antidepressants, such a s the selective serotonin reuptake inhibitors (SSRIs). Depressed individuals can exhibit a significant lift in mood after a night of sleep deprivation.

SSRIs may directly depend on the increase of central serotonergic neurotransmission for their therapeutic effect, the same system that impacts cycles of sleep and wakefulness. Synapses are gaps between nerve cells. These cells convert their electrical impulses into bursts of chemical relayers, called neurotransmitters, which travel across the synapses to receptors on adjacent cells, triggering electrical impulse s to travel down the latter cells. Monoamines are neurotransmitters and neuromodulators that include serotonin, dopamine, norepinephrine, and epinephrine. Many antidepressant drugsincrease synaptic levels of the monoamine neurotransmitter serotonin, but they may also enhance the levels of two other neuro transmitters, norepinephrine and dopamine. The observation of this efficacy led to the mono amine hypothesis of depression, which postulates that the deficit of certain neurotransmitters is responsible for the corresponding features of depression: "Norepinephrine may be related to alertness and energy as well as anxiety, attention, and interest in life; [lack of] serotonin to anxiety, obsessions, and compulsion s; and dopamine to attention, motivation, pleasure, and reward, as w ell as interest in life." The proponents of this hypo thesis recommend choosing the antidepressant with the mechanism of action impacting the most prominent symptoms. Anxious or irritable patients should be treated with SSRIs or norepinephrine reuptake inhibitors, and the ones with the loss of energy and enjoyment of life—with norepinephrine and dopamine enhancing drugs.

Several areas of the brain are implicated in studies seeking to more fully understand the biology of depression:

- *Raphe nuclei:* The sole source of serotonin in the brain is the raphe nuclei, a group of small nerve cell nuclei in the upper brain stem, located directly at the mid-line of the brain. There is some evidence for neuropathological abnormalities in the rostral raphe nuclei in depression. Despite their small size, the y reach very widely through their projections, and are involved in a very diverse set of functions.

- *Suprachiasmatic nucleus (SCN):* The suprachiasmatic nucleus (SCN) is the control center for the body's "biological clock." It contains neurons whose activity waxes and wanes throughout the day. The output from the SCN controls the sleep/wake cycle as well as a number of other biological rhythms, such as fluctuations in body temperature. Disturbances of these cycles are a consistent symptom of depression, especially of the melancholic type.

  The "classic" pattern is for depressed people to have great difficulty falling asleep at night, and then to wakeup right at around 3 AM. The waking is usually preceded by a rise in body temperature, which in non-depressed people does not usually occur until several hours later. It is a common observation that antidepressants produce a return to normal sleep patterns before they produce an improvement in mood: if good sleep does not return, it is a strong sign that the treatment is not going to be effective. Conversely, disruptions to sleep are often the first indication of impending relapse.

  The biological clock exerts a strong influence on the Raphe nuclei: serotonin levels drop during sleep, and fall almost to nothing during REM (dreaming) sleep. It is worth noting that one of the characteristics of sleep in depressed people is that REM tends to appear very soon after sleep onset, whereas in non-depressed people it does not usually dominate sleep until the last hours, in the early morning.

- *Ventral tegmental area (VTA):* The ventral tegmentum (or ventral tegmental area) is a small area in the basal midbrain which is a critical part of the brain's reward system. It sends projections to the nucleus accumbens that use the neurotransmitter dopamine. Addictive drugs universally increase the effects of dopamine in this system, whereas drugs that oppose dopamine produce anhedonia of the sort seen in depressed people. Dopamine-enhancers such as cocaine often relieve the lack-of-pleasure in depression, but the effects only last as long as a drug is present in the body: that is, they temporarily alleviate one of the main symptoms, but do not help to cure the disease.

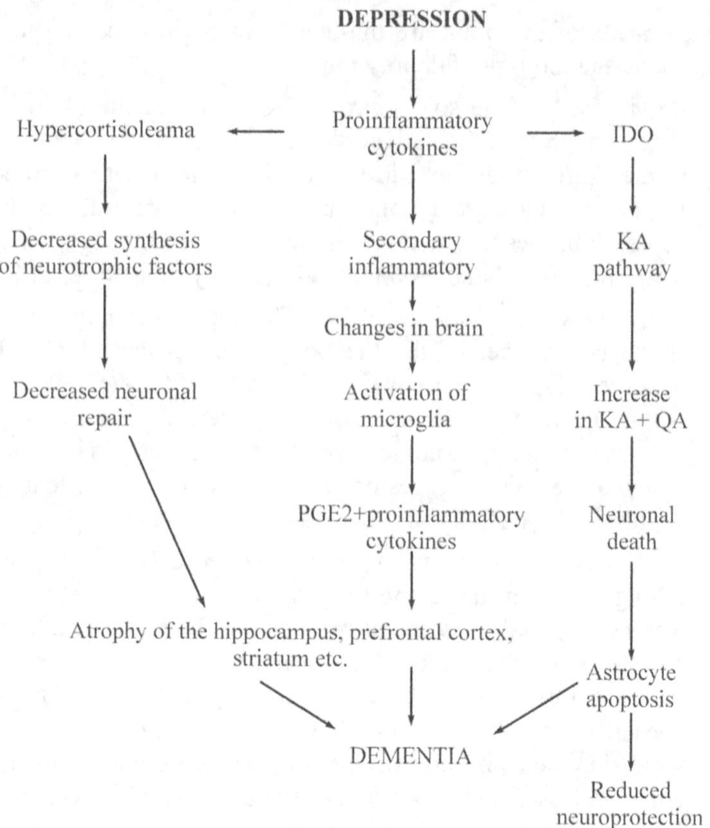

Fig. 9.2 Pathophysiology of depression leading to dementia (Source: www.infostick.in).

Psychotic depression, also known as depressive psychosis, refers to a major depressive episode that is accompanied by psychotic symptoms. It can occur in the context of bipolar disorder or major depressive disorder. It can be difficult to distinguish from schizoaffective disorder; that disorder requires the presence of psychotic symptoms for at least two weeks without any mood symptoms present.

Individuals with psychotic depression experience the symptoms of a major depressive episode, along with one or more psychotic symptoms, including delusions and/or hallucinations. Delusions can be classified as mood congruent or incongruent, depending on whether or not the nature of the delusions is in keeping with the individual's mood state. Common themes of mood congruent delusions include guilt, punishment, personal inadequacy, or disease. Half of patients experience more than one kind of delusion. Delusions occur without hallucinations in about one-half to two-thirds of patients with psychotic depression. Hallucinations can be auditory, visual, olfactory (smell), or haptic (touch). Severe anhedonia, loss of interest, and psychomotor retardation are typically present.

Psychotic symptoms tend to develop after an individual has already had several episodes of depression without psychosis. However, once psychotic symptoms have emerged, they tend to reappear with each future depressive episode. The prognosis for psychotic depression is not considered to be as poor as for schizoaffective disorders or primary psychotic disorders. Still, those who have experienced a depressive episode with psychotic features have an increased risk of relapse and suicide compared to those without psychotic features, and they tend to have more pronounced sleep abnormalities.

Pathophysiology: There are a number of biological features that may distinguish psychotic depression from non-psychotic depression. The most significant difference may be the presence of an abnormality in the hypothalamic pituitary adrenal axis (HPA) axis. The HPA axis appears to be dysregulated in psychotic depression, with dexamethasone suppression tests demonstrating higher levels of cortisol following dexamethasone administration (i.e. lower cortisol suppression).Those with psychotic depression also have higher ventricular-brain ratios than those with non-psychotic depression.

- ***The biogenic amine hypothesis:*** Drugs that decreased monoamines precipitated depression and drugs that increased monoamines relieved depression. It states that depression is caused by a deficiency of monoamines, particularly noradrenaline and serotonin.

- ***Monoamine deficiency:*** Another way to increase monoamines involves blocking the process of reuptake. Blocking reuptake prevents the presynaptic neuron from reclaiming neurotransmitter, which increases the amount of neurotransmitter in the synaptic cleft. Blocking the action of MAO leads to an increased availability of neurotransmitters. When the action of MAO is blocked, neurotransmitters are accumulated in the presynaptic neuron. Drugs which block the metabolism of noradrenaline and serotonin via inhibition of MAO are called MAO inhibitors, or MAOIs. MAOIs were among the first clinically proven antidepressants. Taken chronically, MAOIs also produce desensitization and down-regulation of postsynaptic receptors.

- ***The receptor sensitivity hypothesis:*** The Biogenic Amine Hypothesis alone cannot explain the delay in time of onset of clinical relief of depression of up to 6-8 weeks. Super-sensitivity is acompensatory response of the postsynaptic neuron when it receives too little stimulation. The neuron tries to make up for a lack of stimulation by increasing receptor responsiveness. Over time, the postsynaptic neuron may also compensate for lack of stimulation by synthesizing additional receptor sites. This process is known as up-regulation. Increased neurotransmitter increases stimulation of receptor sites, which prompts the postsynaptic neuron to compensate by decreasing receptor sensitivity, a process known as desensitization. The postsynaptic neuron is also thought to compensate for increasing stimulation by decreasing the number of receptor sites, a process known as down-regulation.

- Antidepressant drugs work by increasing the amount of neurotransmitter in the cleft. They do this by blocking metabolism of monoamines – the MAOIs – or by blocking reuptake – the TCAs. Most TCAs are more effective in blocking noradrenaline reuptake than serotonin reuptake. Chronic administration of TCAs or MAOIs is thought to alter the responsiveness and/or the number of postsynaptic receptor sites. Observation of this long-term effect of antidepressants led to the Receptor Sensitivity Hypothesis.

- This hypothesis proposes that depression is the result of a pathological alteration (supersensitivity and up-regulation) in receptor sites, which results from too little stimulation by monoamines, i.e., a deficiency of noradrenaline and serotonin in the cleft. Chronic administration of TCAs or MAOIs results in increased availability of noradrenaline and serotonin. This causes desensitization (the uncoupling of receptor sites) and possibly down-regulation (a decrease in the number of receptor sites). According to this hypothesis, relief from depression symptoms comes from a normalization of receptor sensitivity.

- According to the Receptor Sensitivity Hypothesis, antidepressant drugs achieve their clinical effect by reducing receptor super sensitivity. This theory is an important step toward understanding the long delay between administration of TCAs and MAOIs and clinical response.

- While TCAs are effective in blocking the reuptake of noradrenaline and serotonin into the presynaptic neuron, they are non-selective: they also block postsynaptic receptor sites, including cholinergic (muscarinic), histaminergic, and adrenergic receptor sites. Blockade of histaminergic receptors can lead to sedation, weight gain, and hypotension. In the elderly, this is a particular problem, since it can result in fainting or falls. TCAs also block muscarinic receptors, which can lead to blurred vision, dry mouth, constipation, urinary retention, confusion, and delirium.

- ***The serotonin-only hypothesis:*** Early in the 1980s, drugs were introduced that selectively blocked serotonin reuptake, resulting in more serotonin available in the cleft. These drugs were known as selective serotonin reuptake inhibitors, or SSRIs. Unlike the TCAs, which are non-selective, the SSRIs may have fewer serious side effects and are therefore easier for patients to tolerate. This has led to the Serotonin-only Hypothesis which emphasizes the role of serotonin in depression and downplays noradrenaline. But the serotonin-only theory has shortcomings:

  1. It does not explain why there is a delay in onset of clinical relief;
  2. It does not explain the role of noradrenaline in depression

- When noradrenergic neurons are destroyed in laboratory animals, drugs that affect serotonin do not have their usual effects. Likewise, when serotonergic neurons are destroyed, drugs that affect noradrenaline do not have their usual effects.

- *The permissive hypothesis:* Current research suggests that mood is controlled by a balance of noradrenaline and serotonin, not by absolute levels of these neurotransmitters or their receptors. According to this hypothesis – the Permissive Hypothesis – the control of emotional behavior results from a balance between noradrenaline and serotonin.

  According to this theory, both the manic phase and the depressive phase of bipolar disorder are characterized by low central serotonin function. Evidence suggests that brain serotonin systems dampen or inhibit a range of functions involving other neurotransmitters. Mood disorders result from the removal of the serotonin damper.

- *The electrolyte membrane hypothesis:* This theory is largely based on state related fluctuations in manic depressive illness such as urine volume and body weight. For example, the lithium-sodium counter flow mechanisms in red cells and protein structural differences between patients with bipolar-polar disorder and controls have been revealed. The mechanism of action of lithium in bipolar disorder is still not understood.

- *The neuroendocrine hypothesis:* According to this hypothesis, pathological mood states are explained or contributed to by altered endocrine function. This theory historically grew out of observations that altered mood states were associated with thyroid or Cushing's disease. Bipolar disorder is characterized by periods of both depressive and manic states, and symptoms may range from euphoria and psychosis to anhedonia and suicidal tendencies. However, a delayed therapeutic effect and propensity to induce mania in bipolar patients often occur upon antidepressant intake. This highlights' both the importance of molecular processes predating monoamine effects, and the need to further understand the etiology of this disorder at the neuroanatomical and cellular levels.

- *Neurotransmitters and hormones:* Bipolar disorder and other mood disorders seem to be associated with an imbalance in brain chemicals known as neurotransmitters, specifically serotonin, norepinephrine, and dopamine. An imbalance in hormone levels may also be present in people with bipolar disorder.

- *Genetics:* There is clearly a hereditary component to bipolar disorder, as people with a close blood relative with bipolar disorder are significantly more likely to develop the disorder themselves. The genetic causes of bipolar disorder are complex, with more than one gene involved in development of the disorder. Past research studies have pointed to a handful of genes that seem to play a role in bipolar disorder, and additional studies are ongoing.

(v) Migraine

A. Vascular Headache

Definition: Headache refers to any kind of pain in or about cranium. Headache is classified into three major categories:

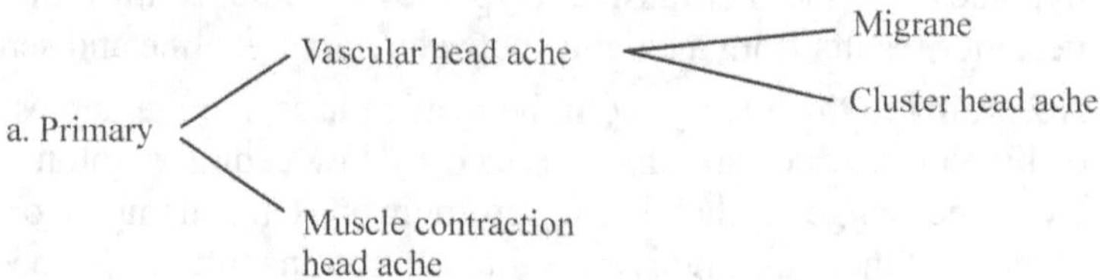

b. Psychogenic

c. Secondary head ache

Fig. 9.3 Vascular headache.

Etiologic agents in migraine:

(a) Psychologic factors – stress– personality

(b) Environmental factors

(c) Physiological factors:

- Autonomic Nervous system dysfunction
- Atherosclerosis
- Epilepsy
- Autosomal trait defect
- Immunologic response
- Allergy
- Hypersensitivity
- Metabolic hormonal abnormality
- Iatrogenic factors
- Dietary factors

Pathophysiology: Migraine headache are usually temporal and unilateral in distribution. It is a progression of vascular events. There appears to be an initial period of vasoconstriction producing an ischaemic area in brain. This neurological ischaemia may correspond to prodrome of classical migraine. Area of ischaemia determines the type and quality of prodrome. Cerebral vasodilation and inflammation usually follow an ischaemic event resulting in pain. The proposed mechanisms include:

- Defective humoral control
- Abnormal platelet function
- Altered calcium homeostasis
- Serotonin (5-hydroxy tryptamine/5 HT) – tyramine
- Nor epinephrine
- Epinephrine

Serotonin is the most important vasoactive amine mediating vascular headaches. Platelet aggregation and 5-HT degradation are abnormal in migrainous patients.

- Decreased vasoactive amine degradation by platelet mono amine oxidase
- Increased platelet sensitivity
- Increased release of 5-HT and prostaglandins

Abnormality in vasoactive amine secretion/response can be identified as common denominator when all these factors are evaluated. Psychological factors/stress, diet may elevate catecholamines (Epinephrine, Norepinephrine). These catecholamines indirectly cause release of platelet vasoactive amines which can mediate migrainous headache.

Dietary factors (e.g.: tyramine, β - phenyl ethyl amine) which can induce migraine include red wine, caffeinated beverages, chocolate etc. Genetic autosomal trait defect in ability to conjugate tyramine.

Iatrogenic agents (drug induced migraine):
- Tryptophan-Serotonin Precursor
- Reserpine & Fenfluramine
- Inhibitor of Reuptake and Storage of 5-HT
- Fluoxetine
- 5-HT Reuptake Blocker
- Ethinyl Estradiol
- Mestranol
- Viloxazine
- Nicotine
- Histamine

These agents induce a transient increase in serotonin, initiating a vasoconstrictive reaction.Physiologic event after vasoconstrictive phase:

- Increased monoamine oxidase enzyme release

- Increased vascular permeability lower the concentration of vasoactive amine (primarily serotonin) without vasoactive amine stimulus, cerebral vasculature dilates producing pain.

Both migraine and cluster headache similarly dilate extra cranial arterial vessels. Migraine additionally dilates intracranial vessels (carotid artery).Unique vascular phenomenon recognised in cluster headache is dilation of ophthalmic artery. The pathophysiology of vasodilation is probably similar for both migraine and cluster headache.

B. Cluster headache

Migraine variant with short severe, episodic, clustering, unilateral pain over orbit and forehead. Factors contributing to the development of cluster headache include:

- Stress/emotion – prolonged strain
- Pharmacologic vasodilators

Pathophysiologic explanation of symptomatology observed during cluster headache is similar to that of migraine. An initial vasoconstriction phase identified in angiography. Thermograms used to localise blood flow showed decreased unilateral circulation in supra orbital and frontal areas prior to the event and subsequent increased blood flow in the same area during attack. Elevated histamine, 5-HT, bradykinin release, increased α-adrenergic and parasympathetic activity are possible cause.

Pain sensation experienced during migraine and cluster headache is due to stimulation of pain nerve fibres, secondary to cranial artery vasodilation. 5-HT depresses the pain threshold. Release of prostaglandins. Oedema around dilated arteries helps to intensify the severity of the headache. Sustained dilation of arterial wall renders them less responsive to treatment. Role of altered calcium homeostasis in constriction of vasculature have recently been investigated. Blockade of calcium channels may prevent the vasomotor effect of vaso-active amines.

Clinical Presentation

Patients with classical migraine experience prodrome-15-30 minutes before headache. Prodrome may be sensory, motor or mood disturbance. Visual scotoma, visual field defect, hemisensory disturbance or aphasia. Patient with complicated migraine, prodromal symptoms persist during/ beyond dilation and headache phase. Migraine headache have onset in child hood or adolescence. Migraine headache usually occur in early morning hours and reach peak intensity within an hour.

Pain is described as severe pounding and throbbing. Migraine headache are temporal unilateral in distribution. Patient has gastro intestinal complication (anorexia, nausea, vomiting).Increased sensitivity to light. Patients are incapacitated (disabled) during attack and seek a dark quiet place to sleep. Post headache characterised by exhaustion, scalp tenderness, recurrence of headache/sudden head movement.

(vi) Epilepsy

Definition: Epilepsy derived from Greek word epilepsia means to attack. Epilepsy is a chronic disorder. Epilepsy is asymptom of disturbed electrical activity of brain caused by wide variety of disorders. Epilepsy implies periodic recurrence of seizure with or without convulsion.

A seizure results from sudden explosive disorderly discharge of cerebral neurons and is characterised by sudden, transient alteration in brain function (electrical activity of brain) –usually involving –motor, sensory, autonomic or psychic/clinical manifestation. Seizure disorder represents a syndrome. There is disturbance in-consciousness, sensory symptoms, motor symptoms, subjective well-being and objective behaviour.

Epilepsy is a collection of many different type of seizure that varies widely in severity, appearance, cause, consequence and management. Seizure is episodic brief and has beginning and end, and may produce post seizure impairment and is involuntary.

Convulsion: (term sometimes applied to seizure): Convulsion is violent involuntary contraction of voluntary muscle. It is a jerky, contract-relax (tonic-clonic) movements associated with some seizures.

Etiology and precipitation of seizure: Anything that disrupts the normal homeostasis of neuronal cell disrupts the stability and trigger abnormal activity and seizure.

Seizure threshold of some persons are genetically lower. Cerebral lesions, biochemical disorder, cerebral trauma etc., resulting from metabolic defect, congenital malformations, genetic predisposition, perinatal injury, post-natal trauma, myoclonic syndrome, infection, brain tumour, vascular disease, fever, drug [Theophylline, anti-depressants etc.], and alcohol.

Seizure may be precipitated by pH of body fluid, by hypoglycaemia, fatigue, lack of sleep, emotional, physical stress, febrile illness, large amount of water ingestion, constipation, use of stimulant drugs, withdrawal from depressant drugs, hyperventilation, some environmental stimuli like blinking lights, poorly adjusted television screen, loud noise, certain music, women have increased seizure activity immediately before or after menses.

Epidemiology: At least 8% of general population have experienced at least one seizure in life time.

Classification of seizure: Seizure may be divided into partial, generalised and unclassified seizure.

(a) *Partial seizure:* [Jacksonian epilepsy, Focal motor Epilepsy] Partial seizure begins in one hemisphere of the brain.

- *Simple partial seizure:* If there is no impairment in consciousness seizure are classified as simple partial seizure.
- *Complex partial* [Temporal lobe, psychomotor seizure]: If there is impairment in consciousness the seizures are described as complex partial seizure.
- *Secondary generalised seizure*: in which complex partial seizure progress to generalised tonic-clonic seizure.

(b) Generalised seizure: Bilaterally symmetric without local onset. Generalised seizure has clinical manifestations that indicate involvement of both hemispheres.

- Absence seizure (petitmal): Is interruption of ongoing activities having sudden onset e.g.: blank stare/brief upward rotation of eye.
- Tonic-clonic seizure (Grandmal epilepsy): Usually preceded by pre-monitory symptoms called aura. The seizure results in sudden sharp clonic contraction of muscle followed by period of rigidity. During the period patient may fall and be injured. During seizure patient may cry or moan, loose sphincter control, bite tongue, develop cyanosis. After seizure, patient may be unconscious and frequently go to deep sleep. Shock like muscle contraction of face, trunk and extremities are known as myoclonic jerk.
- Atonic seizure (drop attack): Sudden loss of muscle tone described as head drop, dropping of limbs, slumping to ground.

(c) *Unclassified seizure:* All seizures that cannot be classified due to inadequate or incomplete data.

(d) *Status epilepticus:* prolonged partial/generalised seizure without recovery between attacks.

Pathophysiology: Epilepsy is thought to be result of genetic mutation that causes abnormalities in brain wiring and/or imbalance in chemical that brain use to send signal or abnormal nerve connections made while attempting to repair itself after injury. Seizure activity is characterised by paroxysmal (sudden) discharges occurring synchronously in a large population of cortical neurons. This is characterised in EEG as a sharp wave or spike. Seizure originates from grey matter of any cortical/sub cortical area.

The basic physiology of seizure episode is traceable to unstable cell membrane or its surrounding supportive cells. A group of neurons exhibit paroxysmal depolarisation shift and function as epileptogenic focus. These neurons are hypersensitive and more easily activated by hyperthermia, hypoxia, hypoglycaemia, hyponatremia, repeated sensory stimulation and certain sleep phase.

Development of an action potential is similar to that in cardiac cell. Major ion species involved in burst of activity is calcium. Generation of epileptogenic discharge depend on three major factors:

Some neurons have inherent ability to elaborate response leading to paroxysmal (sudden) bursts.

Abnormal neurons recruit normal neurons to propagate the discharge. This is augmented by failure of normal inhibitory activities and enhancement of excitatory synaptic activities. [Deficiency of inhibitory neuron transmitter or increased excitatory neurotransmitters promotes abnormal neuronal activity].

Interference with normal metabolic process also promotes seizure activity.

Normal firing of neurons is controlled by excitatory and inhibitory neurotransmitters. Neurotransmitters like acetylcholine, noradrenaline, histamine, corticotrophin releasing factors etc., enhance the excitability and propagation of neuronal activity. Gama amino butyric acid, dopamine etc., inhibits neuronal activity and propagation. Normal neuronal activity also depends on adequate supply of glucose, oxygen, sodium, potassium, calcium and amino acids. Systemic pH also a factor in precipitation of seizure.

Epileptogenic neurons fire more and more often and with greater amplitude. When the intensity reaches a threshold point, cortical excitation spreads. This onset propagates by physiological pathway to adjacent and remote areas. Excitation of subcortical thalamic and brain stem area correspond to tonic phase (muscle contraction with increased muscle tone) and is associated with loss of consciousness.

Clonic phase (alternating contraction and relaxation of muscle) begins when inhibitory neurons in cortex, anterior thalamus and basal ganglia react to cortical excitation. The seizure discharge is interrupted producing intermittent muscle contractions, that gradually decrease and finally cease (epileptogenic neurons are exhausted).

During seizure activity, oxygen consumption is at high rate 60% above normal. Although cerebral blood flow increases, glucose and oxygen rapidly depleted along with lactate accumulation in brain tissue. Continued severe seizure activity causes progressive brain injury and irreversible brain damage. If seizure focus active for prolonged time, minor focus may develop in normal tissue.

Clinical manifestation: The clinical manifestation depends on site of focus, degree of irritability of the surrounding area, and intensity of the impulse. Clinical manifestation associated with seizure depends on its type; two types of symptoms indicate generalised tonic-clonic seizure.

Epileptic aura-a type of simple partial seizure, experienced as a subjective sensation or motor phenomenon that sometimes signals an approaching generalised or complex partial seizure.

Prodroma is an early manifestation occurring hours to days before seizure. (Both may become familiar to a person experiencing recurrent generalised seizure).

Control of abnormal neuronal activity by anti-epileptic drugs accomplished by:

(a) Elevating convulsive threshold of neurons to electrical and chemical stimuli (stabilisation of neuronal membrane)

(b) Limiting the propagation of seizure discharge from its origin. (Depression of synaptic transmission and nerve conduction).

Glaucoma

Definition: Glaucoma is one of the leading causes of blindness. It is a group of ocular disease characterised by increased intraocular pressure (IOP), optic nerve atrophy, optic disc change and loss of visual field. Glaucoma occurs due to impaired out flow of aqueous humour. Obstruction to aqueous flow occurs as a result of:

- Developmental malformation
- Uveitis
- Trauma
- Intra ocular haemorrhage
- Tumour etc.

Classification: Two major type of glaucoma have been identified:

1. Open angle
2. Closed angle glaucoma

In all type of glaucoma degenerative changes appear after gradually and eventually damage to optic nerve and retina occur. In glaucoma, optic disc changes and retinal nerve damage occur from increased intra ocular pressure (normal IOP 15.5 ± 2.5 mmHg by applanation tonometry).

Aqueous humour and intra ocular pressure: Aqueous humour is formed in ciliary body through both ultrafiltration and secretion. Constant inflow of aqueous humour from ciliary body and resistance to outflow result in intra ocular pressure great enough to produce an outflow equal to inflow. Ultrafiltration depends on B.P [blood pressure] and IOP [intraocular pressure]

Osmotic gradient produced by secretion of Na+, bicarbonate and ascorbate into aqueous humour result in movement of water from stromal ultrafiltrate to posterior chamber. Carbonic anhydrase inhibitors like acetazolamide have IOP lowering effect. β-adrenergic agents increase inflow. A-adrenergic and β-adrenergic blockers, dopamine blockers decrease inflow. Pressure in posterior chamber push aqueous humour between iris and lens and through pupil into anterior chamber of eye. Aqueous humour in anterior chamber leave eye by two routes:

- Filtration through trabecular meshwork into Schlemn's canal
- Absorption into iris blood vessels

Cholinergic agents like pilocarpine increase outflow by physically pulling open meshwork pores through ciliary contraction. Increase in IOP in open angle glaucoma result from decreased facility for outflow through trabecular meshwork. Intraocular pressure is measured by tonometry-indentation tonometry, applanation tonometry. IOP between 21-30 mmHg cause optic disc change and visual field loss.

Primary open angle glaucoma [POAG]: Primary open angle glaucoma is bilateral genetically determined disorder. POAG manifest as increase in IOP that result in optic nerve degeneration characterised by disc change and visual field loss. It is chronic, slowly progressive disease. The basic underlying disorder of POAG is decreased outflow facility resulting in imbalance between aqueous production and aqueous outflow. Histological changes in meshwork or Schlemn canal in glaucomatous eye produce increased resistance to out flow.

Secondary open angle glaucoma: Has many causes including systemic disease, trauma, surgery, rubeosis, lens change, ocular inflammatory disease etc. In pre-trabecular form, a membrane overlies the meshwork and does not allow the aqueous outflow. In trabecular form of secondary glaucoma, an alteration in mesh work and accumulation of material in inter trabecular spaces occur. Post trabecular form result from disorder causing increased episcleral venous blood pressure as in Sturge Weber syndrome, retro bulbar tumour, carotid cavernous fistular etc.

Angle closure glaucoma: Angle closure glaucoma results from mechanical blockade trabecular mesh work by iris. Blockade of meshwork occur intermittently resulting in extremely high IOP. Primary angle closure glaucoma occurs in patients with shallow anterior chamber which produce narrow angle between cornea and iris or tight contact between iris and lens (pupillary block).Presence of narrow angle is determined by genioscopy, other test-provocation of angle closure induced IOP increase. Two major types of angle closure are:

- Angle closure with pupillary block which results when iris is in firm contact with lens and this block aqueous flow through pupil to anterior chamber.
- Angle closure without pupillary block which occurs in patients with abnormality called plateau iris.

Prodromal Symptoms

Blurred vision, occasional headache, ocular discomfort, intraocular pressure, oedematous cornea. Prodromal attack last for 1-2hrs. Laser iredectomy produces hole in iris that allow aqueous flow directly from posterior chamber to anterior chamber.

Pathophysiology

The underlying factor in glaucoma is increased intraocular pressure, i.e. ocular hypertension. Intraocular pressure is a function of production of liquid aqueous humor by the ciliary processes of the eye, and its drainage through the trabecular meshwork. Aqueous humor flows from the ciliary processes into the posterior chamber, bounded posteriorly by the lens and the zonules of Zinn, and anteriorly by the iris. It then flows through the pupil of the iris into the anterior chamber, bounded posteriorly by the iris and anteriorly by the cornea. From here, the trabecular meshwork drains aqueous humor via Schlemm's canal into scleral plexuses and general blood circulation.

In open/wide-angle glaucoma, flow is reduced through the trabecular meshwork, due to the degeneration and obstruction of the trabecular meshwork, whose original function is to absorb the aqueous humor. Loss of aqueous humor absorption leads to increased resistance and thus a chronic, painless buildup of pressure in the eye. In close/narrow-angle, the iridocorneal angle is completely closed because of forward displacement of the final roll and root of the iris against the cornea, resulting in the inability of the aqueous fluid to flow from the posterior to the anterior chamber and then out of the trabecular network. This accumulation of aqueous humor causes an acute increase of pressure and pain.

Glaucoma is unique among ophthalmic diseases since its underlying pathophysiology involves structures in both the anterior and posterior segments of the eye. The main problem or pathology in glaucoma is caused by raised intraocular pressure. It is this raised pressure that compresses and damages the optic nerve. Once the optic nerve is damaged, it fails to carry visual information to the brain and this result in loss of vision.

The raised pressure on the retina causes the cells and nerve ganglions in the sensitive retina to die off (retinal ganglion apoptosis) and in addition the small blood vessels of the retina are also compressed depriving it of nutrients. This results in a clinically progressive loss of peripheral visual field and ultimately vision. However, in normal tension glaucoma, there is no rise of intraocular pressure. These patients are said to suffer from a problem in the blood vessels and perfusion. Derangements of the immune system (autoimmune causes) may lead to damage to the optic nerve.

Hypertension

Definition: Hypertension is a disease of vasculature. Hypertension is consistent (steady) elevation of systemic arterial B.P. Pathogenesis of hypertension is due to functional and structural changes in blood vessels. Primary consequences of hypertension:

- Pathological vascular changes
- Accelerated atherosclerosis

- Hyaline and hyperplastic arteriosclerosis
- Arteriolitis

Hypertension is one of the most important risk factor in both coronary heart disease and cerebrovascular accidents. It may also lead to congestive heart failure, aortic dissection and renal failure. A sustained diastolic pressure greater than 90mmHg or sustained systolic pressure greater than 140mmHg is generally considered as hypertension. About 90-95% of hypertension is idiopathic and apparently primary, (essential hypertension).5-10% is secondary to renovascular diseases, primary aldosteronism, Cushing's syndrome, pheochromocytoma, etc.

	Diastolic	Systolic
Normal blood pressure	<85	<130
High normal	85-89	130-139
Mild Hypertension	90-99	140-159
Moderate H.T	100-109	160-179
Severe H.T	110-119	180-209
Very severe	$\geq$120	$\geq$210
Malignant H.T	>140	>200

Etiology (Causes)

Essential hypertension: Genetic defect in renal sodium excretion. Genetic defect in sodium/calcium transport in vascular smooth muscles. Variation in gene encoding angiotensinogen and other protein in renin-angiotensin system. Other factors increase vasoconstrictive influences-behavioural, neurogenic, hormonal.

Secondary hypertension: Renal disease-Increased renin secretion, sodium and fluid retention, decreased vasodilator secretion. Various causes include

- Endocrine causes: Aldosteronism, oral contraceptives, pheochromocytoma, Thyrotoxicosis.
- Vascular causes: Coarctation (narrowing) of aorta, vasculitis.
- Neurogenic causes: Psychogenic, increased intracranial pressure.
- Family History
- Age
- Cigarette smoking
- High dietary sodium intake
- Low dietary intake of K^+, Ca^{++}, Magnesium.

Both essential /secondary Hypertension may be benign or malignant.

Benign hypertension: In most of the cases hypertension remains at a modest level fairly stable over years to decades. Unless myocardial infarction or cerebrovascular accident occurs, it is compatible with long life.

Malignant hypertension: Few persons show a rapidly rising blood pressure which if untreated leads to death within a year/two. This is called accelerated/malignant Hyper Tension. Clinical syndrome of malignant hypertension includes severe hypertension (diastolic pressure over 120mmHg), renal failure, retinal haemorrhage, exudates and papilledema.

Pathogenesis of Hypertension

Regulation of normal blood pressure: Magnitude of arterial pressure depends on two fundamental haemodynamic variables.

- Cardiac output
- Total peripheral resistance

Total peripheral resistance is the resistance of arterioles predominantly related to lumen size. Lumen size determined by thickness of arteriolar wall, neural and hormonal influences Vasoconstrictor agents are angiotensin-II, catecholamines, thromboxane, leukotrienes, endothelin. Vasodilators include Kinins, prostaglandin, nitric oxide.

These mediators act by binding to specific receptor on the smooth muscle cell. Certain metabolic products (lactic acid, hydrogen ion and adenosine) and hypoxia act as local vasodilators. Kidney play important role in blood pressure regulation.

(a) *Renin angiotensin system:* Through release of renin, kidney eventually forms angiotensin-II which alters blood pressure by increasing both peripheral resistance and blood volume. Angiotensin II cause vasoconstriction through direct action on vascular smooth muscles. Stimulation of aldosterone secretion, which increase the distal tubular reabsorption of sodium and water.

(b) *Sodium homeostasis:* Kidney intimately involved in complex process of sod. Homeostasis.

(c) *Glomerular filtration rate (GFR):* When blood volume is reduced GFR falls this in turn lead to increased reabsorption of sodium in proximal tubule in an attempt to conserve sodium and expand blood volume.GRF independent factor include atria natriuretic factor (ANF) or atriopeptin a group of peptides secreted by heart atria in response to volume expansion which inhibit sodium reabsorption in distal tubule and cause vasodilation.

(d) *Renal vasodepressor substance:* Kidney produces a variety of vasodepressor or antihypertensive substance that presumably counter balance the vasopressor effect of angiotensin. These include prostaglandins, urinary kallikrein-kinin system, platelet activating factor, nitric oxide, etc. Abnormalities in these normal mechanisms are implicated in pathogenesis of hypertension in variety of renal diseases.

Mechanism of Essential hypertension: The cause of most cases of hypertension is unknown (essential).The cause must be related either to primary increase in cardiac output or increase in peripheral resistance.

(a) *Increased cardiac output as primary event:*
- Defective renal sodium excretion in the presence of normal arterial pressure.
- Decreased sodium excretion lead to increased fluid volume and rise in cardiac output.

(b) *Vasoconstrictive influence as primary event:* Peripheral vasoconstriction to prevent over perfusion of tissue (autoregulation), which increases peripheral resistance and blood pressure.

(c) *Behavioural/neurogenic factors:* Decrease in blood pressure due to meditation.

(d) *Increased release of vasoconstrictor agent:* renin, catecholamine, endothelin

(e) *Primary increased sensitivity of vascular smooth muscle:* Caused by genetic defect in cell membrane transport of sodium and calcium leading to increased intracellular calcium and contraction in the smooth muscle cells.

Vascular pathology in hypertension: Hypertension accelerates atherogenesis, and cause changes in the structure of wall of blood vessels. Hypertension is associated with two form of small blood vessel disease:
- Hyaline arteriosclerosis
- Hyperplastic arteriosclerosis

Hyaline arteriosclerosis: Condition encountered frequently in elderly patients. More generalised and more severe in patients with hypertension. Vascular lesion consists of homogenous pink hyaline thickening of wall of arterioles with loss of underlying structural features and narrowing of lumen. Hyperplastic arteriosclerosis: Vessel with thickened concentric smooth muscle cell layer and thickened resembling onion -skin, duplicated basement membrane. In malignant hypertension, these hyperplastic changes are often accompanied by fibrinoid necrosis of the arterial intima and media. These changes are most prominent in the kidney and can lead to ischemia and acute renal failure.

Stroke (Ischaemic and Haemorrhage)

DEFINITION: Stroke is referred as sudden onset of focal neurological deficit. Stroke is a syndrome and is manifestation of cerebrovascular disease. Cerebrovascular disease [CVD] refers to any type of pathophysiologic vascular disease of brain. Various pathologic process commonly implicated in cerebrovascular diseases are-thrombosis, embolism, rapture of vessel, hypoxia, hypertensive arteriosclerosis, arteritis, trauma, aneurysm, developmental malformations.

These processes can result in two main type of parenchymal disease:

1. Ischaemic brain damage

2. Intra cranial haemorrhage

Neurological manifestation-depends on location and extend of ischemia, infarct/haemorrhage. Hemiplegia, sensory defect or coma. Intra cranial haemorrhage excruciating generalised head ache with or without unconsciousness. Dysphasia, headache, transient unilateral weakness. Computerised axial tomography (CT/CAT scan) has tremendous importance in diagnosis and assessment of stroke.

Etiology: Major risk factors for ischaemic stroke were identified as transient ischaemic attacks, cerebralinfarction, hypertension, cardiac abnormalities, atherosclerosis, diabetes mellitus. Atherothrombotic infarction Cerebral embolism. Haemorrhage in brain tissue and subarachnoid space.

Singe risk factors:

- Age-above 55 years
- Sex-more in males
- *Hypertension:* is the major predisposing factor for stroke. It causes atherothrombotic brain infarction aswell as cerebral haemorrhage. Elevated systolic B.P closely associated with stroke.
- Environmental factors: high sodium diet
- Diabetes mellitus
- *Impaired cardiac function:* is another important treatable risk factor e.g.: coronary heart disease, CHF, ventricular hypertrophy, arrhythmia etc.
- Transient ischaemic attacks- defined as focal ischaemic neurological deficit lasting less than 24 hrs. Transient ischaemic attack precedes an ischaemic stroke.

Elevated Haematocrit: (percentage volume of erythrocyte in whole blood) It decrease collateral circulation due to increased viscosity of blood. Stroke in patient with elevated haematocrit is due to decreased collateral blood flow (accessory blood flow through small branches). Hyperlipidaemia and hypercholesterolemia may contribute to stroke due to atherosclerosis. Cigarette smoking, alcohol, oral contraceptives etc.

Pathophysiology of acute stroke: Large majority of acute stroke result-either from ischaemic infarctionfrom inadequate blood flow or intracranial haemorrhage.

Atherothrombotic disease [Thrombotic stroke]: Atherosclerosis of brain arteries is a process similar to that found in extra-cranial vessels. Atherosclerosis and subsequent plaque formation results in arterial narrowing or occlusion. Formation of blood clot superimposed on atherosclerotic plaque cause significant stenosis.

Additional factors like blood hypercoagulability, increased platelet count, increased haematocrit also contribute to clotting and sludging (thickening) of blood flow. Platelet play import role in thrombosis. Platelet activation led to formation of thrombus (blood clot). Loss of integrity of endothelial surface of arterial wall (due to trauma/atherosclerosis) exposes blood to vessel collagen which activate platelets which lead to thrombus formation. Embolism-(sudden blocking of artery by clot)-produce stroke when clot/plaque breaks off into circulation and block artery.

Cerebral ischemia: Cerebral ischaemia can be divided into focal or general ischaemia (globalischaemia).

Global ischaemia is associated with lack of collateral blood flow and irreversible brain damage occurs in a short period of time (4-8 min).

In **focal ischaemia** collateral circulation allow survival of brain cells and reverse neuronal damage after period of ischaemia.

Brain is highly aerobic tissue-there is no reserve of oxygen in brain. Normal cerebral function can be continued only 8-10 seconds after cerebral ischemia and irreversible damage follow in 6-8 minutes. Brain ischemia can be due to:

(a) Functional hypoxia [decreased oxygen/oxygen carrying capacity]

(b) Hypotension

(c) Vessel obstruction (Thrombosis/embolism).

- collateral circulation
- duration of ischemia
- degree and rapidity of cessation of blood flow

Two general type of ischaemic (hypoxic) injury are:

(a) *Ischemic encephalopathy:* Ischaemic encephalopathy occurs after episodes of profound hypotension. In mild cases, there may be transient post ischaemic confusional state with complete recovery. Severe global ischaemia due to widespread reduction in cerebral perfusion (resulting from cardio-respiratory arrest)-cause wide spread brain necrosis. Patient who survive this state often severely impaired neurologically and deeply comatose (Persistent vegetative state).

(b) *Cerebral infarction:* Due to reduction/cessation of blood flow to localised area of brain. Clinical signs and symptoms depend on region infarcted. Anatomical location determines whether patient develop hemiplegia, sensory defect, blindness, aphasia /other symptoms.

Lacunar infarcts (Lacunar stroke): Occlusion of small arterial branches of circle of Willis and anterior, middle and posterior cerebral and basilar arteries results in infarct deep in cerebral hemisphere and brain stem. The term lacunar refers to small cavity left after removing necrotic tissue. Arterial hypertension is closely related to occurrence of lacunar infarcts.

Cerebral embolism [Embolic stroke]: Any region of the brain can be affected by embolism. Middle cerebellar artery is commonly involved. Cerebral embolism has rapid onset and not preceded by TIA. There is less time for developing collateral circulation. Embolic strokes are dangerous. Cerebral embolism may develop from heart disease (Cardiogenic embolism), atheromatous plaque, aorta, or air, fat, tumours.

Brain haemorrhage [Haemorrhagic stroke]: This often divided into two broad categories –Intraparenchymal and subarachnoid depending on the site of vascular rapture.

Intraparenchymal haemorrhage [Intracranial haemorrhage]: Although cerebral infarction is more frequent cause of stroke syndrome, intra cerebral haemorrhage is the leading cause of death. Hypertension, rapture of aneurysm, bleeding disorders, arteriovenous malformation, tumour cause haemorrhage. Aneurysm affecting large intracranial arteries-berry aneurysms-are most important and most common. Extravasation of blood into brain tissue forms a tumour. Adjacent brain tissue displaced/compressed producing ischemia/oedema. Clinical outcome of brain haemorrhage depends on position and size of lesion.

Sub arachnoid haemorrhage: Haemorrhage into sub-arachnoid space is caused by rapture of aneurysm or vascular malformation. On rapture, they produce severe generalised head ache suddenly followed by unconsciousness and neurologic defect.

Angina

Angina pectoris: It is chest pain often due to ischemia of the heart muscle, due in general to obstruction or spasm of the coronary arteries. The main cause of angina pectoris is improper contractivity of the heart muscle and coronary artery disease, due to atherosclerosis of the arteries feeding the heart. Angina results when there is an imbalance between the heart's oxygen demand and supply. This imbalance can result from an increase in demand (e.g., during exercise) without a proportional increase in supply (e.g., due to obstruction or atherosclerosis of the coronary arteries).

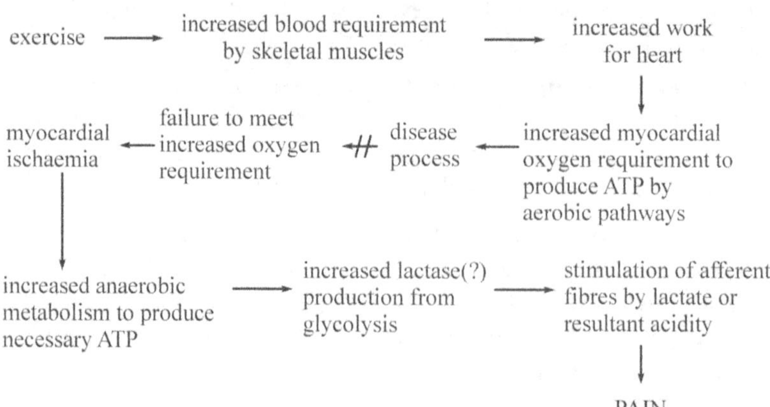

(www.medicinenet.com › ... › heart a-z list › stroke symptoms and treatment index)

Fig. 9.4 Angina and its causes.

Pathophysiology

Instable angina, the relationship between workload or demand and ischemia is usually relatively predictable. However, atherosclerotic arterial narrowing is not entirely fixed; it varies with the normal fluctuations in arterial tone that occur in all people. Thus, more people have angina in the morning, when arterial tone is relatively high. Also, abnormal endothelial function may contribute to variations in arterial tone; eg, in endothelium damaged by atheromas, stress of a catecholamine surge causes vasoconstriction rather than dilation (normal response).

As the myocardium becomes ischemic, coronary sinus blood pH falls, cellular K is lost, lactate accumulates, ECG abnormalities appear, and ventricular function (both systolic and diastolic) deteriorates. Left ventricular (LV) diastolic pressure usually increases during angina, sometimes inducing pulmonary congestion and dyspnea. The exact mechanism by which ischemia causes discomfort is unclear but may involve nerve stimulation by hypoxic metabolites.

Oxygen is delivered to the heart by larger surface vessels (epicardial vessels) and intramyocardial arteries and arterioles, which branch out into capillaries. There is little resistance to blood flow in the epicardial vessels in a healthy heart.

When atherosclerotic plaques are present, blood flow is impeded, but the process of autoregulation can compensate to a degree. Autoregulation is the dilation of the myocardial vessels in response to decreased oxygen delivery. Blood flow to the heart changes rapidly as a result of higher demand.

The most important mediators involved in myocardial perfusion are adenosine (a potent vasodilator), other nucleotides, nitric oxide, prostaglandins, carbon dioxide, and hydrogen ions. A single-cell endothelial layer separates the vascular smooth muscle from the blood. When intact, this vascular endothelium permits vasodilation and prevents thrombus and sclerotic plaque formation.

The coronary artery endothelium synthesizes fibronectin, interleukin-1, tissue plasminogen activator, certain growth factors, prostacyclin, platelet-activating factor, endothelin-1, and nitric oxide (NO). NO is synthesized from L-arginine by nitric oxide synthase. NO then causes relaxation of the arterial smooth muscle. Loss of endothelial layer results in less NO and can occur because of mechanical or chemical assaults or from oxidized low-density lipoprotein (LDL).

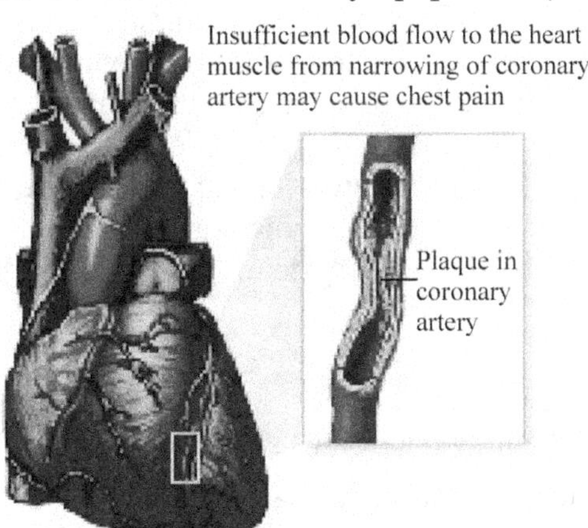

Fig. 9.5 Strokes Syndrome.

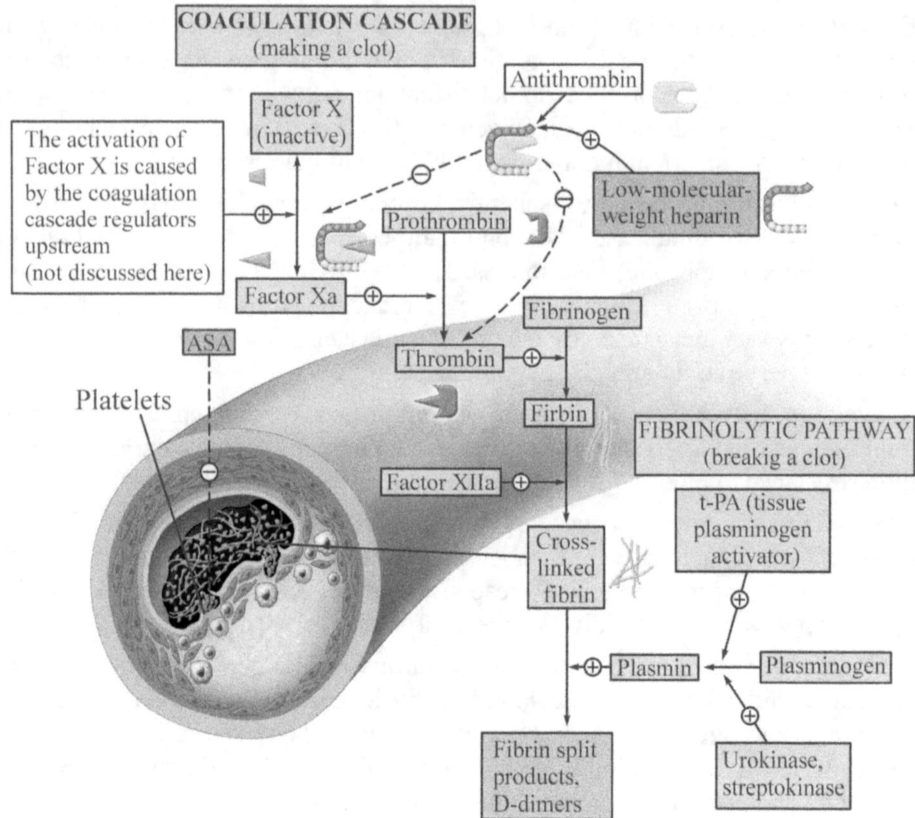

Fig. 9.6 Pathophysiological conditions of Angina Pectoris. (emedicine.medscape.com/article/150215-overview) Images for flowchart of pathophysiology of angina pectoris

Arrhythmia

Cardiac arrhythmias are any abnormality or perturbation in the normal activation sequence of the myocardium. Arrhythmias result from abnormalities of impulse initiation or impulse conduction or a combination of both. Abnormal impulse initiation results from either automaticity or triggered activity. The sinus node, displaying properties of automaticity, spontaneously depolarizes, sending a depolarization wave over the atrium, depolarizing the atrioventricular (AV) node, propagating over the His-Purkinje system, and depolarizing the ventricle in systematic fashion.

Causes

- Failure of automaticity (sick sinus syndrome)
- Overactivity (inappropriate sinus tachycardia)

Ectopic foci prematurely exciting the myocardium on a single or continuous basis results in premature atrial contractions (PACs) and premature ventricular contractions (PVCs). Sustained tachyarrhythmias in the atria, such as atrial fibrillation, paroxysmal atrial tachycardia (PAT), and supraventricular tachycardia (SVT), originate because of micro- or macro re-entry.

Pathophysiology

Three basic mechanisms:

- Enhanced or suppressed automaticity
- Triggered activity
- Re-entry

Automaticity is a natural property of all myocytes. Ischemia, scarring, electrolyte disturbances, medications, advancing age, and other factors may suppress or enhance automaticity in various areas. Enhanced automaticity can result in multiple arrhythmias, both atrial and ventricular. Triggered activity occurs when early after depolarizations and delayed afterdepolarizations initiate spontaneous multiple depolarizations, precipitating ventricular arrhythmias.The most common mechanism of arrhythmogenesis results from re-entry. Requisites for re-entry include bidirectional conduction and unidirectional block.

Automaticity can further be subdivided into (1) automaticity caused by the normal automatic mechanism (a normal property of cardiac cells in the sinus node, in some parts of the atria, in the atrioventricular junctional region, and in the His-Purkinje system) and (2) automaticity caused by an abnormal mechanism (resulting from a decrease in membrane potential of cardiac fibers, which normally have a high level of membrane potential).

Triggered activity is caused by after depolarizations, which are second depolarizations that occur either during repolarization (referred to as early after depolarizations) or after repolarization is complete or nearly complete (referred to as delayed after depolarizations). Abnormal impulse conduction results in reentrant excitation. Automatic tachycardias have the following characteristics:

1. The onset of the tachycardia is not related to an initiating event such as a premature beat.
2. The initiating beat is usually identical to subsequent beats of the tachycardia
3. The tachycardia cannot be initiated by programmed cardiac stimulation
4. Onset of the tachycardia usually is preceded by a gradual acceleration in rate and termination by a deceleration in rate.

Consequence of ischemic or hypoxic damage: The cardiac tissue resorts to anaerobic glycolysis foradenosine triphosphate (ATP) production.

- As high-energy phosphate concentration diminishes, the activity of the transmembrane ion pumps declines, and the resting membrane potential rises.
- This rise in RMP causes inactivation in the voltage dependent sodium channel, and the tissue begins to assume slow conduction characteristics.

- An ischemic, dying cell liberates intracellular potassium, which also causes a rise in the RMP.

Reentrant tachycardias have the following characteristics:

- The onset of the tachycardia is usually related to an initiating event (i.e., premature beat)

- The initiating beat is usually different in morphology from subsequent beats of the tachycardia -Initiation of the tachycardia is usually possible with programmed cardiac stimulation -The initiation and termination of the tachycardia are usually abrupt.

Bradyarrhythmias: Asymptomatic sinus bradyarrhythmias (heart rate less than 60 beats/min) are common especially in young, athletically active individuals. However, some patients have sinus node dysfunction (sick sinus syndrome) because of underlying organic heart disease and the normal aging process, which attenuates SA nodal function.

Congestive Cardiac Failure

Heart failure (HF), often used to mean chronic heart failure (CHF), occurs when the heart is unable to pump sufficiently to maintain blood flow to meet the needs of the body. The terms congestive heart failure (CHF) or congestive cardiac failure (CCF) are often used interchangeably with chronic heart failure.

Signs and symptoms commonly include shortness of breath, excessive tiredness, and leg swelling. Common causes of heart failure include coronary artery disease including a previous myocardial infarction (heart attack), high blood pressure, atrial fibrillation, valvular heart disease, and cardiomyopathy.

Two main types of heart failure:

- Heart failure due to left ventricular dysfunction
- Heart failure with normal ejection fraction

Pathophysiology

Heart failure is caused by any condition which reduces the efficiency of the myocardium, or heart muscle, through damage or overloading, including myocardial infarction (in which the heart muscle is starved of oxygen and dies), hypertension (which increases the force of contraction needed to pump blood) and amyloidosis (in which protein is deposited in the heart muscle, causing it to stiffen). Over time these increases in workload will produce changes to the heart itself:

- Reduced force of contraction, due to overloading of the ventricle. In a healthy heart, increased filling of the ventricle results in increased force of contraction (by the Frank–Starling law of the heart) and thus a rise in cardiac output. In heart failure this mechanism fails, as the ventricle is loaded with blood to the point where heart muscle contraction becomes less efficient. This is due to reduced ability to cross-link actin and myosin filaments in over-stretched heart muscle.

- A reduced stroke volume, as a result of a failure of systole, diastole or both. Increased end systolic volume is usually caused by reduced contractility. Decreased end diastolic volume results from impaired ventricular filling – as occurs when the compliance of the ventricle falls (i.e. when the walls stiffen).

- Reduced spare capacity. As the heart works harder to meet normal metabolic demands, the amount cardiac output can increase in times of increased oxygen demand (e.g. exercise) is reduced.

- Increased heart rate, stimulated by increased sympathetic activity in order to maintain cardiac output. Initially, this helps compensate for heart failure by maintaining blood pressure and perfusion, but places further strain on the myocardium, increasing coronary perfusion requirements, which can lead to worsening of ischemic heart disease. Sympathetic activity may also cause potentially fatal arrhythmias.

- Hypertrophy (an increase in physical size) of the myocardium, caused by the terminally differentiated heart muscle fibres increasing in size in an attempt to improve contractility. This may contribute to the increased stiffness and decreased ability to relax during diastole.

- Enlargement of the ventricles, contributing to the enlargement and spherical shape of the failing heart. The increase in ventricular volume also causes a reduction in stroke volume due to mechanical and inefficient contraction of the heart.

The general effect is one of reduced cardiac output and increased strain on the heart. This increases the risk of cardiac arrest (specifically due to ventricular dysrhythmias), and reduces blood supply to the rest of the body. In chronic disease, the reduced cardiac output causes a number of changes in the rest of the body, some of which are physiological compensations, some of which are part of the disease process:

- Arterial blood pressure falls. This destimulates baroreceptors in the carotid sinus and aortic arch which link to the nucleus tractussolitarii. This center in the brain increases sympathetic activity, releasing catecholamines into the blood stream. Binding to alpha-1 receptors results in systemic arterial vasoconstriction. This helps restore blood pressure but also increases the total peripheral resistance, increasing the workload of the heart. Binding to beta-1 receptors in the myocardium increases the heart rate and make contractions more forceful, in an attempt to increase cardiac output. This also, however, increases the amount of work the heart has to perform.

- Increased sympathetic stimulation also causes the posterior pituitary to secrete vasopressin (also known as antidiuretic hormone or ADH), which causes fluid retention at the kidneys. This increases the blood volume and blood pressure.

- Reduced perfusion (blood flow) to the kidneys stimulates the release of renin – an enzyme which catalyses the production of the potent vasopressor angiotensin. Angiotensin and its metabolites cause further vasoconstriction, and stimulate increased secretion of the steroid aldosterone from the adrenal glands. This promotes salt and fluid retention at the kidneys.

- The chronically high levels of circulating neuroendocrine hormones such as catecholamines, renin, angiotensin, and aldosterone affects the myocardium directly, causing structural remodelling of the heart over the long term. Many of these remodelling effects seem to be mediated by transforming growth factor beta (TGF-beta), which is a common downstream target of the signal transduction cascade. Initiated by catecholaminesand angiotensin II, and also by epidermal growth factor (EGF), which is a target of the signaling pathway activated by aldosterone.

- Reduced perfusion of skeletal muscle causes atrophy of the muscle fibres. This can result in weakness, increased fatigueability and decreased peak strength – all contributing to exercise intolerance.

The increased peripheral resistance and greater blood volume place further strain on the heart and accelerates the process of damage to the myocardium. Vasoconstriction and fluid retention produce an increased hydrostatic pressure in the capillaries. This shifts the balance of forces in favour of interstitial fluid formation as the increased pressure forces additional fluid out of the blood, into the tissue. This results in edema (fluid build-up) in the tissues. In right-sided heart failure this commonly starts in the ankles where venous pressure is high due to the effects of gravity (although if the patient is bed-ridden, fluid accumulation may begin in the sacral region.) It may also occur in the abdominal cavity, where the fluid build-up is called ascites. In left-sided heart failure edema can occur in the lungs – this is called cardiogenic pulmonary edema. This reduces spare capacity for ventilation, causes stiffening of the lungs and reduces the efficiency of gas exchange by increasing the distance between the air and the blood. The consequences of this are dyspnea (shortness of breath), orthopnea and paroxysm al nocturnal dyspnea.

The symptoms of heart failure are largely determined by which side of the heart fails. The left side pumps blood into the systemic circulation, whilst the right-side pumps blood into the pulmonary circulation. Whilst left-sided heart failure will reduce cardiac output to the systemic circulation, the initial symptoms often manifest due to effects on the pulmonary circulation. In systolic dysfunction, the ejection fraction isdecreased, leaving an abnormallyelevated volume of blood in the left ventricle. In diastolic dysfunction, end-diastolic ventricular pressure will be high.

This increase in volume or pressure backs up to the left atrium and then to the pulmonary veins. Increased volume or pressure in the pulmonary veins impairs the normal drainage of the alveoli and favors the flow of fluid from the capillaries to the lung parenchyma, causing pulmonary edema. This impairs gas exchange. Thus, left-sided heart failure often presents with respiratory symptoms such as shortness of breath, orthopnea and paroxysmal nocturnal dyspnea.

In severe cardiomyopathy, the effects of decreased cardiac output and poor perfusion become more apparent, and patients will manifest with cold and clammy extremities, cyanosis, claudication, generalized weakness, dizziness, and syncope. The resultant hypoxia caused by pulmonary edema causes vasoconstriction in the pulmonary circulation, which results in pulmonary hypertension.

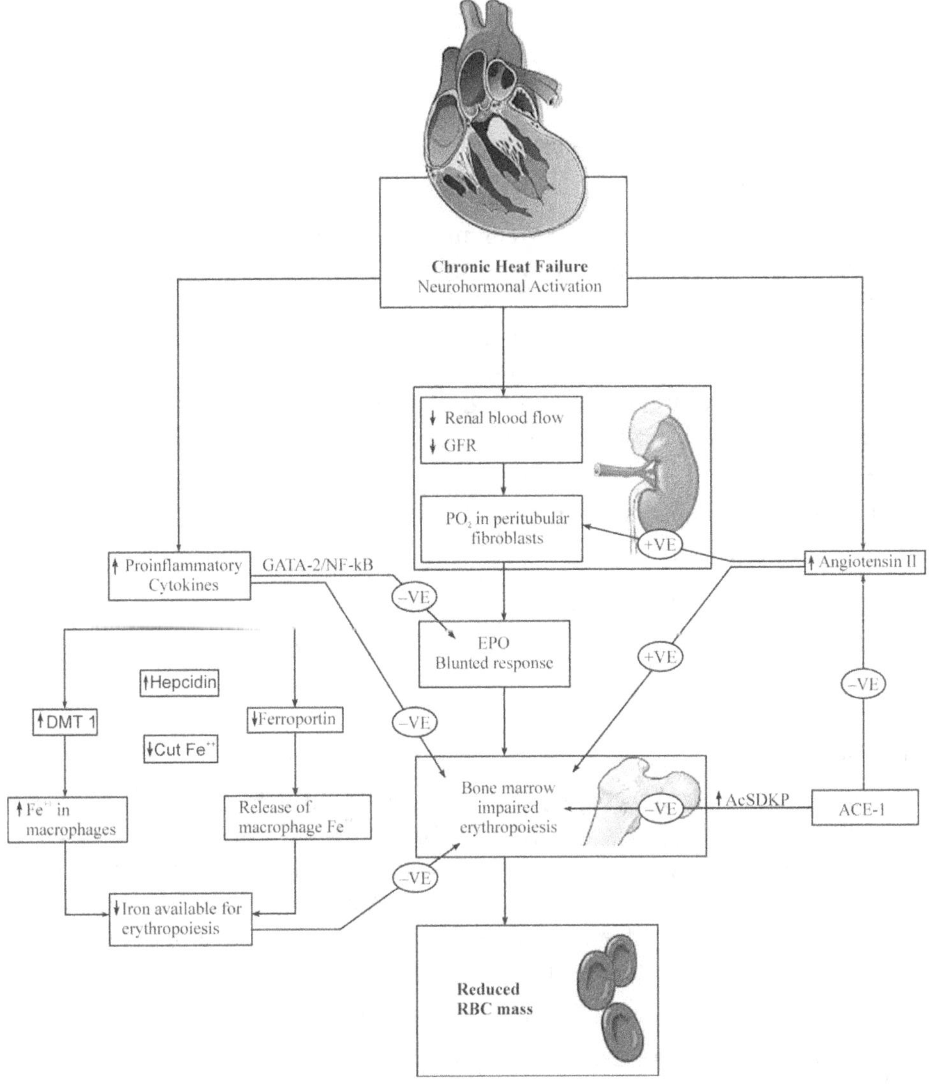

Fig. 9.7 Pathophysiology of congestive heart failure.

Source: acknowledgement:https://www.google.co.in/ search?q=chronic+heart+failure+diagram

Atherosclerosis

Arteriosclerosis is a chronic disease of arterial system characterised by abnormal thickening and hardening of arterial wall. Smooth muscle cell, collagen fibres migrate into tunica intima -causing it to stiffen and thicken-gradually, narrowing the arterial lumen. Changes in lipid, cholesterol and phospholipid metabolism within tunica intima also contribute to arteriosclerosis.

Arteriosclerosis includes:

- Senile arteriosclerosis
- Arteriosclerosis
- Hypertensive arteriosclerosis
- Moncke berg's arteriosclerosis
- Atherosclerosis

Atherosclerosis is the most common and most important form of arteriosclerosis. Atherosclerosis is the specific form of arteriosclerosis affecting primarily the intima of large and medium sized muscular arteries and is characterised by fibro fatty plaque or atheroma. In atherosclerosis, there is soft deposit of intra-arterial fat and fibrin on the wall that harden over time. Any large and medium sized artery may be involved in atherosclerosis. The most commonly affected are -aorta, coronary artery, cerebral arteries. Ischemia due to atherosclerosis cause:

- myocardial infarcts (heart attack)
- cerebral infarcts (stroke)
- peripheral vascular disease Aortic aneurysm
- chronic ischaemic heart disease ischaemic encephalopathy
- mesenteric occlusion

Morphology

Atheroma (Atheromatous plaque): A full developed atherosclerotic lesion is called atheromatous plaque also called fibrous plaque, fibro fatty plaque or atheroma. Atheromatous plaques are yellowish white lesions of varying diameter from 1-2 cm. Atheroma consists of raised focal plaques within intima having core of lipid (mainly cholesterol and cholesterol esters) and a covering fibrous cap. Atherosclerotic plaque has three principal components:

- cells: smooth muscle cell, macrophages, leukocytes
- connective tissue extracellular matrix: (collagen, elastic fibre, proteoglycans) intra or extra cellular lipid deposits
- Fibrous cap consists of smooth muscles cells, macrophages, form cells, lymphocytes, dense connective tissue and is covered by endothelium.
- Central core consists of lipid material, cholesterol clefts, fibrin, form cells (fatty cells).

- Lipid is primarily cholesterol and cholesterol esters.

In small arteries plaques are occlusive, (emboli) and in large arteries they are destructive- weakening the affected vessel wall-causing aneurism, rapture, favour thrombosis.

Complicated lesions: Atherosclerosis has following changes:

- Calcification occurs more commonly in advanced atheromatous plaque
- Focal rapture or ulceration of luminal surface of atheromatous plaque may result in exposure of blood to highly thrombogenic substances that induce thrombus formation (superimposed thrombosis)
- Discharge of debris into blood steam produce micro emboli aneurysmal dilation
- Rapture of artery and haemorrhage
- Fatty streaks are composed of lipid filled form cells

Etiology

- ***Age:*** Atherosclerosis is an age-related disease. Clinically significant lesions are found with increasing age. Fully developed atheromatous plaque usually appears 4th decade and beyond.
- ***Sex:*** Incidence and severity of atherosclerosis are more in men than women. Prevalence of atherosclerotic ischemic heart disease is 3 times higher in men. Lower incidence of ischaemic heart disease (IHD) in women in pre-menopausal age is due to high level of oestrogen and HDL both has anti atherogenic influence.
- ***Genetic factor:*** Play significant role in atherosclerosis.
- ***Geographical factors:*** Significant difference in prevalence of atherosclerosis in different countries has been observed.
- ***Diet:*** Diet, lifestyle and personal habits are important in pathogenesis and progression of atherosclerosis. Diet containing large quantity of saturated fat are harmful (egg, meat, milk etc.), and raise plasma cholesterol level. Diet with low saturated fat and high poly unsaturated fat (fish, fish oil etc.), lower plasma cholesterol level and protective. High intake of total number of calories-carbohydrate, proteins, alcohol, sweet has adverse effect. Omega 3 fatty acids (fish, fish oil) have protective effect.

Hyperlipidaemia: or hypercholesterolemia and other abnormalities in lipid metabolism contribute a major risk factor in atherosclerosis. Atherosclerotic plaques are rich in cholesterol and cholesterol esters derived from lipoproteins.

- Individual with hypercholesterolaemia (above 200mg/dl) due to various causes like diabetes, myxoedema, nephrotic syndrome have increased risk of atherosclerosis and IHD.
- Main lipids in blood are cholesterol (normal 140-240mg/dl) and triglycerides (normal below 160mg/dl).

- Cholesterol level above 260mg/dl has high risk of developing atherosclerosis and IHD.

- Low density lipoproteins (LDL, normal <130mg/dl) are richest in cholesterol and have maximum association with atherosclerosis.

- Hypertriglyceridemia with increased VLDL (very low density lipoprotein, normal <160mg/dl) also increase risk.

- High density lipoprotein (HDL, normal>40mg/dl) are called good cholesterol, and have protective effect.

- Hypertension: This is a major risk factor in development of atherosclerotic IHD and cerebrovascular disease. It acts by mechanical injury to arterial wall due to increased blood pressure. Systolic BP over 160mmHg or diastolic blood pressure over 95mmHg gave high risk of developing atherosclerotic IHD.

- Diabetes mellitus: There is twofold increases in incidence of clinical manifestations of atherosclerosis, (myocardial infarction, cerebral thrombosis and infarction, gangrene of lower extremities) in people with diabetes.

- Cigarette smoking: smoking is firmly established as risk factor in disease caused by atherosclerosis. Cigarette smoking is associated with high risk of atherosclerotic IHD and sudden cardiac death.

Other risk factors:

- Insufficient regular physical activity

- Behavioural pattern-competitive stressful life style obesity

- Oral contraceptives hyper uricaemia

- Hyper homocysteinemia high carbohydrate intake

Pathogenesis

Atherosclerosis is not caused by single etiological factor but is a multi-factorial disease. Anumber of theories have been proposed,

Response to injury hypothesis: **Vascular wall and their response to injury:** Endothelium and smooth muscle cells are the main component of wall of blood vessels-that pay important role in vascular pathology.

Endothelial cell (EC): Endothelial cells form a mono layer that lines the entire vascular system. The structural and functional integrity of endothelial cells (endothelium) is fundamental requirement for maintenance of vessel wall homeostasis and circulatory function. Vascular endothelium is a versatile multi-functional tissue having many synthetic and metabolic functions. Endothelium serves the role of non-thrombogenic blood tissue interface.

Endothelial cell functions: Maintenance of permeability barrier.

- Elaboration of anti-coagulant and anti-thrombic molecule (Prostacyclin, thrombomodulin, Plasminogen activator, Heparin like molecule).

Elaboration of pro thrombic molecule. (Von Willebrands factor, tissue factor, Plasminogen activation inhibitor), Extra cellar matric production (collagen, proteoglycans)

- Modulation of blood flow and vascular reactivity: Vasoconstriction by endothelin, ACE, Vasodilatation by NO/EDRF, Prostacyclin)
- Regulation of inflammation and immunity: (IL-1, 6, 8, Adhesion molecule, Histocompatibility antigen)
- Regulation of cell growth: (growth stimulators-PDRF, CSF, FGF etc.) (Growth inhibitors: heparin, TGF)
- Oxidation of LDL.
- Endothelial injury, inflammation play fundamental role in mediating all the steps in initiation and progression of atherogenesis.

Atherosclerosis begins with injury to endothelial cell that line arterial wall. The possible cause of endothelial injury includes, smoking, hyper tension, diabetes, hyper homocysteinemia, hyperlipidaemia, autoimmune phenomenon, infection, hypoxia, endotoxins, mechanical trauma, haemodynamic forces etc. Injured endothelial cell become inflammed and cannot make normal amount of antithrombotic and vasodilating cytokines.

Inflammed endothelial cells express adhesion molecule that bind macrophages and other inflammatory immune cells. Macrophages adheres to injured endothelium and release enzymes and toxic oxygen radicles that further injure the vessel wall, and result in oxidation of Low density lipoprotein (LDL).

Oxidised LDL is engulfed by macrophages which then penetrate into the intima of the vessel. Lipid laden macrophages are called form cells. They accumulate in significant amount and form a lesion called fatty streak. Fatty streak once formed produce more toxic oxygen radicles and cause immunologic and inflammatory changes. Macrophage derived growth factors stimulate the proliferation fSMCs. Smooth muscle cells shift from contractile phenotype to proliferative and synthetic phenotype.

At this point, smooth muscle cells (SMCs) proliferate; produce collagen. Collagen migrates over fatty streak forming fibrous plaque. This results in further endothelial cell dysfunction, necrosis of underlying vessel tissue and narrowing of vessel lumen.

As the plaque continues, to develop, continued inflammation can lead to instability of the plaque, and can result in ulceration and rapture, resulting in platelet adhesion to the lesion. This is now referred as complicated lesion. Platelet adhesion to the plaque can initiate coagulation cascade and result in rapid thrombus formation (superimposed thrombosis), causing tissue ischemia and infarction. Calcification may occur more commonly in advanced atheromatous plaque.

Monoclonal hypothesis: This hypothesis is based on the postulate that proliferation of smooth musclecells (SMCs) is the primary event and this proliferation is monoclonal in origin (originating from single cell) similar to cellular proliferation in neoplasm. Monoclonal proliferation in smooth muscle cell in atheromatous plaque may be initiated by mutation caused by exogenous chemicals (e.g.: cigarette smoke), endogenous metabolites (e.g.: lipoproteins) and some virus (e.g.: Herpes virus) etc.

Clinical effect: Clinical effect of atherosclerosis depends on size, and type of artery affected.

slow luminal narrowing cause ischemia and atrophy sudden luminal occlusion cause infarction, necrosis

propagation of plaque by formation of thrombi an emboli formation of aneurysmal dilation and rapture of artery

large arteries are affected commonly like aorta, renal, mesenteric and carotid artery small arteries involved are coronaries, arteries of lower limb etc.

Effect of atherosclerosis

- Aorta: aneurysm formation, thrombosis, embolisasion, etc.
- Heart: myocardial infarction, ischemic heart disease (IHD)
- Brain: chronic ischemic brain disease, cerebral infarction (stroke)
- Small intestine: ischaemic bowl disease, infarction
- Lower extremities: Intermittence claudication (lameness) gangrene etc

Myocardial Infarction

Coronary artery disease (CAD): This is any vascular disorder that narrow or occlude coronary arteries. The most common cause of coronary obstruction is atherosclerosis.

Ischaemic heart disease (IHD): is a closely related syndrome resulting from ischaemia. Ischaemic heart disease (IHD) is defined as acute or chronic form of myocardial disability arising from imbalance between myocardial supply and demand for oxygenated blood. Coronary artery disease (CAD) is used synonymously with IHD.

Ischaemia: is a state in which cells are temporarily deprived of blood supply. Ischaemia result from imbalance in supply and demand of blood. Ischaemia cause not only insufficiency of oxygen (hypoxia) but also reduce availability of nutrients and cause inadequate removal of metabolites. Depending upon rate of development, severity of narrowing- four ischaemic syndromes may develop:

- Angina pectoris
- Myocardial infarction
- Chronic ischaemic heart disease
- Sudden cardiac death (Heart attack) (Acute myocardial infarction).

Syndrome of IHD is a late manifestation of coronary atherosclerosis.

Myocardial infarction (MI)

Myocardial infarction is necrosis of heart muscle caused by imbalance between oxygen supply and demand. Most myocardial infarction results from severe narrowing of one of more coronary arteries. The factors that implicated in pathogenesis of Myocardial infarction (MI) include:

- Atherosclerotic Plaque Rapture
- Spasm

Myocardial infarction occurs most commonly at rest/during moderate activity. Severe stress and fatigue increase the precipitation of MI. Acute myocardial infarction or heat attack is the most important form of IHD in industrialised nations.

Etiology (Incidence and Risk Factors): Risk factors associated with development of coronary arterydisease (Myocardial infarction)

- Age (Frequency increase with age)
- Coronary atherosclerosis
- Diabetes mellitus
- Hypoxia
- Hyper lipoproteinemia
- Oral contraceptives
- Oestrogen deficiency
- Physical exertion
- Exposure to cold environment
- Hypertension
- Genetic factors
- Gender
- Direct myocardial injury
- Some drugs-Catechol amines, vasodilators, ergot alkaloids etc.
- Personality: Sedentary life style, Heavy alcohol consumption, Emotional stress, Cigarette smoking etc.

Pathophysiology of Myocardial Ischaemia: Coronary arteries normally supply blood flow sufficient to meet the demand of myocardium. If needs are not met, healthy coronary arteries dilate to increase the flow of oxygenated blood to myocardium. Narrowing of major coronary artery by more than 50%, impair blood flow and hamper cellular metabolism when myocardial demand increases. Atherosclerotic plaques formed in arterial system, occlude vessel depriving myocardium of oxygen and nutrients. Thrombi may form in coronary arteries as a result of ulceration of atherosclerotic plaque (superimposed thrombosis).The growing mass of plaque, platelets, fibrin, cellular debris, eventually can narrow the lumen enough to impede blood flow. Platelet aggregation release thromboxane A2 (a potent vasoconstrictor), that can cause spasm of coronary arteries. Myocardial ischaemia develop if flow/oxygen content of coronary blood is insufficient to meet metabolic demand of myocardial cell.

Role of fixed coronary obstruction: More than 90% of the patients with IHD have advanced stenosing coronary atherosclerosis (fixed obstructions). It can cause 75% reduction in cross sectional area of major epicardial arteries (left anterior descending artery, left cercum flex artery, right coronary artery etc.)

Role of acute plaque change: acute myocardial ischaemia often precipitated by disruption of previously only partially stenosing atherosclerotic plaque with haemorrhage, fissure or ulceration. Such vascular injury is fundamental cause of development of acute coronary syndromes like unstable angina, acute MI, sudden ischaemic death. Slowly developing occlusion stimulates well developed collateral vessels over time that may protect against infarction.

Platelet activation and aggregation increase thromboxane A2 at site of plaque disruption, which promote further platelet aggregation and vasoconstriction. Intermittent fragmentation of thrombus can lead to embolic vascular occlusion.

Pathogenesis: Atherosclerotic coronary artery disease (CAD) is the major underlying cause of myocardial infarction.

Coronary arterial occlusion: At least 90% of transmural acute myocardial infarcts are caused by occlusive intra coronary thrombus overlying an ulcerated or fissured plaque. Acute transmural myocardial infarction occurs due to:

- severe coronary atherosclerosis
- acute atheromatous plaque change (fissuring/ulceration)
- superimposed thrombosis
- platelet activation
- vasospasm

Following sequence of events can be proposed:

- initial sudden change in the morphology of atheromatous plaque (ulceration/fissuring)
- platelets are exposed to sub endothelial collagen and necrotic plaque contents, leading to adhesion, aggregation, activation, which build up platelet mass
- The platelet mass may give rise to emboli/occlusive thrombosis
- simultaneous release of tissue thromboplastin stimulates extrinsic pathway of coagulation
- activated platelets release thromboxane A2, serotonin, platelet factor 3&4 which favour vasospasm Frequently within minutes thrombus evolve to become completely occlusive.

Other causes:

- Vasospasm
- Emboli

Myocardial response: Occlusion of major coronary artery result in ischaemia throughout the anatomical region supplied by that artery (called area of risk), most pronounced is sub endocardium. Ischaemic myocardium undergoes progressive biochemical, functional and morphological changes and the outcome of which depends on severity and duration of flow deprivation (ischaemia). Principal biochemical change is onset of anaerobic respiration. Striking loss of contractility evident in 60 seconds.

Ultra-structural changes (cell and mitochondrial swelling etc.) develop in few minutes. These changes are reversible. Severe ischaemia lasting 20 to 40 minutes or longer leads to irreversible damage. Although function becomes abnormal in one minute, myocardial coagulation necrosis occurs only after 20-40 minutes of severe ischaemia.

Myocardial ischaemia also contribute to arrhythmia and sudden death. A leading cause of mortality in IHD patient is due to ventricular fibrillation. The location, size, and specific morphological features of acute myocardial infarct depend on:

- Location, severity, and rate of development of atherosclerotic obstruction
- Size of vascular bed perfused by obstructed vessel
- Duration of occlusion
- Metabolic, oxygen need of myocardium
- Extend of collateral blood circulation
- Severity of coronary artery spasm
- Other factors- blood pressure, heart rate, rhythm etc.

Repair: Myocardial infarction cause severe inflammatory response that ends in wound repair (scar). The infarcted area becomes fibrous scar tissue within few weeks of acute M.I. The scarred portion of myocardial wall will not function as viable cardiac muscle. It will display:

- Dyskinetic
- Hypokinetic
- Akynetic motion, which will decrease cardiac output

Aneurysm (localised dilation of wall of blood vessel) may also form in the area of infarct. Location of infarct: Infarcts are most frequently located in left ventricle. Atrial infarcts whenever present are more often in right atrium. Region of infarct depends on area of obstructed blood supply. Stenosis of left anterior descending artery cause infarction in anterior left ventricle including apex and anterior 2/3rd of interventricular septum (40-50% chance).

Stenosis of right coronary artery causes infarction in posterior part of left ventricle, posterior 1/3rd of interventricular septum (30-40% chance). Stenosis of circumflex coronary artery cause infarction in lateral wall of left ventricle.

Transmural-Vs-sub-endocardial infarction: There are two types of myocardial infarction, each having different morphology and clinical significance.

(a) *Transmural infarct:* in which the ischaemic necrosis involve full or nearly full thickness of the ventricular wall. This pattern of infarction is commonly associated with atherosclerosis, plaque rapture, superimposed thrombosis etc.

(b) *Sub-endocardial (sub-cardial) infarct (non-trans mural):* A part of myocardial wall is damage. Ischaemic necrosis limited to one third/one half of ventricular wall. Sub-endocardial region is the least well perfused region of myocardium. In sub-endocardial infarct, there is diffuse stenosing coronary atherosclerosis and global reduction in blood flow but neither plaque rapture nor superimposed coronary thrombosis. In sub-endocardial necrosis Q wave failed to develop in ECG (non-Q wave infarction).

Clinical Presentation

Classical symptoms: of myocardial ischaemia include pressure like sub sternal heaviness, chest pain, diaphoresis (sweating), nausea, shortness of breath, sense of impeding (about to happen) doom (death). Pain and pressure may radiate to arms, to back between scapula, neck or jaw. Vomiting and diarrhoea may also be observed. Classical symptoms occur in 50% patients.

Atypical symptoms (25%): present with indigestion, syncope, shock, pulmonary oedema, lethargy, embolic events etc. Asymptomatic M.I occurs in women, older men, diabetics.

Complication of Myocardial Infarction (MI): A significant factor which prevent/ diminish myocardial damage is development of collateral circulation.80-90% cases develop major complications after attack, some of which are fatal:

- Arrhythmia
- Congestive heart failure
- Cardiogenic shock
- Rapture of heart
- Post myocardial infarction syndrome
- Pericarditis

Diagnosis

Detailed history helps to differentiate between myocardial ischaemic pain and non-cardiac chest pain. Shock, weak pulse, systolic blood pressure below 80 mmHg, low grade fever etc. ECG changes:

- ST segment elevation

- T wave inversion
- Wide deep Q wave.

Serum enzyme determination:

- SGOT level rise rapidly
- Creatinine kinase level increase (CK)
- Lactic acid dehydrogenase (LDH) level increase

Treatment objectives:

- Reverse myocardial ischaemia – limit infarct size
- Reduce post myocardial complications – relieve pain and anxiety
- Recognise and control life threatening arrhythmias

Treatment

- Oxygen
- Analgesics
- Sedation (anti-anxiety)
- Vasodilators
- β-blockers
- Thrombolytic agent
- Coronary arteries bypass grafting.

Diabetes Mellitus

Endocrine pancreas: Normal anatomy and function: pancreas consists of 1 million microscopic cellular units called islets of Langerhans. Islets in adult human weigh 1-1.5gm.Islets of Langerhans are scattered throughout pancreas but are most numerous in distal portion (tail).

These round cellular masses contain several types of cells:

- β-cells (70%)-secrete insulin
- α-cells (20%)-secrete glucagon
- Delta cells (5-10%)-secrete somatostatin which suppress both insulin and glucagon release.
- Pancreatic polypeptide cells-which secrete pancreatic polypeptides having some gastrointestinal effect.
- D1-cells which release vasoactive intestinal peptides which induce glycogenolysis and hyperglycaemia
- Enterochromaffin cells-synthesis serotonin

Definition: Diabetes mellitus is characterised by glucose intolerance (hyperglycaemia) and other metabolic derangements, which result from inadequate secretion of insulin or target tissue resistance to its action, lead to vascular changes and neuropathy affecting a number of organs. Diabetes mellitus means primary/ idiopathic diabetes mellitus. Secondary diabetes mellitus means occurrence of hyperglycaemia with some identifiable causes like chronic pancreatitis, post pancreotomy, some drugs, hormonal tumours (pheochro-mocytoma, pituitary tumour), 170owman170s170atosis, genetic disorder etc.

Clinical Features

Primary/idiopathic diabetes: Diabetes mellitus has two principal forms:

 (a)   Insulin dependent diabetes (IDDM), Juvenile onset (Type-I)
 (b)   Non-insulin dependent diabetes mellitus (NIDDM), Maturity onset, (Type-II)
    - Obese NIDDM
    - Non-obese NIDDM
    - Maturity onset diabetes of young

Type I [IDDM]

20 % of the total cases are IDDM. Often begins before patient attains age 15.IDDM is characterised by abrupt onset, weight loss and requirement of insulin injection to prevent ketoacidosis. Difficulty to maintain glucose level in normal limit (brittleness). Histocompatibility antigens, viral illness etc. have important role.

Type II [NIDDM]

Constitute 80% of the cases. Patient need insulin therapy to control the symptoms but does not require it for survival. Principal problem may be in delivery of insulin/resistance to it rather than synthesis.

Comparison between type I and type II

	Type I	Type II
Frequency	10-20%	80-90%
Age of onset	Early, below 40	Late, after 40
Type of onset	Abrupt, severe	Gradual, insidious
Weight	Normal	Obese
HLA	HLA-D linked	No HLA association
Genetic link	20%	60%
Pathogenesis	Autoimmunity, severe insulin deficiency.	Insulin resistance, relative insulin deficiency
Islet cell antibodies	Yes	No
Blood insulin level	Decreased	Normal/increased
Islet cell changes	Insulitis, β-cell depletion	No insulitis, mild β-cell depletion
Clinical management	Insulin, diet	Diet,
Polydipsia, Polyphagia, Polyuria	yes	yes
Metabolic complication (ketoacidosis, hypoglycaemic episodes	Frequent	Less frequent

Symptoms

Classic symptoms of diabetes mellitus are polyuria, polydipsia, polyphagia with paradoxical weight loss etc. In uncontrolled IDDM life threatening ketoacidosis may occur.

- ***Etiology and pathogenesis of type I diabetes (Juvenile onset):*** Caused by absolute deficiency of insulin resulting from reduction in β-cell mass.

- ***Genetic susceptibility:*** familial.

- ***Auto immunity:*** Type I diabetes is believed to be an autoimmune disease that result from specific immunologic destruction of β-cells of islets of Langerhans.

- ***Evidences:***
    - presence of islet cell antibodies in patients
    - lymphocytic infiltration in and around islets
    - association of type I diabetes with other autoimmune disease
    - remission of type I diabetes with immunosuppressive therapy

- ***Environmental factors:*** certain viral infections cause onset of type I diabetes. E.g.: mumps, measles, coxackie B virus, infectious mononucleosis etc.

- Experimental induction of type-I diabetes with certain chemicals are possible e.g.: alloxan, pentamidine, streptozotocin.

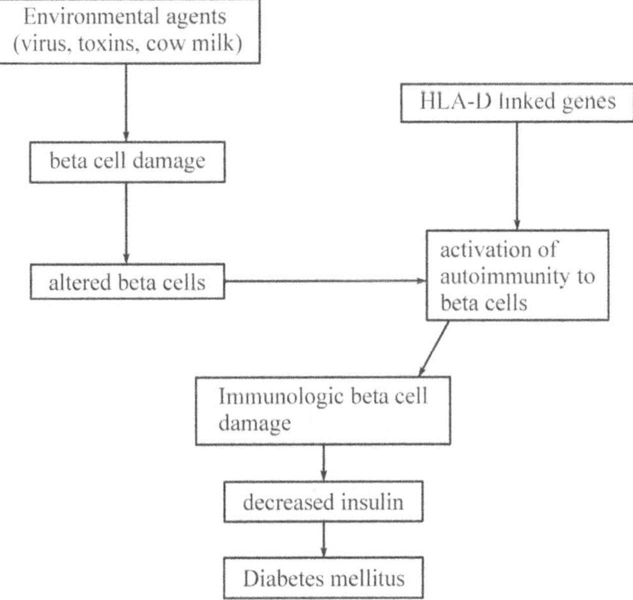

Fig. 9.8 Causes of diabetes mellitus.

Etiopathogenesis of type II diabetes (maturity onset diabetes)

- The basic metabolic defect in type II diabetes is either:
  - delayed insulin secretion relative to glucose load (deranged insulin secretion)
  - peripheral tissue unable to respond to insulin (insulin resistance)
- **Genetic factors:** genetic susceptibility has greater role in pathogenesis of type II diabetes than type I diabetes.

Obesity (Obese type II diabetes)

Obesity is a common finding in type II diabetes. Impaired insulin sensitivity of peripheral tissue such as muscle and fat cells to the action of insulin in obese individuals.

Insulin receptor defect (Non-obese Type II diabetes): Insulin resistance is found in non-obese individuals. In such individuals increased insulin resistance of peripheral tissue is due to either decrease in number of insulin receptors or post receptor defect.

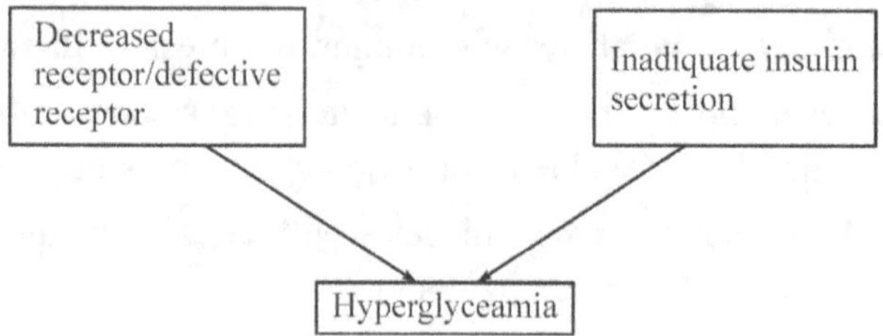

Fig. 9.9 Etiology of hyperglycemia.

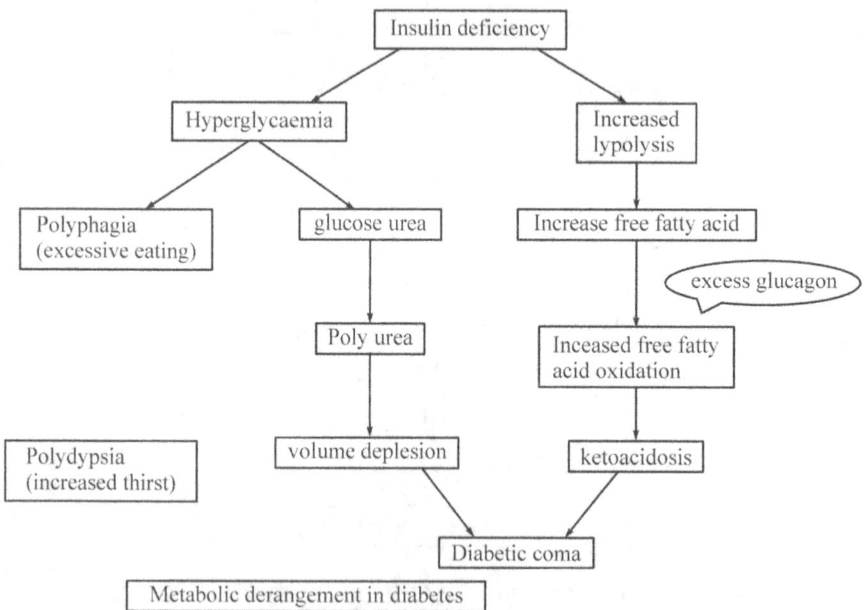

Fig. 9.10 Complications of diabetes.

Complications of Diabetes

A. Acute metabolic complications

Ketoacidosis and hypoglycaemic episodes are primary complication of type I diabetes. Hyperosmolar non-ketotic coma is main complication of type II diabetes. Diabetic ketoacidosis develops in patients with severe insulin deficiency and glucagon excess. Severe lack of insulin causes lipolysis in adipose tissue with release of free fatty acids into plasma. These free fatty acids are oxidised to ketone bodies (aceto acetic acid, β-hydroxy butyric acid) in liver. Such oxidation accelerated in presence of glucagon. It causes ketonaemia and ketonuria.

If urinary excretion is prevented due to dehydration, it causes systemic metabolic ketoacidosis. Clinically this condition is characterised by anorexia, nausea, vomiting, deep and fast breathing and mental confusion.

Hypoglycaemia: Hypoglycaemic episodes may develop in patient of type I diabetes. It may result from excessive administration of insulin, missing meal or due to stress. Hypoglycaemic episodes are harmful as they produce permanent brain damage or result in worsening of diabetic control and rebound hyperglycaemia (called Somogyi effect).

Hyperosmolar non-ketotic coma is usual complication of type II diabetes. It is caused by severe dehydration resulting from sustained hyperglycaemic 174owman174s. Loss of glucose in urine is so severe that patient is unable to drink sufficient water to maintain urinary fluid loss. Blood sugar level is extremely high and plasma osmolarity is high. Thrombotic and bleeding complications are frequent due to high viscosity of blood. Mortality rate is high.

B. Late systemic complications

Non-enzymatic glycosylation: It is a process by which glucose bind with amino group of proteins without aid of enzymes e.g.: Glycosylated Haemoglobin. Glycosylation product (collagen and other protein) accumulate in vessel walls.

Polyol pathway mechanism: Aldose reductase–an enzyme which act on glucose to form sorbitol and fructose in cells of hyperglycaemic patients.

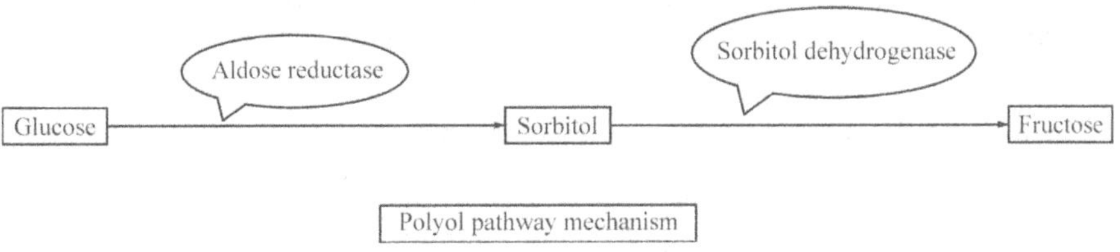

Fig. 9.11 Schematic representation of polyol pathway mechanism.

Intra cellular accumulation of sorbitol and fructose cause entry of water inside the cell, with swelling and cell damage. A number of systemic complications develop after a period of 15-20 years in both type of diabetes.

Atherosclerosis: Diabetes mellitus of both types accelerate development of atherosclerosis. Contributory factors are hyperlipidaemia, reduced HDL level, non-enzymatic glycosylation, increased platelet adhesion, obesity and hypertension.

The ill effects are:

- Coronary artery disease
- Silent myocardial infarction
- Cerebral stroke
- Gangrene of toe and feet

Diabetic microangiopathy: Characterised by basement membrane thickening of small blood vessels and capillaries, of different organs and tissue such as skin, skeletal muscle, eye, kidney. Similar type of basement membrane like material is deposited in non-vascular tissues like peripheral nerves, renal tubule, 175owman's capsule etc.

Pathogenesis of diabetic microangiopathy is increased glycosylation (non enzymatic glycosylation-non enzymatic binding of glucose with amino group of proteins) of haemoglobin and other proteins (like collagen, basement membrane material) resulting in thickening of basement membrane.

Diabetic nephropathy: This is caused by

- Diabetic glomerulosclerosis
- Vascular lesions
- Diabetic pyelonephritis
- Tubular lesion

Diabetic neuropathy: Pathologic changes are-

- Segmental demyelination
- Schwann cell injury
- Axon damage

This is caused by diffuse microangiopathy or accumulation of sorbitol and fructose. Also causes sensory loss, impotence, postural hypotension, constipation, diarrhoea etc.

Diabetic retinopathy:

- Leading cause of blindness
- caused by retinal capillary microangiopathy

Infection: Diabetics have enhanced susceptibility to various infections, such as tuberculosis, pneumonia, pyelonephritis, otitis, diabetic ulcer etc.

Pathological changes:
- *Insulitis:* Lymphocyte infiltration in islets is a feature of type I diabetes.
- *Islet cell mass:* There is reduction in size and number of islets in type I diabetes. In type II, β-cell mass is either normal or mildly reduced.
- *B-cell degranulation and glycogenosis:* Type I diabetics are associated with β-cell degranulation and subsequent deposition of glycogen in these cells.
- *Amyloidosis:* Amyloid deposition around capillaries of islets causes compression and atrophy of islet cell. It is characteristic in chronic type II diabetes.
- *Fibrosis of islets*: Fibro collagenous replacement of islets found in type II diabetes.
- *Small blood vessels*: Diabetic microangiopathy affects small arteries and capillaries. Disappearance of pericytes, thickening of basement membrane is visible in muscle, skin, retina, kidney etc.
- *Medium and large blood vessels:* Arteriosclerosis, lesion common in coronary, cerebral, mesenteric, renal and femoral arteries.
- *Kidney:* Nodular glomerulitis, focal thickening of capillary basement membrane.
- *Eye:* Diabetic retinopathy

Peptic Ulcer

Definition: Peptic ulcers are areas of degeneration and necrosis of gastrointestinal mucosa exposed to acid-peptic secretion. They occur at any level of alimentary tract exposed to hydrochloric acid and pepsin.

Acute peptic Ulcer (Stress ulcers): Multiple, small, mucosal erosions seen most commonly in stomach but occasionally involving duodenum.

Etiology

(a) Psychological stress

(b) Physiological stress as in
- Shock
- Severe trauma
- Septicaemia
- Extensive burn (curling's ulcers)
- Intracranial lesions (cushing's ulcers)
- Drug intake (aspirin, steroids, butazolidine, indomethacin) − local irritants (alcohol, smoking, coffee etc.,)

Pathogenesis

Hyper secretion of gastric acid is demonstrable only in Cushing's ulcer occurring from intracranial conditions like brain trauma, intracranial surgery, brain tumour etc. Ischaemic/hypoxic injury to the mucosal cells. Depletion of gastric mucus barrier rendering mucosa susceptible to attack by acid/pepsin.

Chronic peptic Ulcers (Gastric and duodenal ulcers): It is the two-major form of peptic ulcer disease of upper GI tract. Gastric and duodenal ulcers are two distinct diseases with distinct etiology, pathogenesis and clinical features. Pathological finding in both are similar.

Incidence

Peptic ulcer disease (PUD) is more frequent in middle aged adults. More common in males than female. Duodenal ulcer four times more common than gastric ulcer.

Etiology

Etiology of peptic ulcer disease may not be explained on basis of single factor it is multifactorial. Immediate cause of peptic ulcer disease is disturbance of normal protective mucosal barrier by acid-pepsin resulting in digestion of mucosa.

- *Acid-pepsin secretion:* Patient with gastric ulcer has law/normal gastric acid secretion. Duodenal ulcer occurs due to hyper secretion of acid-pepsin.

- *Mucus secretion:* Any condition that decrease the quantity or quality of normal protective mucous barrier cause development of peptic ulcer.

- *Gastritis:* Some degree of gastritis always present in the region of gastric ulcer. It is not clear that whether it is cause/effect of ulcer.

- *Local irritants:* Pyloric antrum and lesser curvature of stomach are sites most exposed for longer period to local irritants and thus is common site of occurrence of gastric ulcer.

- Some local irritants are-heavily spiced foods, alcohol, cigarette smoking, unbuffered aspirin, NSAIDs.

- *Dietary factors:* Nutritional deficiencies have been regarded as etiologic factor in peptic ulcer.

- *Psychological factors:* Psychological stress, anxiety, fatigue predispose peptic ulcer disease.

- *Genetic factors:* Genetic influence appears to have greater role in duodenal ulcers.

- *Hormonal factors:* Secretion of certain hormones by tumours is associated with peptic ulceration e.g.: elaboration of glucagon by islet cell tumour in Zollinger Ellison Syndrome

- Hyperplasia and adenomas of parathyroid gland, adrenal cortex, anterior pituitary.

Pathogenesis

There is distinct difference in pathogenetic mechanism involved in duodenal and gastriculcers.

- ***Duodenal ulcer:*** High acid-pepsin secretion is the one causative agent of duodenal ulcer.
- ***Other causes:*** hyper secretion of acid in fasting stomach at night which take place under the influence of vagal stimulation.

Patient with duodenal ulcer have rapid emptying of stomach. Food which normally buffer and neutralise gastric acid, pass down leaving duodenal mucosa exposed to aggressive action of gastric acid.

Campylobacter gastritis (caused by Campylobacter pylori/Helicobacter pylori): Seen in 85-100% cases of duodenal ulcer. Mucosal area colonised by this organism are depleted of protective mucous barrier. This exposes the underlying epithelial tissue to injurious effect of acid-pepsin secretion.

Gastric ulcer: Pathogenesis of gastric ulcer mainly due to impaired gastric mucosal defense against acid-pepsin secretion. Patient with gastric ulcer have low to normal gastric acid level. Hyper acidity may occur due to increased serum gastrin level. Normal protective gastric mucous barrier against acid-pepsin is deranged in gastric ulcer. There is depletion of quality as well as quantity of gastric mucus. One mechanism of this depletion is colonisation of *Campylobacter pylori.*

Other factor: gastritis, bile reflex, cigarette smoke etc.

Complications: Acute and sub-acute peptic ulcer heal without any visible scar. Healing of chronic, largerand deeper ulcer may result in complication.

Obstruction: Development of fibrous scar result in pyloric stenosis, duodenal stenosis.

Haemorrhage: Minor bleeding by erosion of small blood vessels occurs in all type of ulcers. Chronic blood loss may cause deficiency anaemia. Erosion of major artery (Left gastric, gastroduodenal, splenic artery may cause massive and severe hematemesis).

Perforation: A perforated peptic ulcer is acute abdominal emergency. Perforation occurs more commonly in chronic duodenal ulcer than chronic gastric ulcer. On perforation content may escape into peritoneal cavity causing acute peritonitis. Sub-phrenic abscess between liver and diaphragm may develop due to infection. Air escape and cause air under diaphragm. Perforation may extend to adjacent organs -liver, pancreas. Malignant transformation: Chronic duodenal ulcer never turns malignant.1% chronic gastric ulcer may transform to carcinoma.

Clinical Features

Peptic ulcers are remitting and relapsing lesions.

- ***Age:*** Peak incidence of duodenal ulcer is 5th decade and gastric ulcer is 6th decade.

- ***People at risk:*** Duodenal occurs more commonly in people faced with more stress. Gastric ulcer more often in labouring group.

- ***Periodicity:*** Attack of peptic ulcer last for 2-6 weeks with 1-6months interval.

- ***Pain:*** In gastric ulcer, epigastric pain occurs immediately/within 2 hrs. after food and never occurs at night. Duodenal ulcer pain severe at late night (hunger pain) and relieved by food.

- ***Vomiting:*** Vomiting which relieve pain is conspicuous feature of gastric ulcer. Duodenal ulcer patient rarely has vomiting but get heart burn.

- ***Hematemesis and melena:*** Hematemesis more in gastric ulcer. Melena (dark stool due to haemorrhage) more in duodenal ulcer.

- ***Weight:*** Weight gain in duodenal, weight loss in gastric.

Inflammatory Bowel Diseases

Definition: The inflammatory bowel disease (IBD) is a group of inflammatory conditions of the colon and small intestine. Crohn's disease and ulcerative colitis are the principal types of inflammatory bowel disease; it can also affect the mouth, oesophagus, stomach and the anus. The chronic inflammatory bowel diseases (IBD), Crohn's disease and ulcerative colitis, are recognized as important causes of gastrointestinal disease in children and adults.

Inflammatory bowel disease (IBD) is an idiopathic disease caused by a dysregulated immune response to host intestinal microflora. The two major types of inflammatory bowel disease are

- Ulcerative colitis (UC), which is limited to the colon,

- Crohn disease (CD), which can affect any segment of the gastrointestinal tract from the mouth to the anus, involves "skip lesions," and is transmural. There is a genetic predisposition for IBD, and patients with this condition are more prone to the development of malignancy.

Collagenous colitis is an inflammatory bowel disease affecting the colon specifically with peak incidence in the 5th decade of life, affecting women more than men. Its clinical presentation involves watery diarrhea, usually in the absence of rectal bleeding. It is often classified under the umbrella entity microscopic colitis, along with a related condition, lymphocytic colitis.

Lymphocytic colitis, a subtype of microscopic colitis, is a rare condition characterized by chronicnon-bloody watery diarrhea. Thecolonoscopy is normal but the mucosal biopsy reveals an accumulation of lymphocytes in the colonic epithelium and connective tissue (laminapropria). Collagenous colitis shares this feature but additionally shows a distinctive thickening of the sub-epithelial collagen table.

Diversion colitis is an inflammation of the colon which can occur as a complication of ileostomy or colostomy, often occurring within the year following the surgery. It can also occur in a neovagina created by colovaginoplasty, sometimes several years after the original procedure. Despite the presence of a variable degree of inflammation the most suggestive histological feature remains the prominent lymphoid aggregates. A foul smelling, mucous rectal discharge may develop from the inflamed mucosa of the distal, unused colon.

Behçet disease, sometimes called Behçet's syndrome or Silk Road disease, is a rare immune-mediated small-vessel systemic vasculitis that often presents with mucous membrane ulceration and ocular problems. It has triple-symptom complex of recurrent oral aphthous ulcers, genital ulcers, and uveitis. As a systemic disease, it can also involve visceral organs such as the gastrointestinal tract, pulmonary, musculoskeletal, cardiovascular and neurological systems.

Hypothesis Regarding Pathogenesis

Pathogenesis of IBD may be due to an autoimmune response to a luminal or mucosal antigen, a dysfunctional immune response to a commensal bacterium, and an infection with a pathogenic organism which remains in the intestinal tissues and results in a chronic inflammatory response.

Autoimmune disease: A destructive inflammatory response directed toward a self-antigen such as mucin, goblet cells, colonocytes, or other cells has been proposed as the underlying basis of IBD, particularly in regard to Ulcerative Colitis (UC).

- Antibodies against neutrophils may be found.
- Levels of antibodies against a human intestinal tropomyosin isoform also have been reported to be increased in UC patients.
- Exposure to microbial peptides that share immunogenic determinants with self-antigens has been suggested as the trigger for the disruption in immune tolerance to endogenous gut antigens.

Infection with a pathogenic organism: The clinical presentation and histologic appearance of IBD has a number of similarities to gastrointestinal infections by known pathogenic organisms. For instance, acutely CD can appear like gastrointestinal disease due to Yersinia or *M. tuberculosis*. Even if an infectious pathogen is involved, genetic factors clearly are important in determining whether IBD subsequently develops.

Dysregulated immune response to commensal role: Intestinal commensal bacteria in the pathogenesis of IBD. Patients may have alterations in the mucus-epithelial layer which allow a more intimate association of gut bacteria with the mucosa. Potentially, the presence of mucosa-associated indigenous bacteria in these patients produces disease despite the absence of more aggressive pathogenic bacteria. The closer proximity of the bacteria to the epithelium may be a crucial component in the initiation of the cycles of inflammation and changes in intestinal permeability that are characteristic of IBD. Genetic factors may contribute to both the increased penetration of the bacteria or bacterial products as well as the pronounced inflammatory response that occurs.

The identities of the commensal bacteria that may be involved in the pathogenesis of IBD are unclear. Some investigations have pointed to a role for anaerobic bacteria such as Bacteroides or *Clostridium spp.* Cell wall components such as lipopolysaccharide and other bacterial products have strong pro-inflammatory effects and mediate intestinal inflammation in animal models.

Cirrhosis and Alcoholic Liver Diseases

Definition: It is characterised by fibrosis and conversion of normal hepatic architecture into structurally abnormal nodules. These events lead to abnormal vascular relationship and portal hypertension. This disorder represents end stage of various chronic diseases that cause diffuse parenchymal damage. It is defined by three characteristics:

- Fibrosis Present in the form of delicate band (portal to central, portal to portal, central to central) or as a broad scar replacing multiple adjacent lobules.
- Parenchymal architecture of entire liver is disrupted by interconnecting fibrous scar.
- Parenchymal nodules (regenerative nodules) are created by regeneration of hepatocytes.

Several features should be underscored:

- Parenchymal injury and consequent fibrosis are diffuse (extending throughout the liver).
- Fibrosis once developed is generally irreversible.
- Vascular architecture is disorganized by parenchymal damage and scarring with formation of abnormal interconnections between vascular inflow and hepatic vein outflow.
- It occurs following hepatocellular necrosis of varying etiology so that there are alternate areas of necrosis and regenerative nodules.

Pathogenesis

Progressive fibrosis is the central feature of cirrhosis. Irrespective of the etiology cirrhosis is initiated by hepatocellular necrosis. Continued destruction of hepatocyte causes collapse of normal lobular hepatic parenchyma, followed by fibrosis around necrotic liver cells and proliferated ductules. There is formation of compensatory regenerative nodules.

In cirrhosis type I and type III collagens are deposited in all portion of the lobule, resulting in severe disruption of blood flow and impaired diffusion of solutes between hepatocytes and plasma. Although hepatocytes are capable of synthesising collagen major source of excess collagen in cirrhosis is Ito cells. Their normal function is fat/Vit-A storage,-they transform to fibroblast like cells.

The stimuli for fibrosis (transformation) - may be inflammatory mediators [TNF-α. TNF-β, Interleukin-I], Kupffer cells (cytokines), distortion normal extracellular matrix etc. The cause of compensatory proliferation of hepatocytes to form regenerative nodules -may be growth factors, hormonal imbalance etc.

Morphological Classification

There are three types of cirrhosis:

    (a) Micro nodular

    (b) Macro nodular

    (c) Mixed nodular

Each of these forms has an active form/inactive form. Active form characterised by continuing hepatocellular necrosis and inflammatory reaction. Inactive form-no evidence of continuing hepatocellular damage.

Micro nodular cirrhosis: Nodules are small, regular and <3mm diameter. It represents impaired capacity of regrowth-as seen in alcoholism, malnutrition, severe anaemia, old age. Micronodular cirrhosis also called portal cirrhosis, nutritional cirrhosis or Laennec's cirrhosis. Nodules are variable size usually larger than 3mm diameter. The pattern of involvement is irregular.

Mixed cirrhosis: Some part of the liver shows micro nodular appearance while other part shows macronodular appearance.

Etiological Classification

Based on cause for cirrhosis following etiologic categories

    1. Alcoholic cirrhosis (60-70%)

    2. Post necrotic cirrhosis (10%)

    3. Biliary cirrhosis (5-10%)

    4. Pigment cirrhosis in hemochromatosis (5%)

    5. Cirrhosis in Wilson's disease

    6. Cirrhosis in α-1 antitrypsin deficiency

    7. Cardiac cirrhosis

    8. Indian childhood cirrhosis (ICC)

    9. Cryptogenic cirrhosis (10-15%)

  10. Miscellaneous forms of cirrhosis.

Clinical Manifestations and Complications

Clinical features of cirrhosis range from asymptomatic state to progressive liver failure and death.

- Loss of functional parenchyma cause major consequence in cirrhosis.
- Hypoalbuminemia, clotting abnormalities, Jaundice
- Impaired drug detoxification.
- High risk of infection.
- Increased risk of developing hepatocellular carcinoma.
- Disorder may affect virtually every organ system.

It causes anaemia, parotid gland enlargement, peptic ulcer disease, fatigue, weight loss, hypogonadism, gynaecomastia, portal hypertension, anorexia, muscle wasting, low grade fever. Abnormal intra-peritoneal accumulation of fluid containing large amount of protein and electrolyte.

Advanced cases develop:

- Portal hypertension
- Progressive hepatic failure
- Hepatocellular carcinoma
- Chronic relapsing pancreatitis
- Steatorrhoea (excretion of fat)
- Gall stone
- Infection

Treatment

- Management of Portal hypertension
- Agent which inhibit collagen synthesis (e.g. colchicine)
- Liver transplantation.

Acute Renal Failure

Definition: Acute renal failure can be defined as an abrupt decrease in renal function/glomerular filtration rate manifested by azotaemia (increased blood urea nitrogen, creatinine) and diminished urine output.

A rise in serum creatinine above 1mg/dl [1mg/100ml] over 2-3 days generally accepted as indicative of acute renal failure. ARF is a severe organ failure which is potentially reversible. Acute tubular necrosis is one of the common types of ARF. Aneuric, oliguric and non-oliguric are other modifiers frequently applied to ARF.

Etiology: Acute renal failure more commonly associated with:

- Acute tubular necrosis
- Trauma, infection, snake bite, pregnancy, poison ingestion etc.

ARF may be divided into three broad categories:

- *Pre-renal:* refers to reduction in glomerular filtration rate that is secondary to diminished renal blood flow. Inadequate cardiac output, hypovolemia, or vascular diseases are causing reduced perfusion of kidney.
- *Post renal:* causes include obstruction of flow of urine anywhere from renal pelvis to distal urethra. This may be caused by mass within lumen (renal calculi, tumour), external compression.
- *Intrinsic renal:* causes are those diseases/processes that directly injure renal parenchyma. e.g.: Vascular disease of arteries and arterioles within kidney, rapidly progressive glomerulonephritis, acute tubular necrosis due to ischaemia or toxins, pyelonephritis etc.

Pathophysiology of Acute Renal Failure [ARF]

The pathogenesis of acute renal failure involves:

(a) ***Decreased ultra-filtration coefficient:*** Reduction in filtration coefficient and alteration in glomerular vascular resistance have been proposed as mechanism for observed decrease in glomerular filtration rate. Renal vasoconstriction, and diminished renal blood flow cause acute tubular necrosis. Angiotensin-II causes reduction in ultra-filtration coefficient and alteration in glomerular vascular resistance.

(b) ***Renal hypo perfusion:*** Renal blood flow under normal condition is 1L/min (25% of cardiac output). When the ability of cardiovascular system to deliver blood to kidney is impaired, result in pre-renal azotaemia. Heart failure, volume depletion, shock is the most common cause. Prolonged and severe renal hypoperfusion result in acute tubular necrosis. Causes of Pre-renal Acute Rena Failure: Decreased cardiac output:

- Cardiomyopathy
- Pericardial tamponade
- Bacterial sepsis/vasodilating drugs
- Decreased intra vascular volume
- Haemorrhage/volume depletion etc.

(c) ***Intrinsic renal causes of ARF:*** Glomerular:

- Glomerulonephritis Tubulointerstitial
- Acute tubular necrosis
- Acute pyelonephritis
- Hypercalcaemia
- Multiple myeloma
- vasculitis
- Malignant nephrosclerosis
- Venous occlusion
- Serum sickness etc.

(d) ***Tubular dysfunction with back leak of filtrate:*** Non-selective back leak of filtrate across damaged renal tubule cause oliguria and azotemia in acute tubular necrosis.

(e) ***Intra tubular obstruction:*** Intra tubular cast (jelly like substance in renal tubule) cause tubular obstruction.

Acute Tubular Necrosis [ATN]

It is a term used for acute renal failure caused by destruction of tubular epithelial cells. It is characterised by sudden cessation of renal function.

(a) ***Ischemic acute tubular necrosis:*** It occurs due to hypoperfusion of kidney resulting in focal damage to tubules.

- Shock (post-traumatic, surgical, burn, dehydration etc.)
- Crush injury
- Rhabdomyolysis (disintegration of striated muscle fibres with excretion of myoglobin in urine.)
- Mismatched blood transfusion
- Arteriolar vasoconstriction induces by renin angiotensin system
- Tubular obstruction by casts (jelly) in lumina or interstitial oedema – Back leak of tubular fluid into interstitium
- Abnormal glomerular permeability

(b) ***Toxic Acute tubular necrosis:*** Due to direct damage to tubular cells by ingestion (taking in), injection or inhalation of toxic agents.

Diagnosis

History and clinical setting are helpful in determining etiology of acute renal failure.

- Physical examination gives valuable diagnostic information
- Urine volume gives another clue to etiology of ARF
- Oliguria is a cardinal feature of ATN
- Examination of urine sediments
- Urine osmolarity
- Concentration of sodium in urine
- Radiologic procedures
- Intravenous urography
- Renal ultrasonography
- Computerised tomography scan
- Renal biopsy

Clinical Features of ARF

Clinical course of acute renal failure varies with etiology of renal dysfunction. Three major patterns are:

1. ***Syndrome of acute nephritis:*** It occurs during, acute streptococcal glomerulonephritis. There is extensive proliferation (multiplication) of epithelial cells of glomeruli with increased glomerular permeability. Characteristic features are mild proteinuria, haematuria, oedema, mild hypertension.

2. ***Pre-renal syndrome:*** Caused by hypovolemia (decreased volume of circulating blood), renal arterial obstruction, hypotension or cardiac insufficiency. Due to depressed in renal blood flow there is decreased in

glomerular filtration rate causing oliguria (diminished urine secretion), azotaemia [increased blood urea nitrogen (BUN), and creatinine], fluid retention and oedema. Glomerulus and tubule are not damaged.

3. ***Syndrome accompanying tubular pathology (necrosis):*** Caused by destruction of tubular cells as inacute tubular necrosis [ATN]. Three characteristic stages occur in ATN:

   (a) *Oliguric phase:* last for 7-10 days characterised by urine output less than 400ml/day. It leads to accumulation of metabolic waste in blood. Symptoms are azotaemia, metabolic acidosis, hyperkalaemia, hypervolemia and pulmonary oedema.

   (b) *Diuretic phase:* occurs with healing of tubule. There is improvement in urinary output. Diuretic phase is characterised by progressive increase in daily urine production. It is a physiologic response, due to excretion of excess solute and water retained during oliguric phase. Also due to inability of healing tubule to appropriately concentrate salt and water.

   (c) *Phase of recovery:* process of healing may take upto 1year with restoration of normal tubular function.

Chronic Renal Failure

Normal human kidney contains approximately two million functionally integrated glomerulotubular units called nephrons. Under normal condition these nephrons work in highly organised fashion to maintain consistency of internal environment of the body [Homeostasis].Kidney plays important role in metabolism of various peptide hormones. It produces biosynthetically renin, ammonia, erythropoietin, 1, 25-Dihydroxy Vitamin-D3.

Renal disease is characterised by disturbance in any of these normal functions. Although whole kidney glomerular filtration rate fall, the glomerular filtration rate of remnant (remaining) nephrons rise.

Definition: Chronic renal failure is a syndrome characterised by progressive and irreversible deterioration of renal function due to slow destruction of renal parenchyma, eventually terminating in death.

For practical purposes, clinical course of progressive renal disease is divided into four stages:

1. ***Decreased of renal reserve:*** This is clinically silent and patient remains asymptomatic except at the time of stress. Damage to renal parenchyma is marginal and kidney remains functional. Glomerular filtration rate may fall to 50%. Blood urea nitrogen (BUN), and creatinine values are normal.

2. ***Renal insufficiency:*** At this stage about 75% functional renal parenchyma, has been destroyed. GFR [Glomerular Filtration Rate] is 25% of normal. Moderate increase in BUN (20-50mg/dl), increase in serum creatinine and mild anaemia. Creatinine clearance of 30-50ml/min. Patients are still asymptomatic but polyuria and nocturia (excessive urination at night) occur

due to tubulointerstitial damage. Sudden stress may precipitate uremic syndrome. A thorough evaluation to determine the etiology of renal impairment is especially critical at this point.

3. ***Renal failure:*** At this stage 90% of functional renal tissue has been destroyed. GFR approximately 10% of normal. Tubular cells are essentially non-functional. Regulation of Na+ and water is lost resulting in oedema, metabolic acidosis, hypocalcaemia and signs and symptoms of uraemia. As creatinine clearance drops below 30ml/min patient develop increased symptom of their renal disease characterised by decreased fatigability, decreased energy, cold intolerance, abnormal taste sensation, anorexia etc.

4. ***End-stage kidney:*** Glomerular filtration at this stage is less than 5%. It is characterised by complex clinical picture of uremic syndrome. It is a clinical syndrome that develops with continued decline in renal function. Ascreatinine clearance drop below 10ml/min the symptom become progressively worse. Severe form of uraemia consists of malaise, lack of energy, generalised pruritus, nausea, vomiting. Neuromuscular irritability, leg cramp, myoclonus, coma, seizure etc. Patient requiring chronic dialysis have end stage renal disease.

Etiology

All chronic nephropathies (disease of kidney) can lead to CRF (Chronic Renal Failure). The disease leading to CRF can be classified into two major groups:

- ***Disease causing glomerular pathology:*** A number of glomerular diseases in CRF have their pathogenesis in immune mechanism. Glomerular destruction results in change in filtration process and lead to nephrotic syndrome characterised by proteinuria, hypoalbuminemia and oedema. Primary glomerular disease: Chronic glomerulonephritis Systemic glomerular disease: Systemic lupus erythematosus, serum sickness, diabetic glomerulosclerosis.

- ***Disease causing tubulointerstitial pathology:*** Damage to tubulointerstitial tissue result in alterations in reabsorption and secretion of important constituents, leading to excretion of large volume of dilute urine.

Nephrosclerosis (hardening of kidney) due to long standing primary hypertension, diabetes. Chronic pyelonephritis (inflammation of renal pelvis).Some toxic substance induces tubular injury e.g.: high dose of analgesics, lead, cadmium, uranium etc. Chronic obstruction in urinary tract like stones, blood clot, tumour, enlarged prostate etc. are some other reasons for CRF.

Pathophysiology

Progressive nature of renal disease: Chronic renal failure is a progressive disease process that cause total destruction of functioning renal mass. Dialysis or renal transplantation is necessary to sustain life. Mechanism responsible for progressive nature of chronic renal failure- metabolic factors like altered calcium and phosphorus metabolism, hyperlipidemia.

Decreased calcium and phosphorus metabolism lead to hyperphosphatemia, secondary hyperthyroidism-result in deposition of calcium and phosphorus in interstitium of kidney. This lead to inflammatory reaction and farther destruction of renal parenchyma. Abnormalities in lipid metabolism accompany renal disease and contribute to progressive glomerular injury. Treatment with lipid lowering agents has beneficial effect. As nephrons are lost, residual nephrons increase both in size and function.

Increased glomerular capillary pressure and flow result in proteinuria. This damage mesangium (membrane supporting capillary loop in glomeruli). Ultimately result in progressive mesangial and glomerular sclerosis (hardening).

The mechanism that induce afferent arteriolar dilation and produce adaptive increase in glomerular filtration rate. Protein loading induces afferent arteriolar dilation and whole kidney glomerular filtration rate. This renal vasodilation is hormonally mediated.

Normal dietary protein intake in reduced renal function results in glomerular capillary hypertension. Restriction of dietary protein intake prevents glomerular hypertension and progressive nephron destruction. Anti-hypertensive drugs also helpful.

Uremic state: A number of organic compounds (toxins) accumulate in uraemia. Toxins in uraemia include urea, creatinine, uric acid, guanides, cyclic AMP, amino acids, Phenols, Insulin and many hormones.

Accumulation result from following mechanism:

1. Decreased excretion
2. Increased secretion of biologically active substances
3. Decreased clearance of endogenous substances normally metabolised by kidney like parathyroid hormone, growth hormone, somatostatin, insulin etc.

Uremic syndrome characterised by prominent alteration in transmembrane transport and cellular water and electrolyte content. Uremic syndrome result primarily from retention of byproducts of protein metabolism. Many manifestation of uremic syndrome can be improved by protein restriction.

- ***Primary uremic manifestations:***
  - Metabolic acidosis Hyperkalaemia
  - Sodium and water imbalance
  - Hyperuricemaia due to excessive accumulation of uric acid

- ***Azotaemia:*** waste products of protein metabolism are unable to be excreted, resulting in high blood urea, creatinine, phenols, guanide etc.

- ***Secondary uremic manifestations:*** Renal excretory and biosynthetic failure affects every organ system in the body:

- ***Cardiovascular system:*** Sodium retention and volume expansion result in volume overload, pulmonary oedema, hypertension, left ventricular hypertrophy, accelerated atherosclerosis, Uremic toxins decreased myocardial contractility Pericarditis, Congestive heart failure.

- *Pulmonary system:* Pulmonary congestion and oedema due to hypervolemia and heart failure.

- *GIT:* Anorexia, hiccups, metallic taste, nausea, vomiting, diarrhoea, abdominal distension.

- *Nervous system:* Neuromuscular irritability, leg cramp, restlessness, peripheral neuropathy, uremic, encephalopathy (degenerative brain disease), Dialysis dementia due to aluminium intoxication.

- *Musculoskeletal system:* Bone disease, Osteomalacia (spongy bone) due to vitamin-D deficiency Osteitis fibrosa (inflammation of bone) due to hyperparathyroidism.

- *Hematologic system:* Anaemia due to decreased erythropoietin production and increased bleeding time.

- *Endocrine system:* Decreased Levothyroxine (T4), Hyperglycaemia due to peripheral resistance to insulin Primary hypogonadism, Deposition of urinary pigments like urochrome in skin causing yellow colour.

Asthma and Chronic Obstructive Airway Diseases

Definition: Asthma is an airway disease that can be classified physiologically as a variable and partially reversible obstruction to air flow, and pathologically with overdeveloped mucus glands, airway thickening due to scarring and inflammation, and bronchoconstriction, the narrowing of the airways in the lungs due to the tightening of surrounding smooth muscle. Bronchial inflammation also causes narrowing due to edema and swelling caused by an immune response to allergens.

Asthma is a common pulmonary condition defined by chronic inflammation of respiratory tubes, tightening of respiratory smooth muscle, and episodes of bronchoconstriction. There are two major categories of asthma, allergic and non-allergic. In both cases, bronchoconstriction is prominent during an asthma episode, inflamed airways react to environmental triggers such as smoke, dust, or pollen. The airways narrow and produce excess mucus, making it difficult to breathe.

Asthma is the result of an immune response in the bronchial airways. In response to exposure to these triggers, the bronchi (large airways) contract into spasm Known as an "asthmatic attack". Inflammation soon follows, leading to a further narrowing of the airways. Excessive mucus production, which leads to coughing and other breathing difficulties.

The normal caliber of the bronchus is maintained by a balanced functioning of the autonomic nervous system, which operates reflexively. The parasympathetic reflex loop consists of afferent nerve endings which originate under the inner lining of the bronchus. Whenever these afferent nerve endings are stimulated (for example, by dust, cold air or fumes) impulses travel to the brain-stem vagal center, then down the vagal efferent pathway to again reach the bronchial small airways.

Acetylcholine is released from the efferent nerve endings. This acetylcholine results in the excessive formation of inositol 1, 4, 5-trisphosphate (IP3) in bronchial smooth muscle cells which leads to muscle shortening and this initiates bronchoconstriction.

The mechanisms behind allergic asthma disease:

- The inhaled allergens find their way to the inner airways.
- They are ingested by a type of cell known as antigen-presenting cells, or APCs.
- APCs then "present" pieces of the allergen to other immune system cells.

In most people, these other immune cells (TH0 cells) "check" and usually ignore the allergen molecules. In asthma patients, however, these cells transform into a different type of cell (TH2), for reasons that are not well understood. A possible reason could be the release of Interleukin-4 by Mast cells that induce differentiation of naive helper T cells (Th0 cells) to Th2 cells.

The resultant TH2 cells activate an important arm of the immune system, known as the humoral immune system. The humoral immune system produces antibodies against the inhaled allergen. Later, when a patient inhales the same allergen, these antibodies "recognize" it and activate a humoral response.

Inflammation results: Chemicals are produced that cause the wall of the airway to thicken, cells which produce scarring to proliferate and contribute to further 'airway remodeling'. Causes mucus producing cells to grow larger and produce more and thicker mucus, and the cell-mediated arm of the immune system is activated.

Inflamed airways are more hyper-reactive, and will be more prone to bronchospasm.

- Allergens from nature, typically inhaled, which include waste from common household pests, the house dust mite and cockroach, as well as grass pollen, mold spores, and pet epithelial cells.
- Indoor air pollution from volatile organic compounds, including perfumes and perfumed products. Examples include soap, dishwashing liquid, laundry detergent, fabric softener, paper tissues, paper towels, toilet paper, shampoo, hairspray, hair gel, cosmetics, facial cream, sun cream, deodorant, cologne, shaving cream, aftershave lotion, air freshener and candles, and products such as oil-based paint.
- Psychological stress: There is growing evidence that psychological stress is a trigger. It can modulate the immune system, causing an increased inflammatory response to allergens and pollutants.
    - Cold weather can make it harder for patients to breathe. Whether high altitude helps or worsens asthma is debatable and may vary from person to person.

10

Infectious Diseases

Sexually Transmitted Diseases

(i) Human Immunodeficiency Virus

Infection occurs via an interaction between glycoprotein 160(gp160) on HIV with CD4 (primary interaction) and chemokine co-receptors (secondary receptors) present on the surface of above mentioned cells. Opportunistic infections in settings without access to antiretroviral drugs are the chief cause of morbidity and mortality associated with HIV infection.

General principles for the management of opportunistic infections include-

- preventing or reversing immunosuppression with antiretroviral therapy
- preventing exposure to pathogens
- vaccination
- prospective immunologic monitoring
- primary chemoprophylaxis
- treatment of acute episodes
- secondary chemoprophylaxis
- discontinuation of such prophylaxis following antiretroviral therapy and subsequent immune recovery

Complete eradication of HIV currently is not possible. Therefore, the goal of antiretroviral therapy is

- to achieve maximal and durable suppression of HIV replication
- Increase CD4 lymphocyte because this closely correlates with the risk for developing opportunistic infections(OIs)

Current recommendations for the initial treatment of HIV advocate a minimum of three active anti-retro agents. The typical regimen consists of two nucleoside analogues with either a protease inhibitor or a non nucleoside reverse transcriptase inhibitor. Clinical use of antiretroviral agents is complicated by drug-drug interactions. Some interactions are beneficial and used purposely; others may be harmful.

Inadequate suppression of viral replication allows HIV to select for antiretroviral resistant HIV variants, the major factor limiting the ability of anti-retroviral drugs to inhibit virus replication and delay disease progression. Current recommendations for treating drug resistant HIV include choosing at least two drugs to which the patients' virus is susceptible.

A retrovirus, human immunodeficiency virus type I (HIV-1), is the major cause of AIDS.A second retrovirus, HIV-2, also recognised to cause AIDS, although it is less virulent transmissible and prevalent than HIV-1.The retroviruses are transmitted primarily by

- Sexual contact
- Blood contaminated needles
- From child bearing women to their offspring.

Combination antiretroviral therapy (ART) consists of combination of anti-retroviral agents that potentially and durably suppress HIV replication, delay onset of AIDS, reverse HIV-associated immunologic deficits, and significantly prolong patient survival. The therapeutic challenges include need for continuous adherence to medication, drug-drug interactions, drug resistant HIV, acute and long-term drug toxicities. No vaccine is available.

Epidemiology: Epidemiological characteristics of HIV infection differ according to geographic region mode of transmission, governmental prevention efforts and resources and cultural factors.

Transmission: Infection with HIV occurs through three primary mode: sexual, parentral and perinatal. Prevention of sexual transmission has focused primarily on

- Education that encourages abstinence (especially for adolescents)
- Use of condoms
- Reduction of high-risk behaviour (anal intercourse and promiscuity)

Additional strategies include

- Intreventional male circumcision
- HIV vaccines
- Topical vaginal microbicides
- Pre-exposure prophylaxis with anti-retroviral agents

Parentral transmission of HIV from, needle stick injury, intravenous injection with used needles, receipt of blood products and organ transplants. Perinatal or vertical transmission, is the most common cause of paediatric HIV infection. Most infection occurs during or near to the time of birth. Factors that increase the likelihood of vertical transmission include genital infection during pregnancy, preterm delivery, vaginal delivery, birth weight less than 2.5Kg, illicit drug use during pregnancy, high maternal viral load, breast feeding.

Persons with HIV infections are broadly categorised as those living with HIV and those with an AIDS diagnosis. An AIDS diagnosis is made when the cluster of differentiation 4 (CD4; T-helper cell) count drops below 200cells/µl or after an AIDS indicator condition is diagnosed.

Etiology: HIV is an enveloped single-stranded RNA virus and a member of the Lentivirinae (lenti, meaning "slow") subfamily of retroviruses. Lentiviruses are characterised by their indolent (lazy) infectious cycle. There are two related but distinct types of HIV: HIV-1 and HIV-2.HIV-2, found mostly in western Africa, consists of seven phylogenetic lineages designated as subtypes (clades) A.B, C. D, E, F, G.HIV-1 also can be categorised based on phylogeny. Three groups of HIV-1 currently are recognised: M (main or major); N (non-M, non-O) and O (outlier). Nine subtypes of HIV-1 group M are identified. Group M, subtype B, is primarily responsible for the epidemic in North America and western Europe.

HIV in humans was the result of a cross-species transmission (zoonosis) from primates infected with simian immunodeficiency virus (SIV). Modern transportation, promiscuity and drug abuse have caused the rapid spread of the virus throughout the world. Detection of HIV and surrogate markers of disease progression:

The most common laboratory method for diagnosing HIV-1 infection is enzyme linked immunosorbent assay (ELIZA), which detect antibodies against HIV-1. ELIZA is both highly sensitive (>99%) and highly specific (>99%) but rarely false positive or false negative result can occur. The minimum time to develop antibodies is 3 to 4 weeks or 6 months in some individuals. Positive ELIZA results are repeated in duplicate, and if one or both tests are reactive, a confirmatory test is performed for final diagnosis.

Western blot is the most commonly used confirmatory test, although an indirect immunofluorescence assay is available. A reactive ELIZA test and positive confirmatory test indicate an established HIV infection. If the confirmatory test is indeterminate, the dilemma can be resolved by retesting the individual after 30 days or performing viral load assay if patient is at high risk or symptomatic.

Once diagnosed, HIV disease is monitored primarily by two surrogate markers, viral load and CD4 cell count. The viral load test quantifies the degree of viremia by measuring the number of copies of viral RNA (HIV-RNA) in the plasma. Viral load is a major prognostic factor for monitoring disease progression and the effect of treatment.

Because HIV attack leads to the destruction of cells bearing the CD4 receptor, the number of CD4 lymphocytes (T-helper cells) in the blood is a critical surrogate marker of disease progression. The normal adult CD4 lymphocyte count ranges from 500to 1,600 cell/mm^3 or 40% to 70% of all lymphocytes (little higher for children). In HIV disease, there is depletion of CD4 cells and associated development of opportunistic infections (OI) and malignancies.

Pathogenesis: Understanding the life cycle of HIV is necessary because the current strategies used for treatment of HIV target various points in this cycle. Once HIV enters the human body, the outer glycoprotein (gp160) on its surface, which is composed of two subunits (gp120 and gp41), has affinity for CD4 receptors bind with cells expressing CD4 receptor protein.

Once initial binding occurs, the intimate association of HIV with the cell is enhanced by further binding to chemokine co-receptors. Two major chemokine co-receptors used by HIV are CCR5 and CXCR4.The HIV strains that preferentially uses CCR5, (R5 viruses) are macrophage tropic and non-syncytium inducing (syncytium is cell clumping). R5 viruses typically implicated in most cases of sexually transmitted HIV.

The HIV strain that targets CXCR4, (designated as X4 viruses) is T-cell tropic and often predominant in the later stage of disease. CD4 and co-receptor attachment of HIV to the cell promotes membrane fusion, which is mediated by gp41, and finally internalisation of the viral genetic material and enzymes necessary for replication.

After internalisation, the viral protein shell surrounding the nucleic acid (capsid) is uncoated in preparation for replication. The genetic material of HIV is positive-sense (5' to 3') single stranded RNA; the virus must transcribe this RNA into DNA (transcription normally occurs from DNA to RNA; HIV works backward, hence named retrovirus).To do so, HIV is equipped with the unique enzyme RNA-dependent DNA polymerase (reverse transcriptase). Reverse transcriptase first synthesises a complementary strand of DNA using the viral RNA as a template.

The RNA portion of this DNA-RNA hybrid is then partially removed by ribonuclease H (RNase H) allowing reverse transcriptase to complete the synthesis of a double stranded DNA molecule. The reliability of the reverse transcriptase is poor, and many mistakes are made during the process. These errors in the final DNA product contribute to the rapid mutation of the virus, which enables the virus to escape the immune response (which complicate vaccine development) and drug resistance to evolve.

Following reverse transcription, the final double stranded DNA product migrate to the nucleus and is integrated in to the host cell chromosome by integrase, another enzyme unique to HIV. HIV can establish a persistent, latent infection, particularly in long lived cells of the immune system such as memory T lymphocytes. The virus is effectively hidden in these cells, and this characteristic has greatly inhibited the ability to cure HIV infection.

Random integration of HIV may cause cellular abnormalities and induce apoptosis. After integration, HIV preferentially replicates in activated cells. Activation by antigen, cytokines or other factors stimulates the cell to produce nuclear factor kappa B (NF-kB), an enhancer binding protein. NF-kB normally regulates the expression of T- lymphocyte genes involved in growth but also can inadvertently (accidentally) activate replication of HIV. HIV encodes six regulatory and accessory proteins which enhance replication.

Assembly of new virion particle occurs in a stepwise manner beginning with the coalescence of HIV proteins beneath the host cell lipid bilayer. The nucleocapsid, subsequently formed with viral single stranded RNA and other components packaged inside. Once packaged, the virion then buds through the plasma membrane, acquiring the characteristics of host lipid bilayer. Within virion protease, another enzyme unique to HIV, begin cleaving a large precursor polypeptide (gag-pol) into functional proteins that are necessary to produce complete virus. Without this enzyme, (protease), the virion is immature and unable to infect other cells.

Infected cells and some uninfected bystander cells will be destroyed by various mechanism

- Cell lysis by newly budding virions
- Cytotoxic T-lymphocyte induced cell killing
- Syncytia formation and apoptosis

Syncytia formation occurs when viral proteins expressed on the surface of the infected cells act as ligand for receptors expressed on uninfected cells. Uninfected cells clump onto the infected cell and fuse into a giant multinucleated cell. The syncytium inducing X4 virus phenotype may develop later in disease and is associated with more rapid disease progression. Destruction of CD4 cells leads to profoundly compromised immune function and consequently AIDS.

Clinical Presentation of Primary Human Immunodeficiency

Symptoms: Fever, sore throat, fatigue, weight loss, myalgia. 40-80% of patients exhibit a morbilliform, maculopapular rash usually involving the trunk. Diarrhoea, nausea, vomiting Lymphadenopathy, might sweats, Aseptic meningitis (fever, head ache, photophobia, stiff neck) may present in 25%of cases. Others include High viral load (may exceed 1,000,000copies/ml), Persistent decrease in CD4 lymphocytes, Symptoms often last for two weeks.

Virus disseminates to and replicates in the lymph tissues (mucosa, lymph node, and gut-associated lymph tissue).Most children born with HIV are asymptomatic. On physical examination, children often present with unexplained physical signs, such as lymphadenopathy, hepatomegaly, splenomegaly, failure to thrive, weight loss, fever etc.

Laboratory findings include: Anaemia, hyper gammaglobulinemia (Ig-A and Ig-M), altered mononuclear cell function, altered T-cell subset ratios. Children have different susceptibility and exposure to opportunistic infections compared with adult. Bacterial infections including Streptococcus pneumoniae, Salmonella species and Mycobacterium tuberculosis, may be more prevalent (predominant) in children with AIDS than in adults with AIDS. Kaposi sarcoma is rare in children.

Children with HIV infection may develop lymphocytic interstitial pneumonitis. Some children present with progressive, unexplained neurologic deterioration including late-onset of seizures, loss of developmental milestones, cessation of brain growth, and diffuse unexplained encephalopathy.

General management of the HIV infected child involves principles similar to those used for the adult, antiretroviral therapy, treatment and prophylaxis of opportunistic infections) and supportive care.

Treatment

From 1996, a new class of antiretrovirals, the protease inhibitors (PIs) was introduced and a new paradigm in HIV treatment was born. A combination of three active antiretroviral agent from two pharmacological classes were shown to profoundly inhibit HIV replication, prevent and reverse immune deficiency and substantially decrease morbidity and mortality-constituting the ART era.

Regular periodic measurement of plasma HIV-RNA levels and CD4 cell counts is necessary to determine risk of disease progression in an HIV infected individual and to determine when to initiate or modify antiretroviral treatment regimen. Treatment decisions should be individualised based on risks indicated by HIV-RNA level, CD4 count, resistant HIV variants, cross resistance, drug interaction etc.

HIV infected persons even those with viral loads below detectable limits, should be considered infections and should be counselled to avoid sexual or drug use behaviours that are associated with transmission or acquisition of HIV and other infectious pathogens.

(ii) Syphilis

Definition: Syphilis is a chronic infection caused by the bacterium Treponema pallidum.

Epidemiology and Etiology: Although the actual number of reported cases is still relatively low (8724 in 2005) the incidence of primary and secondary syphilis has increased in united states by more than 40% since 2001.In addition to being highly contagious syphilis is of major concern because, if left untreated, it can progress to a chronic systemic disease that can be fatal or seriously disabling.

Syphilis usually is acquired by sexual contact with infected mucous membranes or cutaneous lesions although on rare occasions it can be acquired by non-sexual personal contact, accidental inoculation or blood transfusion. The causative organism of syphilis is Treponema pallidum a spirochete.

The risk of acquiring syphilis from an infected individual after a single sexual encounter is approximately 50-60%.After sexual contact, the organism penetrates the intact mucous membrane or a break in the cornified epithelium and spirochetemia occurs.

Evidence of a strong association between syphilis and HIV infection has been noted. Although complex and incompletely understood, it appears that, syphilis, similar to other sexually transmitted genital ulcer diseases, can increase the risk of acquiring HIV in exposed individuals. Immunologic defects in HIV infected individuals can produce an atypical serologic response to syphilis.

Clinical Presentation

Primary syphilis: The primary stage, characterised by the appearance of a chancre on cutaneous ormuco-cutaneous tissue exposed to the organism, is highly infections. Even without treatment, chancres persist only for 1 to 8 weeks before healing spontaneously.

Secondary syphilis: The secondary stage of syphilis is characterised by a variety of mucocutaneous seruptions resulting from widespread haematogenous and lymphatic spread of T. pallidum. Skin lesions can be either generalised or localised to a small portion of the body and with exception of follicular lesions, are non-pruritic. Generalised lymphadenopathy also is seen in most patients. Mild and transitory malaise, fever, pharyngitis, headache, anorexia, and arthralgia. If untreated secondary syphilis disappears in 4 to 10 weeks, however, lesions can reoccur at any time within 4 years.

Latent syphilis: By definition, persons with a positive serological test for syphilis but with no other evidence of disease have latent syphilis. Latent syphilis is further divided into early and late latency. During early latency, the patient is considered potentially infectious, because of 25% risk of spontaneous mucocutaneous relapse. The U.S. Public Health Service defines early latency as 1 year from the onset of infection although other investigators propose a longer interval, such as 2 to 4 years. With the exception of pregnancy in which the mother can pass the disease to the foetus, late latency is considered non-infectious, although the patient remains a host.

Most untreated patients with late latent syphilis have no further sequel; however, approximately 25% to 30% progress either to neurosyphilis or to a late syphilis with clinical manifestation other than neurosyphilis. Treatment of all patents with latent syphilis is essential because there is no way to predict which patients will have progression of their disease.

Tertiary syphilis and Neurosyphilis: If left untreated, syphilis can slowly produce an inflammatory reaction in virtually any organ in the body. Manifestations of this disease progression were referred to previously as tertiary syphilis. These clinical manifestations now are differentiated into two subgroups based on the presence or absence of central nervous system (CNS) involvement of neurosyphilis or tertiary syphilis.

The term neurosyphilis encompasses any patient with cerebrospinal fluid (CSF) abnormalities consistent with CNS infection. Approximately 40% of patients with primary or secondary syphilis exhibit such abnormalities, although most remain asymptomatic. Some investigators suggest that HIV-infected patients are at greater risk of developing symptomatic neurosyphilis than patients with intact immune systems.

The most common manifestations of disease progression from late latency are benign gumma formation and cardiovascular syphilis. The gumma, a nonspecific granulomatous lesion, is the classic lesion of late syphilis and develops in 50% of patients with disease progression. These chronic destructive lesions characteristically infiltrate the skin, bone, soft tissue, liver or any other organ. Gummas of critical organs, such as heart or brain can be fatal.

Congenital syphilis: In pregnant women with syphilis, T. pallidum can cross the placenta at any time during pregnancy. The risk of fatal infection is greatest in pregnant women with primary and secondary syphilis and declines in pregnant women with late disease. Transmission of syphilis during pregnancy occurs primarily transplacentally and can result in foetal death, prematurity, or congenital syphilis.

Symptoms can be seen during the first months of life (early congenital syphilis) or later in childhood or adolescence (late congenital syphilis). Manifestations of early congenital syphilis resemble those of secondary syphilis, whereas that of late congenital syphilis correspond to the tertiary stage in adults.

Presentation of Syphilis Infections

General

- *Primary:* Incubation period 10-90days (mean 21days)
- *Secondary:* Develops 2-8weeks after initial infection in untreated or inadequately treated individuals
- *Latent:* Develops 4 -10weeks after secondary stage in untreated or inadequately treated individuals Tertiary: Develops in approximately 30% of untreated or inadequately treated individuals 10-30years after initial infection.

Site of Infection

- *Primary:* External genitalia, perianal region, mouth, and throat
- *Secondary:* Multi system involvement secondary to haematogenous and lymphatic spread
- *Latent:* Potentially multisystem involvement (dormant)
- *Tertiary:* CNS, heart, eyes, bones, and joints

Signs and Symptoms

- *Primary:* Single, painless, indurated lesion (chancre) that erodes, ulcerates and eventually heals (typical); regional lymphadenopathy is common; multiple, painful, purulent lesions possible but uncommon.

- Secondary: Pruritic or nonpruritic rash, mucocutaneous lesions, flu like symptoms lymphadenopathy
- *Latent:* Asymptomatic
- *Tertiary:* Cardiovascular syphilis (aortitis or aortic insufficiency), neurosyphilis (meningitis, general paresis, dementia, tabes dorsalis, eighth cranial nerve deafness, blindness), gummatous lesions involving any organ or tissue.

(iii) Gonorrhoea

Pathogenesis of Gonorrhea

Gonorrhea is a purulent infection of the mucous membrane surfaces caused by Neisseria gonorrhoeae. N-gonorrhoeae is spread by sexual contact or through transmission during childbirth.

All patients with gonorrheal infection are treated for presumed co-infection with Chlamydia trachomatis. Gonorrhea is caused by a gram-negative diplococcus. Neisseria gonorrhoeae often referred to as gonococcus. The pathogenicity of this organism derives from properties of the surface pili, small hairlike extensions of the surface membrane. The pili of this organism prevent phagocytosis by neutrophils. Also, the pili contain on IgA protease which digests the IgA on the surface of the urethra, fallopian tubes and endocervix.

Adherence to the surface of spermatozoa allows transmission of the organism to the fallopian tube, the presumed mechanism of ascending infection. Initial infection may be asymptomatic, but the organism incites a typical acute inflammatory reaction resulting frequently in a purulent exudate.

The clinical consequences of gonorrhea are due to classic pyogenic infection with resolution by fibrosis. Initial infection is usually seen in the cervical region, but due to the adherence to spermatozoa, the infection may ascend through the uterus into the fallopian tubes and finally out into the peritoneal cavity.

A purulent vaginal discharge is often seen, but frequently the purulent material exudes from the fimbriated end of the fallopian tubes into the peritoneal cavity. Untreated infections may progress to fibrosis. The fibrotic reaction, depending on its location can lead to a variety of complications, such as urethral stricture, fallopian tube stricture; tubo-ovarian abscess, pelvic inflammatory disease (PID) and infertility.

When the infection is confined to the lower genital tract, it is much more responsive to antibiotic therapy. Once the infection ascends and becomes well established, it is difficult to deliver the needed concentrations of antibiotics and the infection is much more difficult to cure with drugs alone. This is due to the lack of blood flow in the walled off areas and is the reason that surgery often becomes necessary. In pregnancy, gonococcus can be transmitted to the foetus at the time of delivery. This results in infection of the conjuctiva of the eye. This appears 1 to 4 days after birth as severe discharge with marked swelling and redness of the eyelids and conjunctiva. This can lead to corneal perforation and blindness. Diagnosis is made by gram stain of the exudate and culture.

The bacteria attach to and spread along the cells of the surface mucous membranes, after which they invade superficially and provoke acute inflammation. However, if treatment is not instituted promptly the organisms extend to the prostate, epididymis, accessory glands, where they cause urethral stricture, epididymitis, orchitis, and sometimes male infertility. In some women (usually during the first menses after exposure), the infection extends to the fallopian tubes, where it produces acute and chronic salpingitis and pelvic inflammatory disease. The fallopian tubes swell with pus, causing acute abdominal pain. Infertility occurs when inflammatory adhesions close the tubes at both ends, blocking the ascent of sperm and the descent of ova.

Infected fallopian tubes ('pus tubes') have the shape of a retort flask. From the fallopian tubes, the infection may spread to the peritoneum, healing as fine adhesions ("violin string" adhesions) between the capsule of the liver and the parietal peritoneum. The vaginal discharge may infect the anal crypts, leading to mucopurulent anal discharge, rectal pruritus, and tenesmus.

Chronic endometritis is a persistent complication of gonococcal infection and is usually a consequence of chronic gonococcal salpingitis. In such cases the endometrium contains many lymphocytes and plasma cells. Women (and to a lesser extent men) may also develop bacteremia, producing disseminated gonococcal infection, which in turn leads to monoarthritis or polyarthritis.

Neonatal infections from infected amniotic fluid or an infected birth canal result in symptoms within a few days after birth. Other sites of neonatal infection are the pharynx, respiratory tract, vagina, anus, leptomeninges, joints, and blood. Uncomplicated gonococcal infections of the urethra and endocervix are treated with penicillin and other antibiotics. Neisseria gonorrhoea is displaying increasing resistance to penicillin.

Urinary Tract Infections

Urinary tract infection (UTI) refers to a symptomatic bacterial infection within the urinary tract. This includes a lower urinary tract infection – cystitis (symptomatic infection of the bladder), or an upper urinary tract infection – acute pyelonephritis (symptomatic infection of the kidney).Asymptomatic bacteriuria is present if a patient has two consecutive urine cultures showing>100000cfu/mL urine, but does not have any symptoms of a UTI.

UTIs may be considered complicated if symptoms of pyelonephritis emerge, or if a UTI is found in certain patient populations, including the immunosuppressed, men, pregnant women, diabetics, those with a history of pyelonephritis, or those with structural abnormalities of the urinary tract.

Table 10.1 Types of UTI and their possible reasons.

Symptom	Reason
Dysuria	Due to acute inflammation of the bladder, resulting in discomfort upon contraction during voiding.
Frequency and urgency	Reduced bladder capacity due to inflammatory edema causing decreased compliance and pain due to bladder distension.
Hematuria	Irritated, edematous urinary tract bleeding with voiding.
Suprapubic tenderness	Due to palpation and compression of an inflamed, edematous bladder.
Chills and sweats	Inflammatory cascade resulting in a febrile response.
Flank pain (may radiate to groin. Dull pain)	Sudden renal edema, resulting in increased pressure and capsular distension.

The pathophysiology of urinary tract infection involves the infection of urinary tract organs such as the urethra, bladder, ureters, and kidneys. Although different microorganisms can cause UTI, the pathophysiology of urinary tract infection is similar for each organism.

Normal urine is sterile, acidic, flow is always toward the external environment and resistant to bacterial growth but when bacterial urinary infection occurs, microorganisms enter through the urethra and may travel up or ascend to other parts of the urinary system. It is important to treat UTI to avoid complications. In all cases, the pathophysiology of urinary tract infection begins with the entry of microorganisms through the outermost part of the urinary system called the urethra.

Other protective mechanisms against bacterial urinary infection include bladder emptying, the presence of contracting muscles called sphincters, and the availability of immune cells and antibodies in the urinary mucosa. In men, secretions of the prostate gland minimize bacterial growth. Bacterial agents, such as Escherichia coli (E. coli), may be transferred from the anus to the urethral opening, leading to urethral infection.

E. coli is an organism that lives in the colon and is passed out in the stools during defecation. The relationship between the anus and the urethra explains why UTI occurs more frequently in women than in men. In women, the anal and urethral openings are closer to each other, and the urethral length is shorter. This leads to easier bacterial translocation and ascension to the upper parts of the urinary tract.

UTI symptoms differ according to what part of the urinary tract is infected. The symptoms of urethra infection or urethritis may be limited to increased frequency of urination as well as burning pain while urinating, called dysuria. With bladder infection or cystitis, there may be additional symptoms of pain over the abdominal and pubic regions, and also a low-grade fever. Kidney infection, or pyelonephritis systemic, symptoms include high fever, chills, nausea, and vomiting. In some cases, blood in the urine and loss of appetite may be experienced.

Different risk factors contribute to the pathophysiology of urinary tract infection. Congenital anatomical abnormalities and acquired diseases, such as kidney stones, can predispose a person to getting UTI. Among sexually active people, the frequency of intercourse and the mode of intercourse increase UTI risk. In elderly men, enlargement of the prostate gland impedes urine flow, leading to increased risk of infection. Immunocompromised states, such as diabetes, contribute to an increased UTI risk because the immune cells of the body are not able to fight against the infection.

Pneumonia (Bronchiectasis)

Definition: Pneumonia is an inflammatory condition of the lung, especially of the alveoli (microscopic air sacs in the lungs) or when the lungs fill with fluid (called consolidation and exudation). Infecting agents can be bacteria, viruses, fungi, or parasites.

Chemical burns or physical injury to the lungs can also produce pneumonia. Typical symptoms include cough, chest pain, fever, and difficulty in breathing. Diagnostic tools include x-rays and examination of the sputum. Treatment depends on the cause of pneumonia; bacterial pneumonia is treated with antibiotics. Pneumonia is a common disease that occurs in all age groups. It is a leading cause of death among the young, the old, and the chronically ill.

Vaccines to prevent certain types of pneumonia are available. The prognosis depends on the type of pneumonia, the treatment, any complications, and the person's underlying health.

Pathophysiology

Bacteria typically enter the lung with inhalation, though they can reach the lung through the bloodstream if other parts of the body are infected. Often, bacteria live in parts of the upper respiratory tract and are continually being inhaled into the alveoli. Once inside the alveoli, bacteria travel into the spaces between the cells and also between adjacent alveoli through connecting pores.

This invasion triggers the immune system to respond by sending white blood cells responsible for attacking microorganisms (neutrophils) to the lungs. The neutrophils engulf and kill the offending organisms but also release cytokines which result in a general activation of the immune system.

This results in the fever, chills, and fatigue common in bacterial and fungal pneumonia. The neutrophils, bacteria, and fluid leaked from surrounding blood vessels fill the alveoli and result in impaired oxygen transportation. Bacteria often travel from the lung into the blood stream and can result in serious illness such as septic shock, in which there is low blood pressure leading to damage in multiple parts of the body including the brain, kidney, and heart.

They can also travel to the area between the lungs and the chest wall, called the pleural cavity. Bronchiectasis is a disease in which there is permanent enlargement of parts of the airways of the lung. Symptoms typically include a chronic cough with sputum production. Other symptoms include shortness of breath, coughing up blood, and chest pain. Wheezing and nail clubbing may also occur. Those with the disease often get frequent lung infections.

Bronchiectasis may result from a number of infective and acquired causes, including pneumonia, tuberculosis, immune system problems, and cystic fibrosis. Cystic fibrosis eventually results in severe bronchiectasis in nearly all cases. The mechanism of disease is breakdown of the airways due to an excessive inflammatory response. Involved bronchi become enlarged and thus less able to clear secretions. These secretions increase the number of bacteria in the lungs; result in airway blockage and further breakdown of the airways.

It is classified as an obstructive lung disease, along with chronic obstructive pulmonary disease and asthma. The diagnosis is suspect based on a person's symptoms and confirmed using computer tomography. Sputum cultures may be useful to determine treatment in those who have acute. Worsening may occur due to infection and in these cases antibiotics are recommended. Bronchiectasis is a result of chronic inflammation compounded by an inability to clear mucoid secretions. This can be a result of genetic conditions resulting in a failure to clear sputum (Primary ciliary dyskinesia), or resulting in more viscous sputum (cystic fibrosis), or the result of chronic or severe infections. Inflammation results in progressive destruction of the normal lung architecture, in particular the elastic fibers of bronchi. Endobronchial tuberculosis commonly leads to bronchiectasis, either from bronchial stenosis or secondary traction from fibrosis.

Typhoid

Definition: Typhoid fever is acute bacterial infection characterised by symptoms like prolonged pyrexia, prostration and involvement of spleen and lymph nodes. It does not cause lifelong or even sufficiently prolonged immunity, second often occurs.

Symptoms

Early symptoms include fever, general ill-feeling, and abdominal pain. High fever (103°F, or 39.5°C) or higher and severe diarrhea occur as the disease gets worse. Some people with typhoid fever develop a rash called "rose spots," which are small red spots on the abdomen and chest.

Other symptoms that occur include:

- Abdominal tenderness
- Agitation
- Bloody stools
- Chills
- Confusion
- Difficulty paying attention (attention deficit)

- Delirium
- Fluctuating mood
- Hallucinations
- Nose bleeds
- Severe fatigue
- Slow, sluggish, lethargic feeling
- Weakness

S. typhi is spread through contaminated food, drink, or water. If you eat or drink something that is contaminated with the bacteria, the bacteria enter your body. They travel into your intestines, and then into your blood. The bacteria travel through the blood to your lymph nodes, gallbladder, liver, spleen, and other parts of the body.

Some persons become carriers of *S. typhi* and continue to release the bacteria in their stools for years, spreading the disease. The earliest pathologic changes are in the stages of bacterial attachment and penetration. Bacteria are firmly attached to intestinal epithelium with an accompanying degeneration of the brush borders. Later as the salmonellae pass to lymphoid follicles of the intestine, there is diffuse enterocolitis and hypertrophy of Peyer's patches.

This is followed by necrosis of intestinal and mesenteric lymphoid tissues, focal granulomas in the liver and spleen, and characteristic mononuclear inflammatory cells ("typhoid nodules") in many organs. Typhoid nodules are primarily aggregates of altered macrophages ("typhoid cells") that phagocytose bacteria, erythrocytes and degenerated lymphocytes. These nodules also contain plasma cells and lymphocytes, but not typically neutrophils. The most common sites for typhoid nodules are the intestine, mesenteric lymph nodes, spleen, liver, and bone marrow. Less commonly, the kidney, testes, and parotid gland are affected.

Although the pathologic changes of typhoid fever may not correlate precisely with the clinical stages, certain patterns are characteristic. During the incubation stage, there is a mild enteritis, mesenteric lymphadenitis, and hyperplasia of intestinal lymphoid tissue, primarily of Peyer's patches of the ileum and solitary lymphoid follicles of the cecum.

The lymphoid hyperplasia may resolve or may progress to capillary thrombosis. Thrombosis causes the adjoining intestinal mucosa to enlarge during the phase of active invasion and then become necrotic. This process gives rise to the characteristic lesions, which are elevated 0.1 to 0.4 cm above adjacent mucosa. While bacilli continue to proliferate, dying bacilli release endotoxins that cause toxemia, beginning during invasion and becoming maximal in fastigium.

The necrotic mucosa sloughs, usually during lysis, producing ulcers that conform to Peyer's patches and are concentrated along the antimesenteric border. The ulcers may bleed or perforate, usually during lysis. Most perforations are near the ileocecal valve, measure less than 1 cm across, and lead to peritonitis.

Interestingly, these areas become repopulated with lymphoid cells and heal without scarring.

During active invasion, the mesenteric lymph nodes enlarge and develop typhoid nodules, focal hemorrhages, and necrosis, changes which resemble those in the intestinal lymphoid tissue. The spleen becomes large and hyperemic and microscopically shows typhoid nodules in the red pulp. The hyperplastic white pulp exhibits areas of focal necrosis. The enlarged liver displays sinusoids lined with swollen Kupffer's cells and histocytes. Focal necrosis of liver cells is common. The lack of neutrophils in typhoid fever is conspicuous.

The intestinal ulcers and focal areas of necrosis are bounded only by chronic inflammatory cells, and the patient is actually leukopenic. Toxemia may cause other complications, including ileus; mild fatty liver; a flabby heart with dilated ventricles, vacuolization of cardiac myocytes, and cardiac arrhythmia that may cause sudden death; mild interstitial pneumonitis; swelling and degeneration of the proximal tubular epithelium of kidney; "ring" hemorrhages in brain; capillary microthrombi; and degeneration of skeletal muscles.

During convalescence, the intestine returns to normal, with minimal scarring of the mucosa. Adhesions are rare. Typhoid nodules in various organs are resorbed without distortion of the architecture. The capsule of the spleen, however, may become fibrotic, giving the appearance of "sugar coating". Skeletal muscles regenerates and toxic changes of heart disappear.

Tuberculosis

Definition: Tuberculosis, MTB, or TB in the past also called phthisis, phthisis pulmonalis, or consumption, is a widespread, and in many cases fatal, infectious disease caused by various strains of mycobacteria, usually Mycobacterium tuberculosis.

Tuberculosis typically attacks the lungs, but can also affect other parts of the body. It is spread through the air when people who have an active TB infection cough, sneeze, or otherwise transmit respiratory fluids through the air.

The classic symptoms of active TB infection are a chronic cough with blood-tinged sputum, fever, night sweats, and weight loss (the latter giving rise to the formerly common term for the disease, "consumption"). Infection of other organs causes a wide range of symptoms. Treatment is difficult and requires administration of multiple antibiotics over a long period of time. Social contacts are also screened and treated if necessary. Antibiotic resistance is a growing problem in multiple drug-resistant tuberculosis (MDR-TB) infections. Prevention relies on screening programs and vaccination with the bacillus Calmette-Guérin vaccine.

Pathogenesis

About 90% of those infected with M. tuberculosis have asymptomatic, latent TB infections (sometimes called LTBI), with only a 10% lifetime chance that the latent infection will progress to overt, active tuberculous disease. In those with HIV, the risk of developing active TB increases. TB infection begins when the mycobacteria reach the pulmonary alveoli, where they invade and replicate within endosomes of alveolar macrophages.

Macrophages identify the bacterium as "foreign" and attempt to eliminate it by phagocytosis. During this process, the entire bacterium is enveloped by the macrophage and stored temporarily in a membrane-bound vesicle called a phagosome. The phagosome then combines with a lysosome to create a phagolysosome. In the phagolysosome, the cell attempts to use reactive oxygen species and acid to kill the bacterium.

M. tuberculosis has a thick, waxy mycolic acid capsule that protects it from these toxic substances. *M. tuberculosis* reproduces inside the macrophage and will eventually kill the immune cell. The primary site of infection in the lungs, known as the "Ghon focus", is generally located in either the upper part of the lower lobe, or the lower part of the upper lobe.

Tuberculosis of the lungs may also occur via infection from the blood stream. This is known as a Simon focus and is typically found in the top of the lung. This hematogenous transmission can also spread infection to more distant sites, such as peripheral lymph nodes, the kidneys, the brain, and the bones. All parts of the body can be affected by the disease, though for unknown reasons it rarely affects the heart, skeletal muscles, pancreas or thyroid.

Tuberculosis is classified as one of the granulomatous inflammatory diseases. Macrophages, T lymphocytes, B lymphocytes, and fibroblasts aggregate to form granulomas, with lymphocytes surrounding the infected macrophages. When other macrophages attack the infected macrophage, they fuse together to form a giant multinucleated cell in the alveolar lumen. The granuloma may prevent dissemination of the mycobacteria and provide a local environment for interaction of cells of the immune system.

However more recent evidence suggests that the bacteria use the granulomas to avoid destruction by the host's immune system. Macrophages and dendritic cells in the granulomas are unable to present antigen to lymphocytes; thus, the immune response is suppressed. Bacteria inside the granuloma can become dormant, resulting in latent infection. Another feature of the granulomas is the development of abnormal cell death (necrosis) in the center of tubercles.

If TB bacteria gain entry to the blood stream from an area of damaged tissue, they can spread throughout the body and set up many foci of infection, all appearing as tiny, white tubercles in the tissues. Tissue destruction and necrosis are often balanced by healing and fibrosis. Affected tissue is replaced by scarring and cavities filled with caseous necrotic material. During active disease, some of these cavities are joined to the air passages bronchi and this material can be coughed up.

Tuberculosis in Relation to HIV

The co -epidemic of tuberculosis (TB) and human immunodeficiency virus (HIV) is one of the major global health challenges in the present time. The World Health Organization (WHO) reports 9.2 million new cases of TB in 2006 of whom 7.7% were HIV-infected. Tuberculosis is the most common contagious infection in HIV-Immunocompromised patients leading to death.

These both diseases become dreadful in combination as HIV declines the human immunity while tuberculosis becomes progressive due to defective immune system. This condition becomes more severe in case of multi -drug (MDRTB) and extensively drug resistant TB (XDRTB), which are difficult to treat and contribute to increased mortality. Tuberculosis can occur at any stage of HIV infection. The risk and severity of tuberculosis increases soon after infection with HIV.

Although tuberculosis can be a relatively early manifestation of HIV infection, it is important to note that the risk of tuberculosis progresses as the CD4 cell count decreases along with the progression of HIV infection. The risk of TB generally remains high in HIV-infected patients above the background risk of the general population even with effective immune reconstitution with ART maintaining high CD4 cell counts.

Pathogenesis of Co-infection of HIV and Tuberculosis

TB can develop either through progression of primary infection or through reactivation of latent infection. Infection with *M. tuberculosis* can occur when an individual is exposed to infectious tubercle bacilli. When the bacilli reach the pulmonary alveoli, they are ingested by alveolar macrophages while other surviving tubercle bacilli multiply within the macrophage and eventually undergo hematogenous spread to other areas of the host body. In HIV infection, defective macrophages function against the TB infection, leading to the progression of TB disease.

Leprosy

Definition: Leprosy, also known as Hansen's disease, is a chronic infectious disease caused by Mycobacterium leprae, a microorganism that has a predilection for the skin and nerves. The disease is clinically characterized by one or more of the three cardinal signs:

- Hypopigmented or erythematous skin patches with definite loss of sensation,
- Thickened peripheral nerves, and acid-fast bacilli detected on skin smears or biopsy material.
- M. leprae primarily infects Schwann cells in the peripheral nerves leading to nerve damage and the development of disabilities.

Leprosy, also known as Hansen's disease, is a chronic infectious disease caused by *Mycobacterium leprae* a microorganism that has a predilection for the skin and nerves. Though nonfatal, leprosy is one of the most common causes of nontraumatic peripheral neuropathy worldwide. The disease has been known to man since time immemorial.

Interaction of M. leprae with Schwann Cells and Macrophages

- Schwann cells (SCs) are a major target for infection by M. leprae leading to injury of the nerve, demyelination, and consequent disability.
- Binding of M. leprae to SCs induces demyelination and loss of axonal conductance It has been shown that *M. leprae* can invade SCs by a specific laminin-binding protein of 21 kDa in addition to PGL-1.
- PGL-1, a major unique glycoconjugate on the M. leprae surface, binds laminin-2, which explains the predilection of the bacterium for peripheral nerves.
- The identification of the *M. leprae*-targeted SC receptor, dystroglycan (DG), suggests a role for this molecule in early nerve degeneration.
- Mycobacterium leprae-induced demyelination is a result of direct bacterial ligation to neuregulin receptor, ErbB2 and Erk1/2 activation, and subsequent MAP kinase signaling and proliferation.

Macrophages are one of the most abundant host cells to come in contact with mycobacteria. Phagocytosis of M. leprae by monocyte-derived macrophages can be mediated by complement receptorsCR1 (CD35), CR3 (CD11b/CD18), and CR4 (CD11c/CD18) and is regulated by protein kinase. Non-responsiveness towards M. leprae seems to correlate with a Th2 cytokine profile.

Disease Classification

Leprosy is classified within two poles of the disease with transition between the clinical forms. Clinical, histopathological, and immunological criteria identify five forms of leprosy:

- tuberculoid polar leprosy (TT),
- borderline tuberculoid (BT),
- midborderline (BB),
- borderline lepromatous (BL),
- lepromatous polar leprosy (LL).

Patients were divided into two groups for therapeutic purposes: paucibacillary (TT, BT) and multibacillary (midborderline (BB), BL, LL).

Histopathological Reactions

Histopathologically, skin lesions from tuberculoid patients are characterized by inflammatory infiltrate containing well-formed granulomas with differentiated macrophages, epithelioid and giant cells, and a predominance of CD4+ T cells at the lesion site, with low or absent bacteria. Patients show a vigorous-specific immune response to M. leprae with a Th1 profile, IFN-γ production, and a positive skin test (lepromin or Mitsuda reaction).

Lepromatous patients present with several skin lesions with a preponderance of CD8+ T cells in situ, absence of granuloma formation, high bacterial load, and a flattened epidermis. The number of bacilli from a newly diagnosed lepromatous patient can reach 1012 bacteria per gram of tissue. Patients with LL leprosy have a CD4: CD8 ratio of approximately 1: 2 with a predominant Th2 type response and high titers of anti-*M. leprae* antibodies. Cell-mediated immunity against *M. leprae* is either modest or absent, characterized by negative skin test and diminished lymphocyte proliferation.

Leprosy reactions: Leprosy reactions are the acute episodes of clinical inflammation occurring during the chronic course of disease. They pose a challenging problem because they increase morbidity due to nerve damage even after the completion of treatment. They are classified as

- Type I (reversal reaction; RR)
- Type II (erythema nodosum leprosum; ENL) reactions.

Type I reaction occurs in borderline patients (BT, midborderline and BL) whereas ENL only occurs in BL and LL forms. Reactions are interpreted as a shift in patients' immunologic status. Chemotherapy, pregnancy, concurrent infections, and emotional and physical stress have been identified as predisposing conditions to reactions. Both types of reactions have been found to cause neuritis, representing the primary cause of irreversible deformities.

Type I reaction is characterized by edema and erythema of existing skin lesions, the formation of new skin lesions, neuritis, additional sensory and motor loss, and edema of the hands, feet, and face, but systemic symptoms are uncommon. The presence of an inflammatory infiltrate with a predominance of CD4+ T cells, differentiated macrophages and thickened epidermis have been observed in RR.

Type II reaction is characterized by the appearance of tender, erythematous, subcutaneous nodules located on apparently normal skin, and is frequently accompanied by systemic symptoms, such as fever, malaise, enlarged lymph nodes, anorexia, weight loss, arthralgia, and edema.

Additional organs including the testes, joints, eyes, and nerves may also be affected. There may be significant leukocytosis that typically recedes after the reactional state. Presence of high levels of proinflammatory cytokines such as TNF-α, IL-6, and IL-1β in the sera of ENL patients suggests that these pleiotropic inflammatory cytokines may be at least partially responsible for the clinical manifestations of a type II reaction.

Immunology of leprosy reactions: Type I reaction is a naturally occurring delayed-type hypersensitivity response to M. leprae immunologically, it is characterized by the development of strong skin test reactivity as well as lymphocyte responsiveness and a predominant Th1 response. RR episodes have been associated with the infiltration of IFN-γ and TNF-secreting CD4+ lymphocytes in skin lesions and nerves, resulting in edema and painful inflammation.

Immunologic markers like CXCL10 are described as a potential tool for discriminating RR. A significant increase in FoxP3 staining was observed in RR patients compared with ENL and patients with non-reactional leprosy, implying a role for regulatory T cells in RR. Pathogenesis of type II reaction is thought to be related to the deposition of immune complexes. Increased levels of TNF-α, IL-1β, IFN-γ, and other cytokines in type II reactions are observed.

- A massive infiltrate of polymorphonuclear cells (PMN) in the lesions is only observed during ENL and some patients present with high numbers of neutrophils in the blood as well.

- Neutrophils may contribute to the bulk of TNF production that is associated with tissue damage in leprosy.

- The mechanism of neutrophil recruitment in ENL involves the enhanced expression of E-selectin and IL-1β, likely leading to neutrophil adhesion to endothelial cells.

TNF-α may augment the immune response towards the elimination of the pathogen and/or mediate the pathologic manifestations of the disease.

Pathophysiology

The precise mechanism of transmission of leprosy is unknown; however, both prolonged close contact and transmission by nasal droplets are thought to be implicated. The bacterium can also be grown in the laboratory by injection into the footpads of mice. Genetic factors have long been thought to play a role, due to the observation of clustering of leprosy around certain families, and the failure to understand why certain individuals develop lepromatous leprosy while others develop other types of leprosy.

This is mostly because the body is naturally immune to the bacteria, and those persons who do become infected experience severe allergic reactions to the disease. Malnutrition and prolonged exposure to infected persons may play a role in development of the disease. The most widely held belief is that the disease is transmitted by contact between infected persons and healthy persons. In general, closeness of contact is related to the dose of infection, which in turn is related to the occurrence of disease.

Two exit routes of *M. leprae* from the human body often described are the skin and the nasal mucosa, although their relative importance is not clear. Lepromatous cases show large numbers of organisms deep in the dermis, but whether they reach the skin surface in sufficient numbers is doubtful. Fairly large numbers of M. leprae were found in the superficial keratin layer of the skin of lepromatous leprosy patients, suggesting the organism could exit along with the sebaceous secretions. The majority of lepromatous patients showed leprosy bacilli in their nasal secretions as collected through blowing the nose.

The entry route of *M. leprae* into the human body is also not definitively known. The skin and the upper respiratory tract are most likely. Entry through the respiratory route appears the most probable route, although other routes, particularly broken skin, cannot be ruled out. In leprosy, both the reference points for measuring the incubation period and the times of infection and onset of disease are difficult to define, the former because of the lack of adequate immunological tools and the latter because of the disease's slow onset. The maximum incubation period reported is as long as 30 years, or over, as observed among war veterans known to have been exposed for short periods in endemic areas, but otherwise living in non endemic areas. The average incubation period is generally believed to be between three and five years.

Malaria

Malaria causes disease through a number of pathways, which depend to a certain extent on the species. Malaria is caused by a single-celled parasite of the genus Plasmodium; there are five species which infect humans, being *Plasmodium faleiparum, P. vivax, P. ovale, P. malariae* and *P. knowlesi.*

All these species are introduced into the human blood stream through the bite of an infected mosquito. The life stage of malaria at this point is called a "sporozoite", and they pass first to the liver, where they undergo an initial stage of replication (called "exo-erythrocytic replication").

Before passing back into the blood and invading red blood cells (called "erythrocytes", hence this is the "erythrocytic" part of the cycle). The malaria parasites that invade red blood cells are known as merozoites, and within the cell they replicate again, bursting out once they have completed a set number of divisions.

It is this periodic rupturing of the red blood cells that causes most of the symptoms associated with malaria, as the host's immune system responds to the waste products produced by the malaria parasites and the debris from the destroyed red blood cells.

Different species of malaria rupture the red blood cells at different intervals, which lead to the diagnostic cycles of fever which characterise malaria; *P. vivax,* for example, tends to produce cycles of fever every two days, whereas *P. malaria* produces fever. In addition, *Plasmodium faleiparum* produces unique pathological effects, due to its manipulation of the host's physiology.

When it infects red blood cells, it makes them stick to the walls of tiny blood vessels deep within major organs, such as the kidneys, lungs, heart and brain. This is called "sequestration", and results in reduced blood flow to these organs, causing the severe clinical symptoms associated with this infection, such as cerebral malaria.

Pathophysiology

Malaria infection develops via two phases:
- One that involves the liver (exoerythrocytic phase),
- One that involves red blood cells, or erythrocytes (erythrocytic phase).

When an infected mosquito pierces a person's skin to take a blood meal, sporozoites in the mosquito's saliva enter the bloodstream and migrate to the liver where they infect hepatocytes.

After a potential dormant period in the liver, these organisms differentiate to yield thousands of merozoites, which, following rupture of their host cells, escape into the blood and infect red blood cells to begin the erythrocytic stage of the life cycle. The parasite escapes from the liver undetected by wrapping itself in the cell membrane of the infected host liver cell. Within the red blood cells, the parasites multiply further, again asexually, periodically breaking out of their host cells to invade fresh red blood cells. Several such amplification cycles occur. Thus, classical descriptions of waves of fever arise from simultaneous waves of merozoites escaping and infecting red blood cells.

Some *P. vivax* sporozoites do not immediately develop into exoerythrocytic-phase merozoites, but instead produce hypnozoites that remain dormant for periods ranging from several months (7–10 months is typical) to several years. After a period of dormancy, they reactivate and produce merozoites. Hypnozoites are responsible for long incubation and late relapses in *P. vivax* infections, although their existence in *P. ovale* is uncertain.

The parasite is relatively protected from attack by the body's immune system because for most of its human life cycle it resides within the liver and blood cells and is relatively invisible to immune surveillance. However, circulating infected blood cells are destroyed in the spleen. To avoid this fate, the *P. falciparum* parasite displays adhesive proteins on the surface of the infected blood cells, causing the blood cells to stick to the walls of small blood vessels, thereby sequestering the parasite from passage through the general circulation and the spleen.

The blockage of the microvasculature causes symptoms such as in placental malaria. Sequestered red blood cells can breach the blood–brain barrier and cause cerebral malaria.

Genetic resistance: The impact of sickle cell trait on malaria immunity illustrates some evolutionary trade-offs that have occurred because of endemic malaria. Sickle cell trait causes a defect in the hemoglobin molecule in the blood. Instead of retaining the biconcave shape of a normal red blood cell, the modified hemoglobin S molecule causes the cell to sickle or distort into a curved shape.

Due to the sickle shape, the molecule is not as effective in taking or releasing oxygen. Infection causes red cells to sickle more, and so they are removed from circulation sooner. This reduces the frequency with which malaria parasites complete their life cycle in the cell. Individuals who are homozygous (with two copies of the abnormal hemoglobin beta allele) have sickle-cell anaemia, while those who are heterozygous (with one abnormal allele and one normal allele) experience resistance to malaria.

Although the shorter life expectancy for those with the homozygous condition would not sustain the trait's survival, the trait is preserved because of the benefits provided by the heterozygous form.

Liver dysfunction: Liver dysfunction as a result of malaria is uncommon and usually only occurs in those with other liver condition such as viral hepatitis or chronic liver disease. The syndrome is sometimes called malarial hepatitis. Liver compromise in people with malaria correlates with a greater likelihood of complications and death.

Dysentery (Bacterial and Amoebic)

Dysentery is characterized by inflammation of the intestine, abdominal pain, and diarrhea with stools that often contain blood and mucus with probability of presence of fever, abdominal pain, and rectal tenesmus (a feeling of incomplete defecation). It is caused by a number of types of infection such as bacteria, viruses, parasitic worms, or protozoa. It is a type of gastroenteritis. The mechanism is an inflammatory disorder of the intestine, especially of the colon.

Amoebic dysentery: Dysentery may be caused by amoebiasis, an infection by the amoeba Entamoeba histolytica, and is then known as amoebic dysentery. Proper treatment of the underlying infection of amoebic dysentery is important; insufficiently treated amoebiasis can lie dormant for years and then lead to severe, potentially fatal, complications. Entamoeba histolytica is mainly found in tropical areas. Inside the bowel of an infected person the organism forms a shell that surrounds and protects them. This group of amoebas is known as a cyst.

The cyst passes out of the person's body in the feces and can survive outside the body. If hygiene standards are poor; for example, if the person does not dispose of the feces hygienically, it can contaminate the surroundings, such as nearby food and water. If another person then eats or drinks food or water that has been contaminated with feces containing the cyst, that person will also become infected with the amoeba.

After entering the person's body through the mouth, the cyst will travel down into the stomach. The amoebas inside the cyst are protected from the stomach's digestive acid. From the stomach, the cyst will travel to the intestines where it will break open and release the amoebas, causing the infection. The amoebas can burrow into the walls of the intestines and cause small abscesses and ulcers to form. The cycle then begins again.

Bacillary dysentery: This is a type of dysentery, and is a severe form of shigellosis. Dysentery may also be caused by shigellosis, an infection by bacteria of the genus Shigella, and is then known as bacillary dysentery (or Marlow Syndrome). Bacillary dysentery, or shigellosis, is caused by bacilli of the genus Shigella. Symptomatically, the disease ranges from a mild attack to a severe course that commences suddenly and ends in death caused by dehydration and poisoning by bacterial toxins. After an incubation period of one to six days, the disease has an abrupt onset with fever and the frequent production of watery stools that may contain blood. Vomiting may also occur, and dehydration soon becomes obvious owing to the copious loss of bodily fluids. In advanced stages of the disease, chronic ulceration of the large intestine causes the production of bloody stools. Enteroinvasive Escherichia coli may also cause a dysentery syndrome.

Pathogenesis

Transmission is fecal-oral and is remarkable for the small number of organisms that may cause disease. Shigella bacteria invade the intestinal mucosal cells but do not usually go beyond the lamina propria. Dysentery is caused when the bacteria escape the epithelial cell phagolysosome, multiply within the cytoplasm, and destroy host cells. Shiga toxin causes hemorrhagic colitis and hemolytic-uremic syndrome by damaging endothelial cells in the microvasculature of the colon and the glomeruli, respectively. In addition, chronic arthritis secondary to *S. flexneri* infection, called Reiter syndrome, may be caused by a bacterial antigen; the occurrence of this syndrome is strongly linked to HLA-B27 genotype, but the immunologic basis of this reaction is not understood.

Infective Hepatitis

Definition: Hepatitis is an inflammatory condition of liver characterised by jaundice, hepatomegaly, anorexia, abdominal gastric discomfort, abnormal liver function, clay coloured stools, dark urine etc. Condition may be caused by bacteria, virus, parasitic infection, alcohol, drugs, toxins, transfusion of incompatible blood etc. It may be

- mild and brief
- severe, fulminant and life threatening
- Severe hepatitis may lead to cirrhosis and hepatocellular carcinoma.

Viral hepatitis: Viral hepatitis refers to infection of liver caused by hepatotrophic viruses [hepatitis virus].

- Hepatitis A virus causing a faecally spread self-limiting disease.
- Hepatitis B virus causing parenterally transmitted disease that may become chronic.
- Hepatitis C virus (HCV) [Non-a Non-B virus (NANB)]-involved in transfusion related hepatitis.
- Hepatitis delta virus (HDV) causes super-infection in hepatitis B patients.
- Hepatitis E virus cause water borne infection.

Liver also infected with Epstein Bar virus, arbovirus (yellow fever), cytomegalovirus, Herpes simplex.

Etiologic Classification

Hepatitis A virus [HAV] (Infectious hepatitis): It is a benign self-limiting disease with incubation period of 14 to 45 days. Usually it spread by faecal or oral route. Parenteral transmission is extremely rare. Overcrowding, poor hygiene, poor sanitation cause spread. Hepatitis A virus (HAV) does not cause chronic hepatitis or carrier stage or fulminant hepatitis. HAV is a small, non-enveloped single stranded RNA picorna virus.

Pathogenesis

Hepatitis is caused by immunological mechanism.

Hepatitis B virus (HBV) (Serum Hepatitis): HBV is the most versatile (able to do many different things/diseases) of hepatotrophic viruses.HBV can produce:

- Acute hepatitis
- Chronic non-progressive hepatitis
- Progressive chronic disease ending in cirrhosis
- Fulminant hepatitis with massive liver necrosis
- Asymptomatic carrier stage with or without progressive disease
- HBV plays important role in development of hepatocellular carcinoma

Transmitted parenterally, by blood transfusion, injection, mother to child, sexually etc. It has longer incubation period (30-180 days). HBV is a DNA virus of hep adenovirus family.

Immunological markers: Immunological markers indicate presence of HBV infection and can be demonstrated in sera and hepatocytes of infected individual.

HBsAg [Australian antigen] (Hepatitis B surface antigen)]: Appear in blood after 6 weeks of infection. Disappear in 3-6 months. Persistence > 6 months indicates carrier stage. Anti-HBs: Ig-M/Ig-G type antibodies appear 3 months after onset of infection. It provides lifelong protection against re-infection. It is the basis for vaccination strategies.

- *HBeAg [Derived from core protein of virus], HBV DNA, DNA polymerase:* all are markers of active viral replication (occur for 3-6 weeks). Persistence beyond 10 weeks indicates chronic liver disease/carrier stage.
- *Anti-HBe:* antibody to HBeAg appears after disappearance of HBeAg. Increased serum anti HBe indicate resolution of infection.
- *HBcAg:* derived from core protein. Cannot be detected in blood but in hepatocytes in carrier stage and in chronic hepatitis patients.
- *Anti HBcAg:* Ig-M /Ig-G type of antibody. High Ig-G indicate recent infection and Ig-M indicate infection in past.

Immunological mechanism is the primary cause of hepatocellular damage. Specifically, cytotoxic T-cells. No cytotoxic effect for virus identified. Delayed hypersensitivity-hepatocellular damage caused by cytotoxic T-lymphocytes.

Immune complex mediated mechanism-formation of immune complex (e.g.: HBsAg-Anti-HBs complex] lead to activation of complement system-and resultant tissue damage. Evidences are:

- Absence of hepatocellular damage in HBV carrier stage
- Presence of specifically sensitised cytotoxic T-lymphocytes at the site of hepatocellular injury
- Patients with depressed cell mediated immunity have high frequency of progression from acute to chronic hepatitis

Hepatitis D: Hepatitis D virus [Hepatitis Delta virus] is unique defective virus which needs genetic information provided by HBV for multiplication-and cause hepatitis only in presence of HBV. Simultaneous co-infection with HBV and HDV result in hepatitis ranging from mild to fulminant. Super infection with HDV in HBV carrier/chronic HBV patient worsens the condition leading to severe fulminant hepatitis/cirrhosis. Hepatitis Delta virus is a single stranded RNA particle. HDV replication and proliferation take place in nuclei of liver cells.

Pathogenesis: HDV is thought to cause direct cytopathic effect on hepatocytes.

- HDV markers: HDV RNA detectable in blood and liver cells.
- HDVAg: detectable in blood.
- Anti-HDVAg: Ig-G/Ig-M anti bodies.
- Ig-M anti body against both HDVAg and HBcAg indicate co-infection.

Hepatitis C: Parenterally transmitted Non-A, Non-B hepatitis. HCV is small enveloped single stranded RNA virus of flavi/pesti virus family. HCV is a major cause of liver disease worldwide. Transmitted by blood transfusion, blood product, parenteral drug abuse, accidental cuts/needle prick in health workers. HCV has high rate of progression to chronic disease and cirrhosis than IIBV. Incubation period 6-12 weeks.

Pathogenesis: Cell mediated immunological destruction of liver cells. HCV markers:

- HCV RNA detected in blood for 1-3 weeks.
- Elevation of serum transaminase.
- Anti-HCV develops after a delay of 4-12 months.

Hepatitis E (HEV): Enterically (orally) transmitted water borne disease.HEV is an unenveloped single stranded RNA virus. In most cases -it is a self-limiting disease. HEV markers:

- HEV RNA
- Anti-HEV antibodies- Ig-G/Ig-M type.
- HEVAg: detected in cytoplasm of hepatocytes.

Hepatitis G: HGV is a single stranded RNA virus. HGV is a blood borne infection and may cause acute to chronic viral hepatitis.

Table: 10.2 Acute viral hepatitis (Comparative feature of 5 hepatotrophic viruses)

Features	HAV	HBV	HCV	HDV	HEV
Family	Picornavirus	Hepadenovirus	Flavivirus	Satellite virus	Calici virus
Particle size	27nm	42nm	30-60nm	40nm	27-32nm
Genome	RNA	DNA	RNA	RNA	RNA
Antigen	HAAg	HBsAg, HBcAg, HBeAg	HCAg	HDAg	HEAg
Antibody	Anti-HDV	Anti-HBsAg, Anti-HBcAg, Anti-HBeAg	Anti-HCV	Anti-HDV	Anti-HEV
Transmission	Faecal, Oral	Perinatal, sexual	Parental, Sexual	Parental, Sexual	Faecal, Oral
Incubation	15-45 days	40-180 days	15-150 days	30-50 days	21-63 days
Mortality	0.2 %	0.2-1 %	0.2 %	2-20 %	0.2 %
Progress to Chronic hepatitis	0 %	5-10 %	50-70 %	2-70 %	0 %
Risk of Hepatocellular Carcinoma	No	Yes	Yes	Possibly	No

(*source:* https://en.wikipedia.org/wiki/Viral_hepatitis with necessary modifications)

Clinicopathologic Syndromes

A number of clinical syndromes may develop after exposure to hepatitis viruses.

1. *Carrier stage:* Asymptomatic individuals without manifestations of disease but harbour the infection with hepatotrophic viruses and are capable of transmitting it.

2. *Acute viral hepatitis:* Most common consequence of all heptotrophic viruses is acute inflammatory involvement of liver. In general type A, B, C, (NANB) run similar clinical course and show identical pathological findings. Clinically acute viral hepatitis is divided into four phases:

   (a) *Incubation period:* Varies among different hepatotrophic viruses:
   - Hepatitis A-4 weeks (15-45 days)
   - Hepatitis B-10 weeks (30-180 days)
   - Hepatitis D-6 weeks (30-50 days)
   - Hepatitis C-7 weeks (20-90 days)
   - Hepatitis E-2-8 weeks (15-160 das)

   (b) Pre-icteric phase

   (c) Icteric phase

   (d) Post-icteric phase

3. *Pre-icteric phase (Prodromal symptoms):* Anorexia, nausea, vomiting, fatigue, malaise (vague feeling of discomfort), arthralgia (Pain in joints), head ache, low grade fever, elevation of transaminases, diarrhoea.

4. ***Icteric phase*** (1-4 weeks) (clinical jaundice): Dark coloured urine due to bilirubinurea, clay coloured stool due to cholestasis, pruritus (itching) due to elevated serum bile acids, loss of weight, abdominal discomfort (due to enlarged tender liver) etc. Deranged liver function test (elevated serum bilirubin, transaminase, alkaline phosphatase, hyperglobulinaemia etc.)

5. ***Post icteric phase (2-12 weeks):*** This is characterised by clinical/biochemical recovery. Recovery phase more prolonged for hepatitis B and C.

Pathologic changes in acute hepatitis: Grossly liver is slightly enlarged, soft and greenish. Hepatocellular injury:

- it is most marked in Zone 3 (centrilobular zone)
- mildly injured hepatocytes appear swollen with granular cytoplasm (ballooning degeneration)
- in acidophilic degeneration-cytoplasm become intensely eosinophilic, the nucleus become small, pyknotic and eventually extruded from the cell leaving an acidophilic mass called councilman body or acidophil body
- in dropping out necrosis isolated small clusters of hepatocyte undergo lysis.
- in bridging necrosis bands of necrosis link portal track to central hepatic vein or on central hepatic vein to another

Bridging necrosis is more severe form of hepatocellular injury in acute viral hepatitis. It may progress to fulminant hepatitis or chronic hepatitis.

- Inflammatory infiltrate -[infiltration of mononuclear inflammatory cells (mainly of lymphocytes and macrophages)].
- Kupffer cell hyperplasia: there is reactive hyperplasia of kupffer cells, many of which contain phagocytosed cellular debris.
- Cholestasis: biliary obstruction
- Regeneration: surviving adjacent hepatocyte undergo regeneration and hyperplasia.

If necrosis cause collapse of reticulin framework of lobules may cause distortion of lobular architecture.

Chronic hepatitis: Chronic hepatitis is a continuing or relapsing hepatic disease for more than 6 months with symptoms and biochemical/serological and histopathological evidence of inflammation and necrosis. Although hepatitis viruses (HBV, HDV, HCV) are the most common causes. There are many other causes-Wilson's disease, α1-antitrypsin deficiency, chronic alcoholism, drugs (α-methyldopa, Isoniazid, methotrexate), autoimmunity. Currently chronic hepatitis classified according to etiologic agent.

Frequency and severity of the disease depends on the organism (virus).The likely hood of chronic hepatitis following acute viral infection:

- HAV-does not produce chronic hepatitis
- HBV-cause chronic hepatitis in 5% cases

- HDV-superinfection on HBV causes chronic hepatitis in 10-40%cases
- HCV (NANBV) post transfusion type account for 40-60% cases
- Enteric type (HEV) case less than 10% cases

Clinical features of chronic hepatitis: Elevation of serum transaminase, hyperglobulinemia, fatigue, malaise, loss of appetite, mild jaundice and immune complex mediated disease. Two important factors which lead to chronic hepatitis are:

- Impaired immunity
- Extreme age

Chronic persistent hepatitis: It is benign self-limiting condition. Here recovery from acute viral hepatitis is delayed beyond six months. The condition may remain asymptomatic/patient may complain fatigue, malaise, poor appetite, intolerance of fat, alcohol, discomfort over liver.

Pathologic changes: Clinical examination reveals normal slightly enlarged and tender liver Laboratory diagnosis reveals-

- elevated transaminase level
- hyperglobulinaemia
- HBsAg

Histologically

- expansion of portal track by mononuclear inflammatory cells (Portal triaditis)
- lobular architecture of hepatic parenchyma preserved
- Necrosis: features of chronic active hepatitis (piecemeal necrosis, bridging necrosis) are absent.

Chronic active hepatitis: Chronic active or chronic aggressive hepatitis is defined as a progressive form of necrotising and fibrosing disease involving portal tract as well as hepatic parenchyma eventually culminating in cirrhosis.

Usual presentation is like features of acute hepatitis-fatigue, anorexia, malaise, mid fever, vague abdominal pain, jaundice. More advanced cases may have portal hypertension, ascites, oesophageal varices. Most common etiologic agents are HBV, HCV (NANBV) and HBV-HDV infection.

Pathological changes: Laboratory diagnosis of chronic active hepatitis is made by elevated serum bilirubin transaminases, gamma globulin, immunological markers.

Microscopic features

- ***Inflammation:*** There is abundant mononuclear inflammatory cell infiltrate that is not confined to portal tract but into periportal hepatic parenchyma.
- ***Necrosis:*** Two type of necrosis is characteristic in chronic active hepatitis:

- *Piecemeal necrosis:* In which case inflammatory infiltrate after eroding limiting plate cause necrosis of small group of hepatocytes in periportal parenchyma.
- *Bridging necrosis:* seen in more severe form of chronic active hepatitis and is characterised by necrosis of tracts of hepatocytes that may bridge portal tract to central hepatic vein, central vein to central vein and portal tract to portal tract.
- *Fibrosis:* Collapsed reticulin frame work left at area of bridging necrosis undergoes fibrous scarring eventually progressing to cirrhosis. The major causes of death are liver failure with hepatic encephalopathy, cirrhosis with hematemesis and hepatocellular carcinoma.

Fulminant hepatitis: Fulminant hepatitis is the most severe form of acute hepatitis in which there is rapidly progressive hepatocellular failure. It culminates in hepatic encephalopathy (hepatic coma).It is caused by viral [HBV, HCV, HBV-HDV, etc.].

Non-viral causes: drugs like acetaminophen, isoniazid, poisoning, hypoxic injury, tumour. Mortality rate is high if hepatic transplantation is not done.

Clinical features [(Hepatic encephalopathy) (Hepatic coma)]: Neuropsychiatric syndrome: Due to toxic product not metabolised by diseased liver like ammonia and other nitrogenous substances from intestinal bacteria. Disturbed consciousness, personality change, intellectual deterioration, law slurred speech, coma, death.

Pathologic changes: Liver is small and shrunken. Capsule is loose and wrinkled. There are extensive areas of muddy red and yellow necrosis and patches of green bile staining.

Histologically two patterns are recognised:
- *Sub massive necrosis:* having less rapid course extending upto 3 months, regeneration orderly. Large group of hepatocytes in Zone 3 (centrilobular area) and zone 2 (mid zone) are wiped out leading to collapsed reticulin frame work. Regeneration in sub massive necrosis is more orderly and may result in restoration of normal architecture.
- *Massive necrosis:* in which liver failure is rapid occurring 2-3 weeks. Entire liver lobules are necrotic. All that left is collapsed and condensed reticulin framework and portal tract with proliferated bile ductules plugged with bile. Regeneration if take place is disorderly forming irregular masses of hepatocytes.

Immunoprophylaxis and hepatitis vaccines: Best prophylaxis against viral hepatitis is prevention of spread to close contacts after detection and identification of its route of contamination (food and water, sexual or parenteral).

Immunoprophylaxis
- Hepatitis B immunoglobulin for HBV.
- Immune serum globulin for HAV.

- It is a passive immunisation given to close contacts of hepatitis patients prophylactically.
- It is administered to sufferers of infection within hours of acquiring viral infection and to neonates born to HBsAg positive mother.
- Hepatitis B vaccines are prepared from outer surface of virus (HBsAg).
- Heat inactivated plasma containing HBsAg.
- Polypeptide vaccines containing antigen determinants of HBsAg.
- Hybrid virus vaccines.
- Synthetic vaccines are available.

Other infections and infestations: Liver is also affected by bacteria, spirochetes, fungi, and some parasitic infestations.

Cholangitis: It is a term used to describe inflammation of extrahepatic/intrahepatic bile duct or both. There are two main types of cholangitis:

- Pyogenic cholangitis
- Primary sclerosing cholangitis

Pyogenic cholangitis: Cholangitis occurring secondary to obstruction of major extrahepatic duct. The obstruction may be from impacted gall stone, carcinoma of extra hepatic duct, carcinoma of head of pancreas, acute pancreatitis, and inflammatory stricture (stenosis/narrowing) of bile duct. Bacteria gain entry into obstructed duct and proliferate in bile. Infection spread along the branches of obstructed duct and reach the liver termed ascending cholangitis. Common infecting bacteria are enteric organisms-E-coli, Klebsiella, Enterobactor.

Pathologic changes: affected ducts show small beaded abscesses accompanied by bile stasis along their course and large abscesses within liver. Abscesses are composed of acute inflammatory cells which are replaced gradually by chronic inflammatory cells and fibrous capsule.

Primary sclerosing (hardening) cholangitis: Chronic fibrosing inflammatory condition of unknown cause. It produces cholestatic syndrome. [cholestasis-stoppage or suppression of bile flow]Patients are generally adult males. About half of the cases have associated chronic ulcerative colitis or some other autoimmune disease. Clinical features include right upper abdominal pain, pruritus and intermittent jaundice. Laboratory investigation reveals cholestasis with elevated serum alkaline phosphatase, bilirubin, high serum copper, ceruloplasmin, lever copper content.

Pathologic changes: marked chronic inflammation involving extrahepatic and intrahepatic bile duct. Fibrosis develops leading to obliteration (destruction) of lumina of intrahepatic ductules. Further progress lead to biliary cirrhosis.

Pyogenic liver abscess: Most of the liver abscesses are pyogenic origin (bacterial origin). Less often amoebic, hydatid, rarely actinomycotic. Pyogenic liver abscesses are classified on the basis of mode of entry:

- *Ascending cholangitis:* Through ascending infection of biliary tract due to obstruction. e.g.: gall stone, cancer, sclerosing cholangitis and biliary strictures. (stenosis/narrowing).
- *Portal pyaemia:* By means of spread of pelvic or gastrointestinal infection resulting in portal pylephlebitis (inflammation of portal vein) or septic emboli. e.g.: from appendicitis, diverticulitis, pancreatitis, infected haemorrhoids, etc.
- *Septicaemia:* Through spread by hepatic artery.
- *Direct infection:* Resulting solitary liver abscess. e.g.: from adjacent periphrenic abscess, secondary infection in amoebic liver abscess, metastasis, formation of haematoma following trauma. Iatrogenic causes: liver biopsy, percutaneous biliary drainage, accidental surgical trauma.
- *Cryptogenic:* From unknown causes.

Commonest infecting organisms are gram negative bacteria, E coli, Pseudomonas, Klebsiella, Enterobactor, anaerobic organisms, Bacteriodes, Actinomyces.

Clinical features: Pain in right upper quadrant, fever, tender hepatomegaly and jaundice. Laboratory examination reveals leucocytosis, elevated serum alkaline phosphatase, hypoalbuminaemia, positive blood culture.

Pathologic changes: they occur as single or multiple yellow abscesses 1cm or more in diameter in and enlarged liver. A singe abscess generally has thick fibrous capsule.

Microscopically: Typical features of abscess are seen. There are areas of extensive necrosis of affected liver parenchyma. Adjacent viable area shows pus, blood clot, in portal vein inflammation, congestion and proliferating fibroblast.

Amoebic liver abscess: Amoebic liver abscess are less common than pyogenic liver abscess. They are caused by spread of Entamoeba histolitica from intestinal lesions. Vegetative trophozoite form of amoeba in colon invades the colonic mucosa forming flask shaped ulcers. From there they are carried to liver via portal venous system. Amoeba multiplies and blocks the small intra hepatic portal radicles resulting in infarction necrosis of the adjacent liver parenchyma.

Pathologic changes: Amoebic liver abscesses are solitary. The centre of abscess contains large necrotic area having reddish brown thick pus. Abscess wall consists of irregular shreds of necrotic liver tissue. Histologically necrotic area consists of liver cells, leucocytes, RBCs, strands of connective tissue and debris. Amoebas are most easily found in liver tissue at margin of abscess.

Hepatic tuberculosis: Tuberculosis of liver occurs as a result of miliary dissemination from primary complex or from chronic adult pulmonary tuberculosis. Diagnosis is possible by liver biopsy. The patient may have unexplained fever, jaundice, hepatomegaly, hepatosplenomegaly. There may be elevated serum alkaline phosphatase level and hyperglobulinaemia.

Pathological changes: Basic lesion is epitheloid cell granuloma characterised by central caseation necrosis with destruction of reticulin frame work and peripheral cuff of lymphocyte.

Hydatid disease (Echinococcosis): Hydatid disease occurs as a result of infection by larval cyst stage of Echinococcus granulosus. Dog is the common definite host while man, sheep and cattle are the intermediate host. Infected faeces of dog contaminate grass and farmland from where ova ingested by sheep, pig and man. Man acquire disease by handling dog/eating contaminated vegetables.

Ova ingested by man are liberated from chitinous wall by gastric juice and pas through intestinal mucosa from where they are carried to liver by portal venous system. They are trapped in hepatic sinusoids where the eventually develop into hydatid cyst. Ova which pass through liver enter right side of heart and are caught in pulmonary capillary blood and form pulmonary hydatid cyst. Some ova which enter systemic circulation form hydatid cyst and reach in brain, spleen, bone, muscles etc.

Complications of hydatid cyst include: secondary infection and hydatid allergy due to sensitisation of host with cyst fluid. The diagnosis is made by:

- Peripheral blood eosinophilia
- Radiological examination
- Serological test like -indirect haemoglobin test, Casoni skin test.

Cystic Fibrosis

Definition: Cystic fibrosis (CF) or mucoviscidosis is an autosomal recessive inherited disease that results from defective epithelial chloride ion transport. It is fundamentally a widespread disorder in the secretory process of all exocrine glands affecting both mucous secreting and exocrine glands though out the body.

Cystic fibrosis (CF), also known as mucoviscidosis, is an autosomal recessive genetic disorder that affects mostly the lung s but also the pancreas, liver, and intestine. Difficulty breathing is the most serious symptom and results from frequent lung infections. Other symptoms —including sinus infections, poor growth, and infertility— affect other parts of the body.

CF is caused by one of many different mutations in the gene for the protein cystic fibrosis transmembrane conductance regulator (CFTR). This protein is required to regulate the components of sweat, digestive fluids, and mucus. Healthy people have two working copies of the CFTR gene.

Carriers have one working copy. People with CF have no working copy. CF therefore has autosomal recessive in heritance. The underlying mechanism is abnormal transport of chloride and sodium across the epithelium, which is the cell layer that covers membranes over organs. This leads to thick, viscous secretions. Individuals with cystic fibrosis can be diagnosed before birth by gen etic testing or by a sweat test in early childhood.

Abnormally viscid mucous secretion due to increased electrolyte concentration lead to obstruction of organ passage, resulting in most of the clinical features of this disease, like recurrent pulmonary infection leading to chronic lung disease, pancreatic insufficiency, stetorrhoea, malnutrition, hepatic cirrhosis, intestinal obstruction, male infertility etc. Manifestation may appear in any point of life from birth, child hood or adolescence.

Etiology and Pathophysiology [Pathogenesis]

Primary defect is in the regulation of epithelial chloridetransport. This is most common inherited disease in whites. The genetic defect responsible for cystic fibrosis resides in long arm of chromosome-7. C.F (cystic fibrosis) gene, located on chromosome 7, encodes for a protein, [cystic fibrosis transmembrane conductance regulator-CFTR), that serves as chloride channel, present in many type of epithelial cells, like air ways, bile duct, pancreas, sweat glands and vas deferens.

Mutation of this gene result in abnormal expression of protein- cystic fibrosis transmembrane conductance regulator-(CFTR) and cause abnormal transmembrane chloride transport. Defective chloride transport in sweat gland produces high concentration of chloride in sweat. In air way lumen, lower the water content of mucus (mucus plugging). Viscid secretion and defective mucociliary action result in recurrent pulmonary infection with Pseudomonas aeruginosa and chronic inflammation.

- In pancreas plugging of duct causes atrophy of exocrine gland and fibrosis.
- In liver, biliary canaliculi plugged by mucinous material. It may lead to biliary cirrhosis.
- In salivary gland, glandular atrophy and fibrosis.

The CFTR protein is a channel protein that controls the flow of H2O and Cl - ions in and out of cells inside the lungs. When the CFTR protein is working correctly, as shown in Panel 1, ions freely flow in and out of the cells. However, when the CFTR protein is malfunctioning as in Panel 2, these ions cannot flow out of the cell due to a blocked channel. This causes cystic fibrosis, characterized by the buildup of thick mucus in the lungs.

The protein created by this gene is anchored to the outer membrane of cells in the sweat glands, lungs, pancreas, and all other remaining exocrine glands in the body. The protein spans this membrane and acts as a channel connecting the inner part of the cell (cytoplasm) to the surrounding fluid. This channel is primarily responsible for controlling the movement of halogens from inside to outside of the cell; however, in the sweat ducts it facilitates the movement of chloride from the sweat duct into the cytoplasm.

When the CFTR protein does not resorb ions in sweat ducts, chloride and thiocyanate released from sweat g lands are trapped inside the ducts and pumped to the skin. Additionally, hypothiocyanite, OSCN, cannot be produced by the immune defense system. Since chloride is negatively charged, this creates a difference in the electrical potential inside and outside the cell causing cations to cross into the cell. Sodium is the most common cation in the extracellular space.

The excess chloride within sweat ducts prevents sodium resorption by epithelial sodium channels and the combination of sodium and chloride creates the salt, which is lost in high amounts in the sweat of individuals with CF. This lost salt forms the basis for the sweat test.

Most of the damage in CF is due to blockage of the narrow passages of affected organs with thickened secretions. These blockages lead to remodeling and infection in the lung, damage by accumulated digestive enzymes in the pancreas, blockage of the intestines by thick faeces, etc.

Clinical Features

Clinical manifestation appears at any stage, at birth, child hood or adolescence. It affects multiple organ and systems. Pancreatic insufficiency, cause stetorrhoea, malabsorption, diabetes mellitus, intestinal obstruction, hepatic cirrhosis, meconeum ileus. In respiratory system, persistent cough, wheeze, recurrent severe pneumonia.

Pathology: Viscid secretion causes inflammation and scarring, which lead to atrophy of ductal and acinar tissue with consequent insufficiency of exocrine function.

Diagnosis: Positive sweat test–increase in concentration of chloride in sweat.

Treatment: Cystic fibrosis is a lifelong disease.

- Nutritional complications are treated by pancreatic replacement therapy and diet.
- Pulmonary complications are managed by antibiotics, expectorants, bronchodilators etc.
- Gene therapy in future.

Hypersensitivity pneumonitis or extrinsic allergic alveolitis isan immunologic inflammatory reaction involving the bronchioles, alveoli, and lung interstitium. Antigens reach the alveoli by inhalation (e.g., organic dusts) or enter the alveolar capillary unit via the bloodstream (e.g., drugs). These agents are usually encountered in work, home, or hobby environments.

Allergic asthma is the most common immunologic pulmonary disease. However, a variety of other inflammatory and genetic lung diseases have immunopathogenic mechanisms. Cystic fibrosis (CF), granulomatous, and interstitial lung disease are important representatives of these immune-mediated diseases.

Ebola Virus

Definition: Ebola virus disease (EVD), formerly known as Ebola haemorrhagic fever, is a severe, often fatal illness in humans. The virus is transmitted to people from wild animals and spreads in the human population through human-to-human transmission. Early supportive care with rehydration, symptomatic treatment improves survival. There is as yet no licensed treatment proven to neutralise the virus but a range of blood, immunological and drug therapies are under development.

Background

The Ebola virus causes an acute, serious illness which is often fatal if untreated. Ebola virus disease (EVD) first appeared in 1976 in 2 simultaneous outbreaks, one in Nzara, Sudan, and the other in Yambuku, Democratic Republic of Congo. The latter occurred in a village near the Ebola River, from which the disease takes its name. The current outbreak in West Africa, (first cases notified in March 2014), is the largest and most complex Ebola outbreak since the Ebola virus was first discovered in 1976.

Transmission

- It is thought that fruit bats of the Pteropodidae family are natural Ebola virus hosts.
- Ebola is introduced into the human population through close contact with the blood, secretions, organs or other bodily fluids of infected animals such as chimpanzees, gorillas, fruit bats, monkeys, forest antelope and porcupines found ill or dead or in the rainforest.
- Ebola then spreads through human-to-human transmission via direct contact (through broken skin or mucous membranes) with the blood, secretions, organs or other bodily fluids of infected people, and with surfaces and materials (e.g. bedding, clothing) contaminated with these fluids.
- People remain infectious as long as their blood and body fluids, including semen and breast milk, contain the virus.
- Men who have recovered from the disease can still transmit the virus through their semen for up to 7 weeks after recovery from illness.

Symptoms of Ebola Virus Disease

The incubation period, that is, the time interval from infection with the virus to onset of symptoms is 2 to 21 days. Humans are not infectious until they develop symptoms.

- First symptoms are the sudden onset of fever fatigue, muscle pain, headache and sore throat.
- This is followed by vomiting, diarrhoea, rash, symptoms of impaired kidney and liver function, and in some cases, both internal and external bleeding (e.g. oozing from the gums, blood in the stools).
- Laboratory findings include low white blood cell and platelet counts and elevated liver enzymes.

Diagnosis

Confirmation that symptoms are caused by Ebola virus infection are made using the following investigations:

- antibody-capture enzyme-linked immunosorbent assay (ELISA)
- antigen-capture detection tests
- serum neutralization test
- reverse transcriptase polymerase chain reaction (RT-PCR) assay
- electron microscopy
- Virus isolation by cell culture.

Samples from patients are an extreme biohazard risk; laboratory testing on non-inactivated samples should be conducted under maximum biological containment conditions.

Ebola Virus GP and Viral Pathogenesis

The Ebola virus genome is 19 kb long, with seven open reading frames encoding structural proteins, including the virion envelope glycoprotein (GP), nucleoprotein (NP), and matrix proteins VP24 and VP40; nonstructural proteins, including VP30 and VP35; and the viral polymerase. Unlike that of Marburg virus, the GP open reading frame of Ebola virus gives rise to two gene products, a soluble 60- to 70-kDa protein (sGP) and a full-length 150- to 170-kDa protein (GP) that inserts into the viral membrane through transcriptional editing.

The Ebola virus GP is synthesized in a secreted (sGP) or full-length transmembrane form, and each gene product has distinct biochemical and biological properties. Preferential binding of Ebola virus GP to the endothelium was demonstrated by use of two independent methodologies as follows:

- Direct binding was assessed by fluorescence-activated cell sorter analysis,
- Pseudotyping experiments were performed in which virus titers, cell numbers were carefully determined the viral GP plays a key role in the manifestations of Ebola virus infection.

The transmembrane form of GP targets the Ebola virus to cells that are relevant to its pathogenesis. GP allows the virus to introduce its contents into monocytes and/or macrophages, where cell damage or exposure to viral particles may cause the release of cytokines associated with inflammation and fever, and into endothelial cells, which damages vascular integrity.

Thus, sGP may alter the immune response by inhibiting neutrophil activation, while the transmembrane GP may contribute to the hemorrhagic fever symptoms by targeting virus to cells of the reticuloendothelial network and the lining of blood vessels. Both the adaptive immune and inflammatory systems respond to infection at the same time that some cell types, specifically monocytes and macrophages, are targets relevant to disease pathogenesis.

This feature of the infection was initially suggested by the immune histochemical localization of Ebola virus in vivo: endothelial cells, mononuclear phagocytes, and hepatocytes are the main targets of infection.

Pathophysiology

Replication of the virus in monocytes triggers the release of high levels of inflammatory chemical signals. Once infected, endothelial cells (cells lining the inside of blood vessels), liver cells, and several types of immune cells such as macrophages, monocytes, and dendritic cells are the main targets of infection.

Following infection with the virus, the immune cells carry the virus to nearby lymph nodes where further reproduction of the virus takes place. From there, the virus can enter the bloodstream and lymphatic system and spread throughout the body. Macrophages are the first cells infected with the virus, and this infection results in programmed cell death.

After infection, a secreted glycoprotein, small soluble glycoprotein (sGP) (or Ebola virus glycoprotein [GP]), is synthesized. EBOV replication overwhelms protein synthesis of infected cells and the host immune defenses. The GP forms a trimeric complex, which tethers the virus to the endothelial cells.

The sGP forms a dimeric protein that interferes with the signaling of neutrophils, another type of white blood cell, which enables the virus to evade the immune system by inhibiting early steps of neutrophil activation. The presence of viral particles and the cell damage resulting from viruses budding out of the cell causes the release of chemical signals (such as TNF-α, IL-6 and IL-8), which are molecular signals for fever and inflammation.

The damage to human cells, caused by infection of the endothelial cells, decreases the integrity of blood vessels. This loss of vascular integrity increases with the synthesis of GP, which reduces the availability of specific integrins responsible for cell adhesion to the intercellular structure and causes damage to the liver, leading to improper clotting.

Ebola virus enters the body through mucous membranes, breaks in the skin, or parenterally. The pathogen infects many cell types, including monocytes, macrophages, dendritic cells, endothelial cells, fibroblasts, hepatocytes, adrenal cortical cells, and epithelial cells.

Cell entry and tissue damage: whatever the point of entry into the body, macrophages and dendritic cells are probably the first cells to be infected. Spread to regional lymph nodes results in further rounds of replication, followed by dissemination of virus to dendritic cells and fixed and mobile macrophages in the liver, spleen, thymus, and other lymphoid tissues. Rapid systemic spread is aided by virus-induced suppression of type I interferon responses as the disease progresses, hepatocytes, adrenal cortical cells, fibroblasts, and many other cell types also become infected, resulting in extensive tissue necrosis.

Systemic inflammatory response: In addition to causing extensive tissue damage, filoviruses also induce a systemic inflammatory syndrome by inducing the release of cytokines, chemokines, and other proinflammatory mediators from infected macrophages and other cells. Macrophages infected with Ebola Zaire virus produce tumor necrosis factor (TNF)-alpha, interleukin (IL)-1beta, IL-6, macrophage chemotactic protein (MCP)-1, and nitric oxide (NO). Breakdown products of necrotic cells also stimulate the release of the same mediators. It is thus the host response to infection, rather than any toxic effect of the virus, that is responsible for the fever, malaise, vasodilatation, increased vascular permeability, hypotension, and shock.

Coagulation defects: the coagulation defects seen in Ebola and Marburg virus disease are also induced indirectly. Virus-infected macrophages synthesize cell-surface tissue factor (TF), triggering the extrinsic coagulation pathway. Proinflammatory cytokines also induce macrophages to produce TF. The simultaneous occurrence of these two stimuli helps to explain the early appearance, rapid development, and ultimate severity of the coagulopathy. As the disease progresses, hepatic injury may also cause a decline in plasma levels of certain coagulation factors.

Impairment of adaptive immunity: Failure of adaptive immunity, through impaired dendritic cell function and lymphocyte apoptosis, helps to explain how these viruses are able to cause severe, frequently fatal illness. Filoviruses act both directly and indirectly to disable antigen-specific immune responses. Dendritic cells, which have primary responsibility for the initiation of adaptive immune responses, are a major site of filoviral replication. In vitro studies have shown that infected cells fail to undergo maturation and are unable to present antigens to naive lymphocytes, potentially explaining why patients dying from Ebola hemorrhagic fever do not develop antibodies to the virus.

Symptoms and signs: Patients with Ebola virus disease initially present with non-specific influenza-like symptoms.

Laboratory findings: Leukopenia, thrombocytopenia, transaminase elevations, as well as renal and coagulation abnormalities are often observed in patients with Ebola or Marburg virus disease. Other laboratory findings include a marked decrease in total plasma protein (reflective of a capillary leak syndrome) and elevated amylase levels.

- Leukopenia — Leukopenia usually presents as lymphopenia and is then followed by an elevated neutrophil count, with an increased percentage of immature forms. Immature granulocytes and abnormal lymphocytes, including plasmacytoid cells and immunoblasts, were seen in blood smears.

- Thrombocytopenia — Platelet counts are usually in the range of 50,000 to 100,000/microL.

- Transaminitis — because filoviruses can cause multifocal hepatic necrosis, blood chemistry tests usually demonstrate elevated serum aspartate aminotransferase (AST) and alanine aminotransferase. (ALT) levels, with the former typically increasing more than the latter.

- Coagulation abnormalities — Prothrombin (PT) and partial thromboplastin times (PTT) are prolonged and fibrin degradation products are elevated, consistent with disseminated intravascular coagulation (DIC). These changes are most prominent in severe and fatal cases.

- Renal abnormalities — Proteinuria is a common finding, and renal insufficiency occurs with progression of illness.

In summary, an understanding of the mechanisms underlying Ebola virus-induced cytopathic effects has facilitated the process of vaccine and antiviral therapy development, which has in turn provided new information about pathogenesis and the immune response.

Ebola virus does not exhibit the high degree of variability that other enveloped viruses may employ to evade host immunity, but Ebola virus GP alters target-cell function and exemplifies a novel strategy for immune evasion that may have arisen through the evolution of Ebola virus with its natural host. The cytotoxic effects of GP on macrophage and endothelial cell function disrupt inflammatory cell function and the integrity of the vasculature.

In addition, by altering the cell surface expression of adhesion proteins and immune recognition molecules, Ebola virus may disrupt processes critical to immune activation and cytolytic-T-cell function. These phenomena likely account for the dysregulation of the inflammatory response and the vascular dysfunction characteristic of lethal Ebola virus infection, providing a rationale for focusing on GP as a target for a preventative vaccine and providing leads for other clinical interventions.

Laboratory Reference Ranges in Healthy Adults
The Values Listed below are Generalizations

Electrolytes
- Ammonia: 15-50 µmol/L
- Ceruloplasmin: 15-60 mg/dL
- Chloride: 95-105 mmol/L
- Copper: 70-150 µg/dL
- Creatinine: 0.8-1.3 mg/dL
- Blood urea nitrogen: 8-21 mg/dL
- Ferritin: 12-300 ng/mL (men), 12-150 ng/mL (women)
- Glucose: 65-110 mg/dL
- Inorganic phosphorous: 1-1.5 mmol/L
- Ionized calcium: 1.03-1.23 mmol/L
- Magnesium: 1.5-2 mEq/L

- Phosphate: 0.8-1.5 mmol/L
- Potassium: 3.5-5 mmol/L
- Pyruvate: 300-900 µg/dL
- Sodium: 135-145 mmol/L
- Total calcium: 2-2.6 mmol/L
- Total iron-binding capacity: 45-85 µmol/L
- Total serum iron: 65-180 µg/dL (men), 30-170 µg/dL (women)
- Transferrin: 200-350 mg/dL
- Urea: 1.2-3 mmol/L
- Uric acid: 0.18-0.48 mmol/L
- Zinc: 70-100 µmol/L

Hematology

- Hemoglobin: 13-17 g/dL (men), 12-15 g/dL (women)
- Hematocrit 40%-52% (men), 36%-47% (Women)
- Glycosylated hemoglobin 4%-6%
- Mean corpuscular volume (MCV): 80-100 fL
- Red blood cell distribution width (RDW): 11.5%-14.5%
- Mean corpuscular hemoglobin concentration (MCHC): 30-35 g/dL
- Reticulocytes 0.5%-1.5%
- White blood cells (WBC) 4-10 x 10^9/L
- Neutrophils: 2-8 x 10^9/L
- Lymphocytes: 1-4 x 10^9/L
- Monocytes: 0.2-0.8 x 10^9/L
- Eosinophils: < 0.5 x 10^9/L
- Platelets: 150-400 x 10^9/L
- Prothrombin time: 11-14 sec
- International normalized ratio (INR): 0.9-1.2
- Activated partial thromboplastin time (aPTT): 20-40 sec
- Fibrinogen: 1.8-4 g/L
- Bleeding time: 2-9 min

Lipids

- Triglycerides: 50-150 mg/dL
- Total cholesterol: 3-5.5 mmol/L
- High-density lipoprotein (HDL): 40-80 mg/dL
- Low-density lipoprotein (LDL): 85-125 mg/dL

Acid Base Values

- pH: 7.35-7.45
- Base excess: (–3)-(+3)
- H+: 36-44 nmol/L
- Partial pressure of oxygen (pO2): 75-100 mm Hg
- Oxygen saturation: 96%-100%
- Partial pressure of carbon dioxide (pCO2): 35-45 mm Hg
- Bicarbonate (HCO3): 18-22 mmol/L

Gastrointestinal Function

- Albumin: 35-50 g/L
- Alkaline phosphatase: 50-100 U/L
- Alanine aminotransferase (ALT): 5-30 U/L
- Amylase: 30-125 U/L
- Aspartate aminotransferase (AST): 5-30 U/L
- Direct bilirubin: 0-6 µmol/L
- Gamma glutamyl transferase: 6-50 U/L
- Lipase: 10-150 U/L
- Total bilirubin: 2-20 µmol/L
- Total protein: 60-80 g/L

Cardiac Enzymes

- Creatine kinase: 25-200 U/L
- Creatine kinase MB (CKMB): 0-4 ng/mL
- Troponin: 0-0.4 ng/mL

Hormones

- 17 hydroxyprogesterone (female, follicular): 0.2-1 mg/L
- Adrenocorticotropic hormone (ACTH): 4.5-20 pmol/L
- Estradiol: 1.5-5 ng/dL (male), 2-14 ng/dL (female, follicular), 2-16 ng/dL (female, luteal), < 3.5 ng/dL (postmenopausal)
- Free T3: 0.2-0.5 ng/dL
- Free T4: 10-20 pmol/L
- Follicle-stimulating hormone (FSH): 1-10 IU/L (male), 1-10 IU/L (female, follicular/luteal), 5-25 IU/L (female, ovulation), 30-110 IU/L (post menopause)
- Growth hormone (fasting) : 0-5 ng/mL
- Progesterone: 70-280 (ovulation), ng/dL
- Prolactin: < 14 ng/mL

- Testosterone (male): 10-25 nmol/L
- Thyroxine-binding globulin: 12-30 mg/L
- Thyroid-stimulating hormone (TSH): 0.5-5 mIU/L
- Total T4: 4.9-11.7 mg/dL
- Total T3: 0.7-1.5 ng/dL
- Free T3: 0.6-1.6 ng/mL

Vitamins

- Folate (serum) : 7-36 nmol/L
- Vitamin A: 30-65 µg/dL
- Vitamin B12: 130-700 ng/L
- Vitamin C: 0.4-1.5 mg/dL
- Vitamin D: 5-75 ng/mL

Tumor Markers

- Alpha fetoprotein: 0-44 ng/mL
- Beta human chorionic gonadotropin (HCG): < 5 IU/I
- CA19.9: < 40 U/mL
- Carcinoembryonic antigen (CEA): < 4 ug/L
- Prostatic acid phosphatase (PAP): 0-3 U/dL
- Prostate-specific antigen (PSA): < 4 ug/L

Miscellaneous

- Alpha 1-antitrypsin: 20-50 µmol/L
- Angiotensin-converting enzyme: 23-57 U/L
- C-reactive protein: < 5 mg/L
- D-dimer: < 500 ng/mL
- Erythrocyte sedimentation rate (ESR): Less than age/2 mm/hour
- Lactate dehydrogenase (LDH): 50-150 U/L
- Lead: < 40 µg/dL
- Rheumatoid factor: < 25 IU/ml

Value courtesy http://emedicine.medscape.com/article/2172316-overview

ECF and ICF Composition

Distribution of Ions in Body Compartments	ICF/Intracellular (MEQ/L)	Tissue fluid / interstitial (MEQ/L)	Blood plasma (MEQ/L)
Na^+ Cations	10	147	142
K^+ Cations	140	4.0	5.0
Ca^{++} Cations	5	2.5	5.0

Table *Contd...*

Distribution of Ions in Body Compartments	ICF/Intracellular (MEQ/L)	Tissue fluid / interstitial (MEQ/L)	Blood plasma (MEQ/L)
Mg+Cations	27	2.0	3.0
$HCO3^-$ Anions	10	30	27
Cl^- Anions	25	114	103
$PO4^-$	80	2.0	2
$SO4^-$ Anions	20	1.0	1
Organic acids	–	7.5	6
Proteins	47	0	16

These are the actual quantitative numbers. The units are in milliequivalents per liter (mEq/L.)
https://en.wikipedia.org/wiki/Extracellular_fluid/Intracellular Fluid